Pharmacology
for
Massage Therapy

Pharmacology
for
Massage Therapy

Jean M. Wible
RN, BSN, NCTMB, CHTP

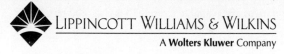
LIPPINCOTT WILLIAMS & WILKINS
A **Wolters Kluwer** Company

Philadelphia • Baltimore • New York • London
Buenos Aires • Hong Kong • Sydney • Tokyo

Editor: Peter Darcy
Development Editor: David Payne
Senior Project Editor: Karen Ruppert
Marketing Manager: Christen DeMarco
Designer: Doug Smock
Compositor: Maryland Composition
Printer: R.R. Donnelley

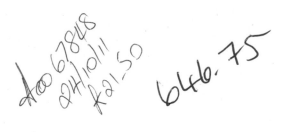

Printed in China

Library of Congress Cataloging-in-Publication Data

Wible, Jean M.
   Pharmacology for massage therapy / Jean M. Wible.
     p. ; cm.
   Includes bibliographical references and index.
   ISBN 0-7817-4798-8
    1. Pharmacology. 2. Massage therapy. I. Title.
   [DNLM: 1. Pharmacology—Case Reports. 2. Drug Therapy—Case Reports. 3. Drug
   Therapy—Adverse Effects—Case Reports. 4. Massage—Case Reports. QV 4 W632p 2005]
   QM125.W534 2005
   615.8′22—dc22

                                                    2004048438

To purchase additional copies of this book, call our customer service department at **(800) 638-3030** or fax orders to **(301) 824-7390**. International customers should call **(301) 714-2324**.

Visit Lippincott Williams & Wilkins on the Internet: *http://www.LWW.com*. Lippincott Williams & Wilkins customer service representatives are available from 8:30 am to 6:00 pm, EST.

DEDICATION

*To my parents, who started me on the path, and
to the Healing Touch Community in Baltimore, who
taught me to go with the flow and find my power and energy within.*

Preface

Overview

In teaching massage therapy students and professionals over the years, I, like most instructors in the field, have always stressed the importance of conducting a thorough initial and on-going health assessment for each client to ensure safety and to individualize the massage session. A complete listing of medications taken by the client is always a part of this assessment. Other than pointing out a few "red flag" drugs, though, I typically would not give any further instruction concerning drugs, their effects on the body, or their effects on massage. I have found, however, that students inevitably want more information, asking me, "What do I do with the medication list?" or "I look up the drugs, but what does it mean for my massage?" This textbook will help to answer these questions.

Organization

With content arranged in easy-to-follow chapters organized by body system and/or symptom, this text explores how to assess the effects of drug treatment on the body and the associated implications for massage. Some drugs presented have no significant implications for massage, in which case only basic pharmacologic information is given. Other drugs listed, however, have physiologic effects on the body that require modification in how massage is given or even contraindication; for these, specific massage-related directions are provided in a special section titled, "Massage Implications and Assessment." Thus, this text, the first of its kind to my knowledge, will help massage therapists to assess their clients on the basis of medications taken and adjust their techniques accordingly.

The first chapter concisely outlines the physiologic effects that massage has on the healthy body and introduces the deductive reasoning process that is the core of this text. The second chapter introduces the key concepts of pharmacology that will be used throughout the chapters to help understand the effects of each category of drugs on the body. Pharmacokinetics (how the drug is absorbed, distributed, and excreted from the body), pharmacodynamics (how the drug produces its effects in the body), and pharmacotherapeutics (how the drug is used to treat disease or symptoms) are explained.

The following chapters cover a wide variety of drug categories, including drugs that affect the nervous system, respiratory system, gastrointestinal system, endocrine system, cardiovascular system, and the blood. In addition, there are chapters covering drugs for pain control, infections, inflammation and allergies, fluid and electrolytes balance, psychiatric conditions, and cancer. The final chapter discusses the most common over-the-counter supplements that are used by so many of our massage clients today.

Key Features

Each chapter is set up in a common format allowing easy access to key information for each category of drug. Chapter features include:

- Lists of Common Drug Names at the beginning of each drug group feature both generic and brand names

- The Massage Implications and Assessment section, highlighted in a box with a blue background, discusses the effects of the drugs, the changes that may be needed in applying massage, contraindications, and the effects of adverse reactions the client may experience while taking the drug
- Adverse Reactions sidebars outline the most common side effects and adverse reactions associated with a given drug or drug group
- Quick Quizzes at the end of each chapter provide application-oriented questions to help students integrate what they have learned into practice
- Case Studies included in Appendix A also give students the opportunity to apply information in real-world scenarios
- A Drug Index at the end of the book, in addition to a general index, is included as a convenient reference for quickly finding information on specific drugs

Drug Regimen Assessment Process for Massage Therapy

The Drug Regimen Assessment Process for Massage Therapy is a deductive reasoning model introduced in Chapter 1 and used throughout the text. It is a step-by-step process that helps therapists to consider the drugs each client is taking and to determine cautions, contraindications, effects on massage, and the best massage strokes to use with each client. It is this assessment model that will enable readers to apply the information they have read to real-life situations, in which clients are often taking multiple drugs, and to truly individualize their massage sessions. Thus, the assessment model makes this text a dynamic assessment tool and not simply a repository of pharmacologic facts.

Closing Thoughts

I hope that those who read and use this textbook will find the information they need to know clearly presented and that they can easily apply it in their massage practices. Although massage therapists do not prescribe drugs and should never presume to be experts in pharmacology, knowledge about drugs and their effects on how the body receives and is affected by massage is critical. Furthermore, as massage becomes more and more integrated with the medical system and as the clients who come to us are more and more those with chronic conditions, I hope this text will assist us in working with our clients holistically and individually, maintaining our focus on the client and not on the disease.

Jean M. Wible, RN, BSN, NCTMB, CHTP

Acknowledgments

My special thanks to Peter Darcy, David Payne, Eric Branger, and all the staff at Lippincott Williams & Wilkins who patiently guided me at each step of publication.

Reviewers

Laura Allen, LMBT
Instructor, The Whole You School of Massage
Rutherfordton, North Carolina

Kate Anagnostis, LATC, LMT
Instructor, Downeast School of Massage
Waldoboro, Maine

Glen E. Farr, PharmD
Professor of Pharmacy and Associate Dean
University of Tennessee College of Pharmacy
Knoxville, Tennessee

Kay S. Peterson
Wisconsin Certified Massage Therapist
Altoona, Wisconsin

Contents

Pharmacology and Massage Therapy

1

Pharmacology and massage may, at first glance, seem to be two topics that have nothing in common. Pharmacology is the mainstay of traditional allopathic medicine. Massage is a wholly natural modality (usually grouped with alternative and complimentary medicine) that does not include prescribing or using drugs. The reality, however, is that many clients coming to receive massage therapy are also receiving some kind of drug therapy and/or using over-the-counter medications and supplements on a regular basis. This is true whether the work is done in a medical setting, in a salon or spa setting, or in private practice and wellness centers. Recognizing that drug therapy of any kind brings about physiologic and chemical changes in the body as well as that massage therapy also brings about these changes in the body, it is more than reasonable to explore these effects together. The knowledge that the effects of drug therapy may enhance/increase or disrupt/decrease the effect of massage can and should lead to changes in how we apply massage therapy in individual situations. This chapter explores the physiologic and chemical effects of massage therapy.

Physiologic Effects of Massage

As with any discipline, massage therapy utilizes basic tools to achieve its effects. These include effleurage, pétrissage, vibration, friction, tapotement, traction, and movement/stretching. Variations in how these are applied (such as speed, depth, direction, and intention) can and will change the physiologic effects of the massage.

General Effects

The general effects traditionally associated with massage therapy are those of relaxation. Muscles warm and relax, blood circulation to the areas massaged increases, cardiac and respiratory rates decrease, and the parasympathetic nervous system is activated through neurotransmitter and endocrine substances released into the bloodstream. However, other modalities in massage have different goals. In these cases (such as sports massage and deep tissue massage), the above tools are applied differently, the physiologic effects may be more stimulating, and different chemicals may be released to engage the sympathetic nervous system. These differences in goals and application must be taken into account when determining whether drug therapy will affect the desired outcomes of the work.

Body System Effects

The effects of massage come from a combination of mechanical factors acting locally and nervous system reflex reactions. The mechanical methods of manipulation directly affect local soft tissue and fluid movement. The nervous system reflex reactions affect local tissue and also systemically stimulate changes in neural and chemical substances, which bring about widespread changes in the body. Knowledge of how these changes react in each body system will help in understanding how drugs can change these responses.

Nervous System

The nervous system consists of the central nervous system (CNS) (brain and spinal cord) and the peripheral nervous system (cranial, spinal, and peripheral nerves). The peripheral nervous system is separated into the somatic, sensory, and autonomic divisions. The autonomic division is subdivided into the sympathetic nervous system (which activates, stimulates, and expends energy) and the parasympathetic nervous system (which restores, rests, repairs, stores, and builds up energy reserves) (Fig. 1-1).

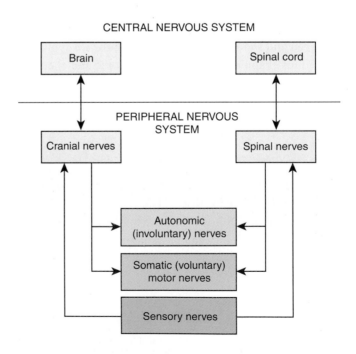

Figure 1-1 Divisions of the Nervous System. (Adapted from Thibodeau GA, Patton KT. The Human Body in Health and Disease. 2nd Ed. St. Louis: Mosby, 1997.)

As soon as massage begins, the sensory nerves are stimulated and send messages to the CNS. The method and speed of the application will be read by the CNS, which in turn sends neurotransmitters to the autonomic division of the peripheral nervous system. All body systems then follow the new rhythms produced by this massage through the systemic effects of changes in the neuroendocrine chemicals of the body (see "Neuroendocrine System" below).

There is an initial stimulation of the sympathetic nervous system in all cases of massage. Then, depending on the application of the massage techniques, the body will stay in sympathetic activation or fall into the slower rhythm of the parasympathetic nervous system. Both will relax a client, the latter to a deep state of rest and the former to an alert state, where stress hormones are used up or dissipated, bringing the body to homeostasis.

The effects that come through the somatic nervous system are based on reflex arcs (fast and predictable responses to change in the "environment" inside and outside the body). Muscle spindles, tendon organs, and joint receptors are stimulated. The somatic nervous system responds to maintain balance and protect muscles, tendons, and ligaments from damage. Some bring about muscle contraction; others bring about muscle relaxation. Both sides of the body are affected together to allow balance and control. Reflex arcs also cause relaxation of the antagonist muscles when agonist muscles are contracted, and vice versa (i.e., hamstring muscles—antagonists—relax when quadriceps muscles—agonists—are contracted).

Neuroendocrine System

The effects on the endocrine system are closely linked to the neurologic system. Both neurotransmitters and hormone levels can be changed by massage (see Box 1-1).

Cardiovascular and Respiratory Systems

Massage does have direct mechanical effects on the cardiovascular system. Most massage strokes manipulate local tissue and bring increased blood and fluid circulation to the area. Some strokes move fluid and blood enough to directly increase systemic blood flow, leading to slight increases in heart rate and respiratory rate. However, most of the reactions of the cardiovascular and respiratory systems are mediated through the nervous system. The sympathetic nervous system will increase heart rate, blood pressure, and respiratory rate as well as dilate skeletal muscle blood vessels while constricting others. The parasympathetic nervous system will decrease heart rate, blood pressure, and respiratory rate as well as increase blood flow through the internal organs.

Other Body Systems

Massage has direct effects on the skin, mainly through mechanically removing dead skin cells and increasing blood and warmth to the surface. Connective tissue is also directly affected by the mechanics of massage. Warmth and fluids are brought to the local area by standard massage strokes as well as by specific connective tissue and myofascial techniques.

Box 1-1

Neurotransmitters and Hormones Influenced by Massage

The combination of these changes in the chemicals active in the body at any given time allows massage to bring relaxation and balance.

Neurotransmitters

Dopamine: Influences fine motor activity and coordination, increases concentration, and improves mood. Increased by massage.

Serotonin: Regulates mood and ability to act appropriately; subdues irritability; and may play a role in regulating hunger, cravings, and sleep/wake cycles. Increased by massage.

Hormones

Epinephrine/norepinephrine (also called adrenaline/noradrenaline): Activates arousal, alertness, and fight-or-flight alarm functions of the sympathetic nervous system. Increased or decreased by massage depending on what the body needs to reach balance and homeostasis at the time of the massage.

Endorphins/enkephalins: Improve mood and modulate pain perception. Increased by massage.

Oxytocin: Believed to aid in bonding, attachment, and feelings of connection with self and others. Increased by massage.

Cortisol: Sustains sympathetic nervous system arousal, suppresses immune function, and increases substance P (which increases pain perception). Decreased by massage.

Growth hormone: Promotes cell division, replication, repair, and regeneration. Increased by massage.

The resultant loosening and softening of the ground substance leads to loosening of tissues and muscles as well as ease of movement.

The effects on the lymphatic system are derived from the mechanical movement of lymph. This movement of fluid enhances the function of the immune system. In addition, the balance of the sympathetic and parasympathetic nervous systems will increase the restorative effects of the immune system and its defenses against infection.

The digestive system is affected only indirectly, again through the nervous system. The sympathetic nervous system slows the activity of the digestive system; the parasympathetic nervous system increases its activity.

The kidneys are indirectly affected by the increase in cellular metabolism, the release of waste into body fluids and the bloodstream, and the increase in systemic circulation that can occur with massage.

The mental/emotional effects are highly individual. In general, mental focus and concentration, as well as creative and logical thinking, are improved. Most clients find massage relaxing and nurturing, creating feelings of well-being. However, the client's past experiences and current emotional state can have a very strong influence that may even completely override all the other effects previously discussed.

Massage Strokes and Their Effects

Massage, like any other discipline, has a variety of tools. The incredible number of different modalities and types of massage applications can be traced back to a limited number of basic massage strokes. These are touch/compression, vibration/shaking, tapotement, friction, pétrissage, effleurage, stretching, and traction. The effects of these strokes are greatly changed by varying the depth, direction, speed, time, and intention with which they are applied to the body. All the above strokes will have local effects in the skin, connective tissue, and cardiovascular system. Those that work best for these local, mechanical results are pétrissage, friction, and effleurage. The strokes whose efficacy relies strongly on local (somatic) reflex nervous system mechanisms are friction, vibration/shaking, touch/compression, stretching, and traction. Strokes that have a strong systemic reflex action are effleurage, friction, rocking, and tapotement. Strokes that have a strong mechanical systemic effect on one or more of the individual body systems are effleurage (cardiovascular system) and tapotement (nervous system) (Table 1-1). Again, the variations in applying these strokes can modify or increase these effects. Knowledge of how individual strokes create their effects is essential to individualizing a session for the client receiving drug therapy (Table 1-2).

General Effects of Drug Therapy on Massage

Each drug category has an effect on massage based on how the drug acts on the body. Many drugs used today have actions that work through the nervous system (even when the drug therapy is for another body system). To the extent that a drug would change the reflexive reactions of the nervous system or slow the activity of the CNS, the drug will change how a client's body reacts to massage. Other drugs may work on a cellular level,

Table 1-1 Summary of Massage Stroke Actions

Massage Action/Effects	Strongest Strokes for This Effect	How Effect Works Physiologically
Mechanical	Effleurage Pétrissage Friction	Warms local area Softens tissue Brings blood/lymph circulation to the area
Local (somatic) reflex	Touch/compression Friction Vibration/shaking Stretching/traction	Stimulates local sensory receptors in muscles, tendons, and ligaments CNS reflex response to above causes muscle tonus (contraction and relaxation) to change
Systemic reflex	Effleurage Friction Rocking Tapotement	Stimulates ANS to change levels of neuroendocrine substances These chemical changes affect whole body systems
Mechanical systemic effects	Effleurage (cardiovascular) Tapotement (nervous)	Physically increases systemic blood and lymph flow Physically stimulates the peripheral and central nervous systems

change tissue, increase toxins, or work on a specific body system. In some cases, the drug will have little or no effect on how massage works. In others, the drug may have a significant effect. The majority of drugs will fall in between; that is, the effect will be small but will be enough that minor changes in how massage is applied will allow the practitioner to better meet the goals of the session.

General Cautions and Contraindications for Drugs and Massage Therapy

Although individual drug actions, the effect of different massage strokes, and the goal of a massage session all must be taken into account in individualizing the massage session, several general cautions do apply.

Most drugs are taken orally (by mouth), and their absorption rates will not be greatly affected by massage. In the case of medications delivered by subcutaneous or intramuscular injection, as well as topical drugs, massage can change the rate of absorption. Depending on how quickly the drug is absorbed, no massage should be performed on the local area of injection or application for several to 24 hours after the application or injection. Onset, peak, and duration times for individual drugs provide a more exact time frame.

Another contraindication is any drug that is related to blood clotting. This is a red flag that always needs further investigation before proceeding to massage. Drugs such as warfarin (Coumadin) could indicate the presence of blood clots, which is a contraindica-

Table 1-2 Physiologic Actions of Individual Massage Strokes

Massage Stroke	Means of Action	Systems Acted on Directly	Effects	Summary
Touch/ compression	Mechanical and somatic reflex	Skin, connective tissue, and muscle	Warms Increases blood to local area Relaxes muscles	Mostly a local effect, only indirectly affects other body systems
Effleurage (gliding)	Mechanical, systemic reflex, and some somatic reflex Direct mechanical effects on the cardiovascular system	Skin, connective tissue, muscle, cardiovascular, and lymphatic	Moves fluid and blood through the body, warming local area tissues and muscles, increasing heart rate and blood pressure initially, then slowing and lowering them (unless done rapidly) Brings about changes in the neuroendocrine chemicals	Very strong systemic effect on cardiovascular system Strong local effects and strong systemic effects Indirectly increases then decreases respiratory rate Increases gastrointestinal and genitourinary activity Increases immune function
Pétrissage	Mechanical and somatic reflex	Skin, tissue, and muscles	Warms and brings blood circulation to the local area Relaxes muscles Softens connective tissue	Mostly local effects Indirect and minimal effects on other body systems
Friction	Mechanical, somatic reflex, and some systemic reflex	Skin, tissue, and muscles	Warms and brings blood circulation to the local area Softens connective tissue as well as tendons, ligaments, and muscles	Mostly local effect Some changes in the neuro-endocrine chemicals, but slight Increasing the time and depth can activate the nervous system and affect all other systems through it

continued

Table 1-2 Continued

Massage Stroke	Means of Action	Systems Acted on Directly	Effects	Summary
Vibration/ shaking/ rocking	Somatic and systemic reflex	Autonomic nervous system, muscles, and mental/emotional	Relaxes muscles Activates parasympathetic nervous system, feelings of well-being	Vibration has a local effect Shaking and rocking have a systemic effect through the changes in neuroendocrine chemicals
Tapotement (percussion)	Systemic reflex	Central and peripheral nervous system, muscles, skin, and tissue	Warms and brings blood to the area muscles and tissues Stimulates the CNS and through it, the sympathetic nervous system	Strong systemic effect on nervous system and indirectly on other body systems through the activation of the sympathetic division
Movement/ stretching/ traction	Somatic reflex	Muscles, tendons, ligaments, and connective tissue	Softens tissues, especially connective tissue, tendons, and ligaments, and relaxes muscles	Mostly local effects

tion for massage therapy. A call to the client's physician is always warranted in this case. Only the physician can tell you if a blood clot is present or if the risk of a blood clot is high. A physician's release is required. Sometimes these drugs are used long term and for prevention; in such cases, a modified massage may be appropriate. Only the physician can determine this.

A massage therapist should always review the drugs, both prescription and over-the-counter, that a client is taking before performing massage. This allows the therapist to determine what types of medical conditions the client may have and whether there are any dangers to the client in receiving massage. A call to the physician is appropriate to determine safety and the best way to apply massage in any case in which multiple drugs or a serious medical condition make safety uncertain. Do not be afraid to discuss with the physician the details of massage and the effects of each of the massage strokes you wish to use. Many physicians do not have a clear idea of the broad effects of massage on the body and will appreciate your input in determining safety for their patients.

Another general caution concerns any medication that would slow the nervous system response to stimuli or slow the CNS response time. In these cases, greater care must be taken in the depth of massage strokes given and in recognizing that response may take more time. Pain receptors will not allow the client to give accurate feedback on depth in these cases; therefore, less pressure should be applied as a matter of course.

Side Effects and Adverse Effects

When considering the effects of drug therapy, side effects of the drug will need to be looked at closely. In general, side effects and adverse reactions may be terms used to describe effects of drugs that are other than the desired effect. However, most of the time (and for the purposes of this text) side effects are milder and occur frequently, and adverse effects are more severe and serious but occur less frequently. Adverse effects are brought to a physician's attention as soon as possible and, when present, are a contraindication for massage.

Client Drug Regimen Assessment Process

What do you do with the list of drugs your client gives you before making an appointment for massage? Many massage therapists have been taught to obtain this list of medications and have no idea of what to do with it. Several questions need to be answered and several steps taken to determine if the client's drug therapy regimen requires any change in the way massage therapy is applied. Using a deductive reasoning process is the best approach. This allows for application to a variety of clients and situations as well as individualization of sessions. Simply giving protocols for each drug will not address clients who have multiple drugs, dosages, and goals for their massage sessions.

The first question to be answered is, "What is the stated goal of the massage session for this client?" The second is, "What type of massage and what strokes would the therapist normally use to achieve these results for a client who was healthy and taking no medications?" The deductive process can now begin.

The massage therapist must first determine if there are any immediate red flags that indicate massage could be harmful. If so, consult the client's physician. Next, determine if the absorption of the drug is likely to be affected by massage. If yes, determine what local contraindication exists and the time frame in which it exists. (For example, insulin given by subcutaneous injection into the left thigh would contraindicate massage in that thigh. The time frame is determined by the absorption rate of the insulin and can be determined by looking up the onset and peak effect times in a drug book.) Each drug needs to be evaluated with regard to the strokes and goals. How does this drug achieve its effects in the body? What is its action? What are the side effects of this drug? See if the body's reaction to each stroke would be affected by the action of the drug in question. Then look at the desired effect of the stroke and see if the action or the side effects of the drug would increase or decrease this desired effect. Ask the following questions: Will the body's reaction to massage be altered, and will the drug's action and side effects be increased or decreased? If the answers are no, then proceed with massage as planned. If the answers are yes, look at each individual stroke and determine if it should be modified to achieve the desired effects, should not be used at all, should be replaced by another stroke that could

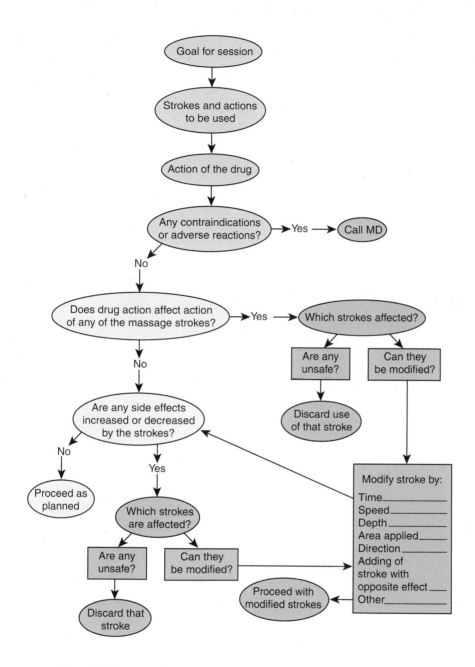

Figure 1-2 Drug Regimen Assessment Process for Massage Therapy.

bypass the drug effects, or should be paired with another stroke to modify the amount of effect the drug would have.

Once this is done for each stroke and each medication, put together the massage session using the strokes least affected and best suited to the goal of the session. This process is not as complicated as it may seem and depends on both knowledge and common sense. Many times the answers will be no to all questions and the massage can proceed as planned. When the answer is yes to any of the questions, a better massage, one that meets the goals of the client, can be achieved by taking the time to examine how to apply massage in these situations. An outline of the deductive process is found in Figure 1-2.

In going through this text and looking at each category of drug, information is provided to help clarify this process. Massage implications are highlighted along with the common drug names. Also, case studies have been added to give examples of the use of this process and its application to massage therapy.

Quick Quiz

1. A client comes to you and says she took her long-acting insulin, Novolin-N, 2 hours ago by subcutaneous injection in her left thigh. What does this mean for your massage?

2. A new client calls and asks for an appointment for massage. She is very stressed at work and is looking for relaxation mainly. She lists her medications as Synthroid, a birth control pill, and a multivitamin. What does this mean for your massage?

Fundamentals of Clinical Pharmacology

2

This chapter focuses on the fundamental principles of pharmacology. It discusses basic information, such as how drugs are named, how they are created, and the different routes by which drugs can be administered. The chapter also discusses what happens when a drug enters the body. This involves three main areas:

1. Pharmacokinetics (the absorption, distribution, metabolism, and excretion of a drug)
2. Pharmacodynamics (the biochemical and physical effects of drugs and the mechanisms of drug actions)
3. Pharmacotherapeutics (the use of drugs to prevent and treat disease)

This chapter also provides an introduction to adverse drug reactions.

Pharmacology Basics

Drug Nomenclature

Drugs have a specific kind of nomenclature; that is, a drug can go by three different names:

1. The chemical name is a scientific name that precisely describes its atomic and molecular structure.
2. The generic, or nonproprietary, name is an abbreviation of the chemical name and is commonly used.
3. The trade name (also known as the brand name or proprietary name) is selected by the drug company selling the product. Trade names are protected by copyright. Inserting the symbol ® after the trade name or capitalizing the drug name indicates that the name is registered by and restricted to the drug manufacturer. In this text, trade names are indicated by capitalization (e.g., chemical name, acetylsalicylic acid; generic name, aspirin; trade name, Bayer).

In 1962, the federal government mandated the use of official names so that only one official name would represent each drug. The official names are listed in the *United States Pharmacopeia* and *National Formulary*.

Drug Class

Drugs that share similar characteristics are grouped together as a pharmacologic class (or family). Beta-adrenergic blockers are an example of a pharmacologic class. A second grouping is the therapeutic classification, which groups drugs by therapeutic use. Antihypertensives are an example of a therapeutic class.

Where Drugs Come From

Traditionally, drugs have been derived from natural sources such as plants, animals, and minerals. Today, however, laboratory researchers have used traditional knowledge, along with chemical science, to develop synthetic drug sources. One advantage of chemically developed drugs is that they are free from the impurities found in natural substances. In addition, researchers and drug developers can manipulate the molecular structure of substances, such as antibiotics, so that a slight change in the chemical structure makes the drug effective against different organisms. The first-, second-, third-, and fourth-generation cephalosporins are an example. The earliest drug concoctions from plants used everything—the leaves, roots, bulb, stem, seeds, buds, and blossoms. Subsequently, harmful substances often found their way into the mixture. As the understanding of plants as drug sources became more sophisticated, researchers sought to isolate and intensify active components while avoiding harmful ones.

Plant Sources

The active components of plants consist of several types and vary in character and effect.

1. Alkaloids, the most active component in plants, react with acids to form a salt that is able to dissolve more readily in body fluids. The names of alkaloids and their salts usually end in "-ine." Examples include atropine, caffeine, and nicotine.
2. Glycosides are other active components found in plants. Names of glycosides usually end in "-in," such as digoxin.
3. Gums constitute another group of active components. Gums give products the ability to attract and hold water. Examples include seaweed extractions and seeds with starch.
4. Resins, of which the chief source is pine tree sap, commonly act as local irritants or as laxatives and caustic agents.
5. Oils, thick and sometimes greasy liquids, are classified as volatile or fixed. Examples of volatile oils include peppermint, spearmint, and juniper. Fixed oils, which are not easily evaporated, include castor oil and olive oil.

Animal Sources

The body fluids or glands of animals can also be drug sources. The drugs obtained from animal sources include hormones, such as insulin; oils and fats (usually fixed), such as cod liver oil; enzymes, which are produced by living cells and act as catalysts, such as pancreatin and pepsin; and vaccines, which are suspensions of killed, modified, or attenuated microorganisms.

Mineral Sources

Metallic and nonmetallic minerals provide various inorganic materials not available from plants or animals. The mineral sources are used as they occur in nature or are combined with other ingredients. Examples of drugs that contain minerals are iron, iodine, and Epsom salts.

Modern Drugs

Today, most drugs are produced in laboratories and can be natural (from animal, plant, or mineral sources), synthetic, or a combination of the two. Examples of drugs produced in the laboratory include thyroid hormone (natural), cimetidine (synthetic), and anistreplase (a combination of natural and synthetic).

Recombinant deoxyribonucleic acid (rDNA) research has led to another chemical source of organic compounds. For example, the reordering of genetic information enables scientists to develop bacteria that produce insulin for humans. In the future, human DNA may become a source to develop new drugs.

New Drug Development

In the past, drugs were found by trial and error. Now, they are developed primarily by systematic scientific research. The Food and Drug Administration (FDA) carefully monitors new drug development, which can take many years to complete. The FDA approves an application for an investigational new drug (IND) only after reviewing extensive animal studies and data on the safety and effectiveness of the proposed drug (see Box 2-1).

Exceptions to the Rule

Although most INDs undergo all four phases of clinical evaluation mandated by the FDA, a few can receive expedited approval. For example, because of the public health threat posed by acquired immune deficiency syndrome (AIDS), the FDA and drug companies agreed to shorten the IND approval process for drugs to treat that disease. This allows physicians to give "treatment INDs," which are not yet approved by the FDA, to qualified patients with AIDS. Sponsors of drugs that reach phase II or III clinical trials can apply for FDA approval of treatment IND status. When the IND is approved, the sponsor supplies the drug to physicians whose patients meet appropriate criteria.

Methods of Administration

The routes through which drugs are administered (enter the body) are many and varied. Within each route there are further divisions in the

---

Box 2-1

Phases of New Drug Development

When the FDA approves the application for an investigational new drug, the drug must undergo clinical evaluation involving human subjects. This clinical evaluation is divided into four phases.

1. Phase I. The drug is tested on healthy volunteers.
2. Phase II. Phase II involves trials with human subjects who have the disease for which the drug is thought to be effective.
3. Phase III. Large numbers of patients in medical research centers receive the drug. This larger sampling provides information about infrequent or rare adverse effects. The FDA will approve a new drug application if phase III studies are satisfactory.
4. Phase IV. Phase IV is voluntary and involves postmarket surveillance of the drug's therapeutic effects at the completion of phase III. The pharmaceutical company receives reports from physicians and other health care professionals about the therapeutic results and adverse reactions of the drug. Some medications have been found to be toxic and have been removed from the market after their initial release.

types of carriers used (the packaging for delivery). The following discussion will touch on all of these.

Routes

The main routes for administering drugs are enteral, parenteral, transdermal, inhalation, and topical.

Enteral

The enteral route is the one most commonly used. It utilizes the gastrointestinal (GI) tract for absorption of the drug. Giving the drug orally (by mouth) and having the patient swallow it into the stomach is one enteral method. This requires that the drug be broken down for absorption and pass through the liver detoxification system before entering the bloodstream. This is a slower way of absorption. Other enteral routes that try to bypass the liver initially but still utilize the GI tract are sublingual (dissolved under the tongue), buccal (dissolved in the side of the mouth, the cheek area), and rectal/vaginal/urethral (dissolved in the opening of the rectum, vagina, or urethra). When these routes are used, drugs are absorbed through the mucous membranes that line these areas and from the tissues into the bloodstream. Drugs given in this manner are more rapidly absorbed than those administered by mouth.

Parenteral

Parenteral routes allow the drug to enter the bloodstream directly. They are intravenous (IV; directly into a vein), intramuscular (IM; into the deep muscles for absorption into the blood capillaries), subcutaneous (SC; into the layer of tissue and fat under the skin for absorption into the blood capillaries), subdermal (just under the epidermis or first layer of the skin for absorption into the blood capillaries), and intrathecal (directly into the spinal fluid bathing the spinal cord). These routes have a faster absorption and bypass the liver initially. IV is the fastest.

Transdermal, Inhalation, and Topical

The transdermal route involves application of a drug to the skin. The drug will transverse the skin and go into the deeper layers of tissue for absorption through the fluid in the tissues. Only certain medications are appropriate for this route. Inhalation routes allow drugs to be delivered directly into the respiratory system. Many of these have some systemic absorption, but a few have a local effect on respiratory tissue only. The topical route is application of a drug to the outer layer of the skin. The drug only absorbs into the skin and not into the deeper tissues. This route is used for treatment of skin diseases.

Carriers

The type of packaging of a drug for administration is called its carrier. Carriers include tablets, capsules, solutions, suspensions, patches, ointments, creams, aerosols, and suppositories.

Tablets are small disc-like masses of medicinal powders. They easily dissolve and crumble and are used for the oral, buccal, and sublingual routes. Capsules are drugs in liquid or powder form encased in a gelatin container that may be hard or soft (gelcaps). They are used for oral routes. Solutions are liquid preparations of drugs that do not separate. They can be used for oral or parenteral routes. Suspensions are liquid preparations of drugs that are not stable. They will separate into different elements if left to stand and require being shaken or mixed before administration. These are used for oral and parenteral routes. Patches are types of bandages that contain drugs. They are used on the skin for transdermal administration. Ointments and creams are topical drug carriers. Aerosols are for inhalation drugs. Suppositories are medicines in soft molded form for rectal, vaginal, or urethral routes.

Pharmacokinetics

Kinetics refers to movement. Pharmacokinetics deals with a drug's actions as it moves through the body. Therefore, pharmacokinetics discusses how a drug is absorbed (taken into the body), distributed (moved into various tissues), metabolized (changed into a form that can be excreted), and excreted (removed from the body). This branch of pharmacology is also concerned with a drug's onset of action, peak concentration level, and duration of action.

Absorption

Drug absorption covers the progress of a drug from the time it is administered, through the time it passes to the tissues, until it becomes available for use by the body. On a cellular level, drugs are absorbed by several means, primarily through active or passive transport.

Cellular Transport

Passive transport requires no cellular energy because the drug moves from an area of higher concentration to one of lower concentration. It occurs when small molecules diffuse across membranes. Diffusion (movement from a higher concentration to a lower concentration) stops when drug concentrations on both sides of the membrane are equal.

Active transport requires cellular energy to move the drug from an area of lower concentration to one of higher concentration. Active transport is used to absorb electrolytes, such as sodium and potassium, as well as some drugs, such as levodopa.

Pinocytosis is a unique form of active transport that occurs when a cell engulfs a drug particle. Pinocytosis is commonly employed to transport fat-soluble vitamins (vitamins A, D, E, and K).

Speed of Absorption

If only a few cells separate the active drug from the systemic circulation, absorption will occur rapidly and the drug will quickly reach therapeutic levels in the body. Typically, drug absorption occurs within seconds or minutes when administered sublingually, intravenously, or by inhalation.

Absorption occurs at a slower rate when drugs are administered by the oral, IM, or SC routes because the complex membrane systems of GI mucosal layers, muscle, and skin delay drug passage. At the slowest absorption rates, drugs can take several hours or days to reach peak concentration levels. A slow rate usually occurs with rectally administered or sustained-release drugs.

Other factors can affect how quickly a drug is absorbed. For example, most absorption of oral drugs occurs in the small intestine. If a patient has had large sections of the small intestine surgically removed, drug absorption decreases because of the reduced surface area and the reduced time a drug is in the intestine.

Other Factors Affecting Absorption

Drugs absorbed by the small intestine are transported to the liver before being circulated to the rest of the body. The liver may metabolize much of the drug before it enters circulation. This mechanism is referred to as the first-pass effect. Liver metabolism may inactivate the drug; if so, the first-pass effect lowers the amount of active drug released into the systemic circulation. Therefore, higher drug dosages must be administered to achieve the desired effect.

Increased blood flow to an absorption site improves drug absorption, whereas reduced blood flow decreases absorption. More rapid absorption leads to a quicker onset of drug action. For example, the muscle area selected for IM administration makes a difference in the drug absorption rate. Blood flows faster through the deltoid muscle (in the upper arm) than through the gluteal muscle (in the buttocks). The gluteal muscle, however, accommodates a larger volume of drug than does the deltoid muscle.

Pain and stress can decrease the amount of drug absorbed. This may be because of a change in blood flow, reduced movement through the GI tract, or gastric retention triggered by the autonomic nervous system response to pain.

High-fat meals and solid foods slow the rate at which contents leave the stomach and enter the intestines, delaying intestinal absorption of a drug. In addition, drug formulation (such as tablets, capsules, liquids, sustained-release formulas, inactive ingredients, and coatings) affects the drug absorption rate and the time needed to reach peak blood concentration levels. Finally, combining one drug with another drug, or with food, can cause interactions that increase or decrease drug absorption, depending on the substances involved.

Distribution

Drug distribution is the process by which the drug is delivered to the tissues and fluids of the body. Distribution of an absorbed drug within the body depends on several factors, including blood flow, solubility, and protein binding.

After a drug has reached the bloodstream, its distribution in the body depends on blood flow. The drug is quickly distributed to organs with a large supply of blood. These organs include the heart, liver, and kidneys. Distribution to other internal organs, skin, fat, and muscle is slower. The ability of a drug to cross a cell membrane depends on whether the drug is water-soluble or lipid (fat)-soluble. Lipid-soluble drugs easily cross through cell membranes, whereas a water-soluble drug cannot. Lipid-soluble drugs can also cross the blood–brain barrier and enter the brain. As a drug travels through the body, it comes in contact with proteins such as the plasma protein albumin. The drug can remain free or bind to the protein. The portion of a drug that is bound to a protein is inactive and cannot exert a therapeutic effect. Only the free, or unbound, portion remains active. A drug is said to be highly protein-bound if it is more than 80% bound to protein.

Metabolism

Drug metabolism, or biotransformation, refers to the body's ability to change a drug from its dosage form to a more water-soluble form that can then be excreted. Drugs can be metabolized in several ways. Most commonly, a drug is metabolized into inactive metabolites (products of metabolism), which are then excreted. Other drugs can be converted to metabolites that are active, meaning they are capable of exerting their own pharmacologic action. Metabolites may undergo further metabolism or may be excreted from the body unchanged. Still other drugs can be administered as inactive drugs, called prodrugs, and do not become active until they are metabolized.

The majority of drugs are metabolized by enzymes in the liver; however, metabolism can also occur in the plasma, kidneys, and membranes of the intestines. In contrast, some drugs inhibit or compete for enzyme metabolism. When such drugs are administered together, accumulation of the drugs occurs. This accumulation increases the potential for an adverse reaction or drug toxicity. Finally, some drugs (such as penicillins) remain unmetabolized. They exert their action and are excreted unchanged.

Factors Affecting Metabolism

Certain diseases lower a person's metabolic rate. These diseases include cirrhosis (liver disease) and heart failure, which reduce circulation to the liver. Genetic factors allow some people to metabolize drugs rapidly, whereas others metabolize them more slowly. Environment also alters drug metabolism. For example, if a person is surrounded by cigarette smoke, the rate of metabolism of some drugs may be affected. A stressful environment also changes how a person metabolizes drugs. Finally, developmental changes affect drug metabolism. For example, because infants have immature livers, they have reduced rates of metabolism. Elderly patients experience a decline in liver size, blood flow, and enzyme production; this also slows metabolism.

Excretion

Drug excretion refers to the elimination of drugs from the body. Most drugs are excreted by the kidneys and leave the body through the urine. Drugs can also be excreted through the lungs, exocrine glands (sweat, salivary, or mammary), skin, and intestinal tract.

Half-Life Equals Half the Drug

The half-life of a drug is the time it takes for half of the drug to be eliminated by the body. Factors that affect a drug's half-life include its rate of absorption, metabolism, and excretion. Knowing how long a drug remains in the body helps determine how frequently a drug should be taken.

A drug that is given only once is eliminated from the body almost completely after five half-lives. A drug that is administered at regular intervals, however, reaches a steady concentration (or steady state) after approximately five half-lives. Steady state occurs when the rate of drug administration equals the rate of drug excretion.

Onset, Peak, and Duration

In addition to absorption, distribution, metabolism, and excretion, the following three factors play important roles in a drug's pharmacokinetics: onset of action, peak concentration, and duration of action.

Onset of Action

Onset of action refers to the time interval that starts when the drug is administered and ends when the therapeutic effect actually begins. Rate of onset varies depending on the route of administration and on other pharmacokinetic properties.

Peak Concentration

As the body absorbs more drug, blood concentration levels rise. The peak concentration level is reached when the absorption rate equals the elimination rate. However, the time of peak concentration is not always the time of peak response.

Duration of Action

The duration of action is the length of time the drug produces its therapeutic effect.

Pharmacodynamics

Pharmacodynamics is the study of the drug mechanisms that produce biochemical or physiologic changes in the body. The interaction at the cellular level between a drug and cellular components, such as the complex proteins that make up the cell membrane, enzymes, or target receptors, represents drug action. The response resulting from this drug action is the drug effect.

Ways Drugs Work

A drug can modify cell function or the rate of function, but a drug cannot impart a new function to a cell or to target tissue. Therefore, the drug effect depends on what the cell is capable of accomplishing. A drug can alter the target cell's function by (1) modifying the cell's physical or chemical environment or (2) interacting with a receptor (a specialized location on a cell membrane or inside a cell).

Many drugs work by stimulating or blocking drug receptors. A drug attracted to a receptor displays an affinity (attraction) for that receptor. When a drug displays an affinity for a receptor and stimulates it, the drug acts as an agonist. The drug's ability to initiate a response after binding with the receptor is referred to as intrinsic activity.

If a drug has an affinity for a receptor but displays no intrinsic activity (in other words, it does not stimulate the receptor), then it is called an antagonist. The antagonist prevents a response from occurring. Antagonists can be competitive or noncompetitive. A competitive antagonist competes with the agonist for receptor sites. Because this type of receptor binds reversibly to the receptor site, giving larger doses of an agonist can overcome the antagonist's effects. A noncompetitive antagonist binds to receptor sites and blocks the effects of the agonist. Giving larger doses of the agonist cannot reverse its action.

Receptors

If a drug acts on a variety of receptors, it is said to be nonselective and can cause multiple and widespread effects. In addition, some receptors are classified further by their specific effects. For example, beta receptors typically produce increased heart rate and bronchial relaxation as well as other systemic effects. Beta receptors are divided into beta$_1$ receptors (which act primarily on the heart) and beta$_2$ receptors (which act primarily on smooth muscles of the lungs and gland cells).

Potency

Drug potency refers to the relative amount of a drug required to produce a desired response. Drug potency is also used to compare two drugs. If drug X produces the same response as drug Y but at a lower dose, then drug X is more potent than drug Y.

As its name implies, a dose-response curve is used to graphically represent the relationship between the dose of a drug and the response it produces (Fig. 2-1).

Maximum Effect

On the dose-response curve, a low dose usually corresponds with a low response. At a low dose, an increase in dose produces only a slight increase in response. With further increases in dose, there is a significant rise is drug response. After a certain point, an increase in dose yields little or no increase in response. At this point, the drug is said to have reached maximum effectiveness.

Therapeutic Index

Most drugs produce multiple effects. The relationship between a drug's desired therapeutic effects and its adverse effects is called the drug's therapeutic index. It is also referred to as its margin of safety. The therapeutic index usually measures the difference between an effective dose for 50% of patients treated and the minimal dose at which adverse reactions occur. Drugs with a low therapeutic index have a narrow margin of safety. This means that there is a narrow range of safety between an effective dose and a lethal one. On the other hand, a drug with a high therapeutic index has a large margin of safety and less risk of toxic effects.

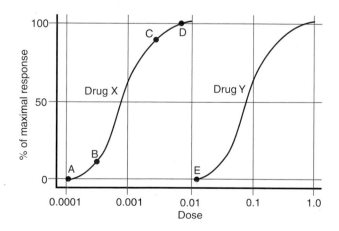

Figure 2-1 Dose-Response Curve. This curve show the drug-response curve for two different drugs. At low doses of each drug, a dosage increase results in only a small increase in drug response (e.g., from point A to point B). At higher doses, an increase in dosage produces a much greater response (from point B to point C). As the dosage continues to climb, an increase in dose produces very little increase in response (from point C to point D). This graph also shows that drug X is more potent than drug Y because it results in the same response but at a lower dose (compare point A with point E).

Pharmacotherapeutics

Pharmacotherapeutics is the use of drugs to treat disease. When choosing a drug to treat a particular condition, health care providers consider not only the drug's effectiveness but also other factors, such as the type of therapy the patient will receive.

Types of Drug Therapy

The type of therapy a patient receives depends on the severity, urgency, and prognosis of the patient's condition and can include:

- Acute therapy, if the patient is critically ill and requires acute intensive therapy.
- Empiric therapy, based on practical experience rather than on pure scientific data.
- Maintenance therapy, for patients with chronic conditions that do not resolve.
- Supplemental or replacement therapy, to replenish or substitute for missing substances in the body.
- Supportive therapy, which does not treat the cause of the disease but maintains other threatened body systems until the patient's condition resolves.
- Palliative therapy, used for end-stage or terminal diseases to make the patient as comfortable as possible.

Response

A patient's overall health as well as other individual factors can alter that patient's response to a drug. Coinciding medical conditions and personal lifestyle characteristics must be considered when selecting drug therapy (see Sidebar 2-1: *Factors Affecting a Patient's Response to a Drug*).

In addition, it is important to remember that certain drugs have a tendency to create drug tolerance and drug dependence. Drug tolerance occurs when a patient has a decreased response to a drug over time. The patient then requires larger doses to produce the same response.

Drug Dependence

Tolerance differs from drug dependence, in which a patient displays a physical or psychological need for the drug. Physical dependence produces withdrawal symptoms when the drug is stopped, whereas psychological dependence results in drug-seeking behaviors.

Drug Interactions

Drug interactions occur between drugs or between drugs and foods. They can interfere with the results of a laboratory test or produce physical or chemical incompatibilities. The more drugs a patient receives, the greater the chances are that a drug interaction will occur.

Factors Affecting a Patient's Response to a Drug

Because no two people are alike physiologically or psychologically, patient response to a drug can vary greatly, depending on such factors as:

- Age
- Cardiovascular function
- Diet
- Disease
- Drug interactions
- Gender
- GI function
- Hepatic function
- Infection
- Renal function

Potential drug interactions include additive effects, potentiation, antagonistic effects, decreased or increased absorption, and decreased or increased metabolism and excretion.

Additive Effects

An additive effect occurs when two drugs with similar actions are administered to a patient. The effects are equivalent to the sum of the effects of either drug administered alone in higher doses.

Giving two drugs together such as two analgesics (painkillers) has several potential advantages: lower doses of each drug, decreased probability of adverse reaction, and greater pain control than from one drug given alone (probably because of different mechanisms of action).

Potentiation

A synergistic effect, also called potentiation, occurs when two drugs that produce the same effect are given together and one drug potentiates (enhances the effect) of the other drug. This produces greater effects than each drug taken alone.

Antagonistic Effects

An antagonistic drug interaction occurs when the combined response of two drugs is less than the response produced by either drug alone.

Absorption Problems

Two drugs given together can change the absorption of one or both of the drugs. For example, drugs that change the acidity of the stomach can affect the ability of another drug to dissolve in the stomach. Some drugs can interact and form an insoluble compound that cannot be absorbed. After a drug is absorbed, the blood distributes it throughout the body as a free drug or one that is bound to plasma protein.

When two drugs are given together, they can compete for protein-binding sites, leading to an increase in the effects of one drug as that drug is displaced from the protein and becomes a free, unbound drug.

Toxic drug levels can occur when a drug's metabolism and excretion are inhibited by another drug. Some drug interactions affect excretion only. Drug interactions can also alter laboratory test results and produce changes on a patient's electrocardiogram.

Food Interactions

Interactions between drugs and food can alter the therapeutic effects of the drug. Food can also alter the rate and amount of drug absorbed from the GI tract, affecting bioavailability (i.e., the amount of a drug dose available to the systemic circulation). Drugs can also impair vitamin and mineral absorption.

Some drugs stimulate enzyme production, increasing metabolic rates and the demand for vitamins that are enzyme cofactors (which must unite with the enzyme for the enzyme to function). Dangerous interactions can also occur. For instance, when food that contains tyramine (such as aged cheddar cheese) is eaten by a person taking a monoamine oxidase inhibitor, hypertensive crisis can occur.

Adverse Drug Reactions

A drug's desired effect is called the expected therapeutic response. An adverse drug reaction (also called a side effect or adverse effect) is a harmful, undesirable response. Adverse drug reactions can range from mild ones that disappear when the drug is discontinued to debilitating diseases that become chronic.

Dose-Related Effects

Adverse drug reactions can be classified as dose-related or patient-sensitivity–related. Most adverse drug reactions result from the known pharmacologic effects of a drug and are typically dose-related. These types of reactions can be predicted in most cases.

Dose-related reactions include secondary effects, hypersusceptibility, overdose, and iatrogenic effects.

Secondary Effects

A drug typically produces not only a major therapeutic effect but also additional, secondary effects that can be beneficial or adverse. For example, morphine used for pain control can lead to two undesirable secondary effects: constipation and respiratory depression. Diphenhydramine used as an antihistamine is accompanied by the adverse reaction of sedation and is sometimes used as a sleep aid.

Hypersusceptibility

A patient can be hypersusceptible to the pharmacologic actions of a drug. Even when given a usual therapeutic dose, a hypersusceptible patient can experience an excessive therapeutic response or secondary effects. Hypersusceptibility typically results from altered pharmacokinetics (absorption, metabolism, and excretion), which leads to higher than expected blood concentration levels. Increased receptor sensitivity also can increase the patient's response to therapeutic or adverse effects.

Overdose

A toxic drug reaction can occur when an excessive dose is taken, either intentionally or accidentally. The result is an exaggerated response to the drug that can lead to transient changes or more serious reactions, such as respiratory depression, cardiovascular collapse, and even death. To avoid toxic reactions, chronically ill or elderly patients often receive lower drug doses.

Iatrogenic Effects

Some adverse drug reactions, known as iatrogenic effects, can mimic pathologic disorders. For example, drugs such as antineoplastics, aspirin, corticosteroids, and indomethacin commonly cause GI irritation and bleeding. Other examples of iatrogenic effects include induced asthma with propranolol, induced nephritis with methicillin, and induced deafness with gentamicin.

Sensitivity Reactions

Patient-sensitivity–related adverse reactions are not as common as dose-related reactions. Sensitivity-related reactions result from a patient's unusual and extreme sensitivity to a drug. These adverse reactions arise from a unique tissue response rather than from an exaggerated pharmacologic action. Extreme patient sensitivity can occur as a drug allergy or an idiosyncratic response.

Drug Allergy

A drug allergy occurs when a patient's immune system identifies a drug, a drug metabolite, or a drug contaminant as a dangerous foreign substance that must be neutralized or destroyed. Previous exposure to the drug or to one with similar chemical characteristics sensitizes the patient's immune system, and subsequent exposure causes an allergic reaction (hypersensitivity).

An allergic reaction not only directly injures cells and tissues but also produces broader systemic damage by initiating cellular release of vasoactive and inflammatory substances. The allergic reaction can vary in intensity from an immediate, life-threatening anaphylactic reaction with circulatory collapse and swelling of the larynx and bronchioles to a mild reaction with a rash and itching.

Idiosyncratic Response

Some sensitivity-related adverse reactions do not result from pharmacologic properties of a drug or from allergy but are specific to the individual patient. These are called idiosyncratic responses. A patient's idiosyncratic response sometimes has a genetic cause.

Quick Quiz

1. While teaching a patient about drug therapy for diabetes, you review the absorption, distribution, metabolism, and excretion of insulin and oral antidiabetic agents. Which principle of pharmacology are you describing?

   A. Pharmacokinetics
   B. Pharmacodynamics
   C. Pharmacotherapeutics

2. Which type of drug therapy is used for patients who have a chronic condition that cannot be cured?

   A. Empiric therapy
   B. Palliative therapy
   C. Maintenance therapy

3. Which branch of pharmacology studies the way drugs work in living organisms?

   A. Adverse reactions
   B. Pharmacokinetics
   C. Pharmacodynamics

Autonomic Nervous System Drugs

Drugs that affect the autonomic nervous system include those that stimulate or block the actions of both the sympathetic and parasympathetic branches of this system. These drugs include cholinergics, cholinergic blockers, adrenergics, and adrenergic blockers. The actions of the sympathetic and parasympathetic branches of the autonomic nervous system are outlined in Figure 3-1.

Cholinergic Drugs

Cholinergic drugs promote the action of the neurotransmitter acetylcholine. These drugs are also called parasympathomimetic drugs because they produce effects that imitate parasympathetic nerve stimulation.

There are two major classes of cholinergic drugs: cholinergic agonists and anticholinesterase drugs. Cholinergic agonists mimic the action of the neurotransmitter acetylcholine. Anticholinesterase drugs work by inhibiting the destruction of acetylcholine at the cholinergic receptor sites (Fig. 3-2).

Cholinergic Agonists

Common Drug Names

acetylcholine: Miochol-E, Miochol (optic)

bethanechol: Duvoid, PMS-Bethanechol Chloride, Urecholine

carbachol: Carbastat, Carboptic, Isopto Carbachol (topical), Miostat (intraocular)

pilocarpine: Diocarpine, Isopto Carpine, Miocarpine, Ocusert Pilo, Pilocar, Pilopine, Piloptic, Salagen

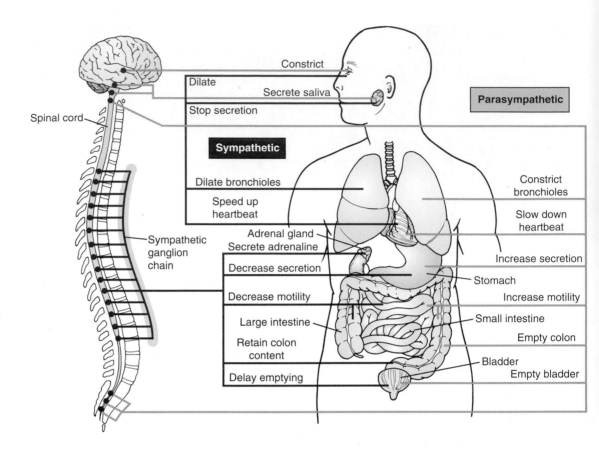

Figure 3-1 Autonomic Nervous System: Sympathetic and Parasympathetic Branches. The sympathetic pathways are highlighted with dark blue, and the parasympathetic pathways are highlighted with light blue. (Adapted from Thibodeau GA. Structure and Function of the Body. 11th Ed. St Louis: Mosby, 2000.)

Pharmacokinetics (how drugs circulate)

The action and metabolism of the cholinergic agonists vary widely. Acetylcholine poorly penetrates the central nervous system (CNS), and its effects are primarily peripheral, with a widespread action. The drug is rapidly destroyed in the body.

The cholinergic agonists rarely are administered by intramuscular (IM) or intravenous (IV) injection because they are almost immediately broken down by cholinesterases in the interstitial spaces between tissues and inside the blood vessels. Moreover, they begin to work rapidly and can cause a cholinergic crisis (a drug overdose resulting in extreme muscle weakness and possible paralysis of the muscles used in respiration). Cholinergic agonists are usually administered topically (via eye drops), orally, or by subcutaneous (SC) injection. SC injections begin to work more rapidly than oral doses. In addition, their response is often more effective.

All cholinergic agonists are metabolized by cholinesterases (enzymes that break down acetylcholine). All drugs in this class are excreted by the kidneys.

Pharmacodynamics (how drugs act)

Cholinergic agonists work by mimicking the action of acetylcholine on the neurons in certain organs of the body, called target organs. When cholinergic agonists combine

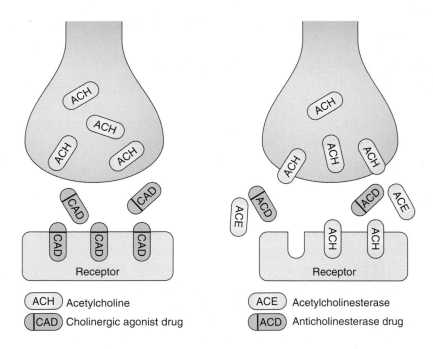

Figure 3-2 Action of Cholinergic Drugs.

Cholinergic drugs fall into one of two major classes: cholinergic agonists and anticholinesterase drugs. These drugs achieve their effects in the following ways.

Cholinergic agonists. When a neuron in the parasympathetic nervous system is stimulated, the neurotransmitter acetylcholine is released. Acetylcholine crosses the synapse and interacts with receptors in an adjacent neuron. Cholinergic agonist drugs work by stimulating cholinergic receptors, mimicking the action of acetylcholine.

Anticholinesterase drugs. After acetylcholine stimulates the cholinergic receptor, it is destroyed by the enzyme acetylcholinesterase. Anticholinesterase drugs produce their effects by inhibiting acetylcholinesterase. Acetylcholine is not broken down and begins to accumulate; therefore, the effects of acetylcholine are prolonged.

with receptors on the cell membranes of target organs, they stimulate the muscle and produce salivation, bradycardia (slow heart rate), dilation of blood vessels, constriction of the bronchioles of the lungs, increased activity of the gastrointestinal (GI) tract, increased tone and contraction of the muscles of the bladder, and constriction of the pupils.

Pharmacotherapeutics (how drugs are used)

Cholinergic agonists are used to treat atonic (weak) bladder conditions and postoperative and postpartum urine retention; to treat GI disorders, such as postoperative abdominal distention and GI atony (lack of muscle tone); to reduce eye pressure in patients with glaucoma and during eye surgery; and to treat salivary gland hypofunction caused by radiation therapy and Sjögren's syndrome.

MASSAGE IMPLICATIONS AND ASSESSMENT

In general, massage itself is used to stimulate the parasympathetic nervous system and to bring about relaxation. If the client is taking a drug whose main action is to stimulate this same system, then the effects of the massage will be greatly increased and could lead to problems. The systemic reflexive strokes (such as effleurage and friction) also can increase acetylcholine as well as increase endorphins and enkephalins. These also "turn on" the parasympathetic system. Cholinergics that are given as eye drops to treat glaucoma have little systemic effect and are therefore not of major concern.

Any cholinergic drug given by mouth or injection will have systemic effects. During the massage, limiting the use of systemic reflexive strokes and utilizing more mechanical and somatic reflex strokes (pétrissage, vibration, compression) minimize the additive effect of the drugs and still provide muscle relaxation effects.

Side Effects

These drugs have many side effects. Stimulation of the parasympathetic nervous system has effects throughout the body. The main side effects that a massage therapist should be aware of are low blood pressure and orthostatic hypotension (drop in blood pressure when changing positions). These conditions can lead to dizziness and fainting. The above changes in the type of massage strokes used can help prevent a worsening of these effects. In addition, using stimulating strokes at the end of the massage, such as rapid effleurage and tapotement, prevents a possible drop in blood pressure. Always stay with the client while he or she sits up to ensure that there is no dizziness. Let the client sit on the side of the table for a few minutes.

Using more rapid effleurage strokes throughout the massage may also be helpful. This gives the mechanical effects of the stroke (rather than the systemic reflex effects) more strength. If the goal of the massage is not relaxation but stimulation, more effort will be required. The drugs will act against you in this case, requiring the sedation and relaxation effects of the drug to be overcome. Stimulating strokes may need to be applied for a longer time than usual to obtain the desired effects. The more severe adverse reactions that can occur with cholinergic drugs must be reported to the physician, and massage is contraindicated (see Sidebar: *Adverse Reactions to Cholinergic Agonists*).

Adverse Reactions to Cholinergic Agonists

Side Effects
- Hypotension
- Nausea
- Increased salivation and sweating
- Urinary frequency

Adverse Effects
- Nausea and vomiting
- Cramps and diarrhea
- Blurred vision
- Decreased heart rate
- Severely low blood pressure
- Shortness of breath

Anticholinesterase Drugs

Common Drug Names

ambenonium: Mytelase

donepezil: Aricept, Ezozo

echothiophate: Phospholine Iodide

edrophonium: Enlon, Reversol, Tensilon,

galantamine: Reminyl

neostigmine: Prostigmin

physostigmine salicylate: Antilirium

pyridostigmine: Mestinon, Mestinon-SR, Regonol, Timespan

rivastigmine: Exelon

tacrine: Cognex, tetrahydroaminoacrine, THA

Anticholinesterase drugs block the action of the enzyme acetylcholinesterase (which breaks down acetylcholine) at cholinergic receptor sites, thus preventing the breakdown of the neurotransmitter acetylcholine. As acetylcholine builds up, it continues to stimulate the cholinergic receptors. Anticholinesterase drugs are divided into two categories—reversible and irreversible. Reversible anticholinesterase drugs have a short duration of action.

Irreversible anticholinesterase drugs have long-lasting effects and are used primarily as toxic insecticides and pesticides or as nerve gas in chemical warfare. Only echothiophate (Phospholine Iodide) has therapeutic usefulness.

Pharmacokinetics

This section briefly describes how anticholinesterase drugs move through the body. Many of the anticholinesterase drugs are readily absorbed from the GI tract, the skin, and mucous membranes. Because neostigmine is poorly absorbed from the GI tract, higher doses are necessary when this drug is taken orally. However, because the duration of action for an oral dose is longer, the patient does not need to take the drug as frequently. When a rapid effect is needed, the drug is given intramuscularly or intravenously. Most anticholinesterase drugs are metabolized in the body by enzymes in the plasma and excreted in the urine. Donepezil and tacrine are metabolized in the liver.

Pharmacodynamics

Anticholinesterase drugs, like cholinergic agonists, promote the action of acetylcholine at receptor sites. Depending on the site and the drug's dose and duration of action, they can produce a stimulant or depressant effect on cholinergic receptors.

Reversible anticholinesterase drugs block the breakdown of acetylcholine for minutes to hours. The blocking effect of the irreversible anticholinesterase drugs lasts for days or weeks.

Pharmacotherapeutics

Anticholinesterase drugs have a variety of therapeutic uses. They are used to reduce eye pressure in patients with glaucoma and during eye surgery, to increase bladder tone, to improve tone and peristalsis (movement) through the GI tract in patients with reduced motility and paralytic ileus (paralysis of the small intestine), to promote muscular contraction in patients with myasthenia gravis, to diagnose myasthenia gravis (neostigmine and edrophonium are used for this purpose), and to treat mild to moderate dementia of the Alzheimer's type. They also serve as an antidote to cholinergic blocking drugs (also called anticholinergic drugs), tricyclic antidepressants, belladonna alkaloids, and narcotics.

MASSAGE IMPLICATIONS AND ASSESSMENT

Anticholinesterase drugs stimulate the parasympathetic nervous system by preventing the breakdown of the neurotransmitter acetylcholine, rather than by directly stimulating the receptors themselves (as in the case of cholinergic drugs). The effects, however, are very similar. Massage increases parasympathetic activity and so do anticholinesterase drugs. The same changes in the approach to massage that were needed with cholinergic drugs are therefore needed with anticholinesterase drugs. More mechanical and somatic reflex strokes and less systemic reflex strokes are used.

Side Effects

As with the cholinergic drugs, anticholinesterase drugs have many systemic side effects when taken orally or by injection. Lower blood pressure, orthostatic hypotension, and dizziness can all be problematic. Again, the use of stimulating systemic strokes such as tapotement, deep compression, or rapid effleurage should be used at the end of a session. Stay with clients as they sit up, and have them sit on the side of the table for a few minutes to ensure safety. Stimulation may take longer than usual owing to the effects of the drug. Severs adverse reactions must be reported to the physician, and massage is contraindicated (see Sidebar: *Adverse Reactions to Anticholinesterase Drugs*).

Adverse Reactions to Anticholinesterase Drugs

Side Effects

- Hypotension
- Muscle cramps and fasciculation
- Urinary frequency
- Increased saliva and sweat

Adverse Effects

- Nausea and vomiting
- Diarrhea
- Shortness of breath, wheezing, or tightness in the chest
- Seizures

Cholinergic Blocking Drugs

Common Drug Names: Alkaloids

atropine: Atropisol, Isopto-Atropine, Sal-Tropine

belladonna

homatropine: Isopto-Homatropine

hyoscyamine sulfate: Anaspaz, A-Spas, Cystospaz, Hyosine, Levbid, Levsinex, Spacol, Symax (with other compounds: Antispas, Domapine)

scopolamine hydrobromide: Isopto Hyoscine, Scopace, Transderm Scōp, Transderm-V

Common Drug Names: Synthetics

clidinium: Librax

glycopyrrolate: Robinul

propantheline: Propanthel

Common Drug Names: Tertiary Amines

benztropine: Apo-Benztropine, Cogentin

dicyclomine: Bentylol, Bentyl, Dicyclocot, Formulex, Lomine

ethopropazine: Parsitan

oxybutynin: Ditropan, Gen-Oxybutynin, Novo-Oxybutynin

tolterodine: Detrol, Detrol LA

trihexyphenidyl: Apo-Trihex, Artane

Cholinergic blocking drugs interrupt parasympathetic nerve impulses in the central and autonomic nervous systems. These drugs are also referred to as anticholinergic drugs because they prevent acetylcholine from stimulating cholinergic receptors. The major cholinergic blocker drugs are the belladonna alkaloids.

Because benztropine, ethopropazine, and trihexyphenidyl are almost exclusively treatments for Parkinsonism, they are discussed fully in Chapter 4, "Neurologic and Neuromuscular Drugs."

Pharmacokinetics

This section briefly describes how cholinergic blockers move through the body. The belladonna alkaloids are absorbed from the eyes, GI tract, mucous membranes, and skin. They are metabolized in the liver and excreted by the kidneys as unchanged drug and metabolites. When administered intravenously, cholinergic blockers such as atropine begin to work immediately.

The synthetic drugs are a bit more complicated. The synthetic derivatives are absorbed primarily through the GI tract, although not as readily as the belladonna alkaloids. Hydrolysis occurs in the GI tract and the liver; excretion is in feces and urine.

How dicyclomine is metabolized is unknown, but it is excreted equally in feces and urine.

Pharmacodynamics

Cholinergic blockers can have paradoxic effects depending on the dosage and condition being treated. These drugs can produce a stimulating or depressing effect, depending on the target organ. For example, when targeting the heart, the drugs have a stimulating effect. When targeting the GI tract, the drugs have a depressant effect. In the brain, cholinergic blockers produce both effects—low drug levels stimulate the brain and high drug levels depress it.

The effects of a drug are also determined by a patient's disorder. Parkinsonism, for example, is characterized by low dopamine levels that intensify the stimulating effects of acetylcholine. Cholinergic blockers, however, depress this effect. In other disorders, these same drugs stimulate the CNS.

Pharmacotherapeutics

Cholinergic blockers are often used to treat GI disorders and complications. All cholinergic blockers are used to treat spastic or hyperactive conditions of the GI and urinary tracts because they relax muscles and decrease GI secretions. The quaternary ammonium compounds, such as propantheline, are the drugs of choice for these conditions because they cause fewer adverse reactions than the belladonna alkaloids.

Cholinergic blocking drugs are given by injection before such diagnostic procedures as endoscopy or sigmoidoscopy to relax the GI smooth muscle. Cholinergic blockers such as atropine are given before surgery to reduce oral and gastric secretions, to reduce secretions in the respiratory system, and to prevent a drop in heart rate caused by vagal nerve stimulation during anesthesia. Cholinergic blockers are used to treat Parkinson's disease and the extrapyramidal (Parkinson-like) symptoms caused by drugs. They are also used as cycloplegics. This means that they paralyze the ciliary muscles of the eye (used for fine focusing and accommodation) and alter the shape of the lens of the eye. Moreover, cholinergic blockers act as mydriatics to dilate the pupils of the eye, making it easier to measure refractive errors during an eye examination or to perform eye surgery.

The belladonna alkaloids are used with morphine to treat biliary colic (pain caused by stones in the bile duct). Atropine is the drug of choice to treat symptomatic sinus bradycardia (when the heart beats too slowly, causing low blood pressure or dizziness) (Fig. 3-3). The belladonna alkaloids, particularly atropine and hyoscyamine, are effective antidotes to cholinergic and anticholinesterase drugs. Atropine is the drug of choice to treat poisoning from organophosphate pesticides. Atropine and hyoscyamine also counteract the effects of the neuromuscular blocking drugs by competing for the same receptor sites.

Scopolamine, given with the pain medications morphine or meperidine, causes drowsiness and amnesia in patients undergoing surgery. Scopolamine is also used to treat motion sickness.

MASSAGE IMPLICATIONS AND ASSESSMENT

In theory, the action of the cholinergic blockers is to decrease parasympathetic actions. However, these drugs tend to have different effects depending on what organ is targeted, the dose and frequency of the medication, and the route of administration. Effects on the brain are dose related. High dosages stimulate the parasympathetic response, and low dosages decrease this response. Because these drugs affect only the muscarinic receptors but not all receptors of the parasympathetic system, the response of the target organ may be to block the parasympathetic stimulation, but the rest of the body may experience side effects of stimulation of the parasympathetic system. This makes working with clients taking these drugs very confusing. A discussion with the client, physician, or pharmacist concerning the drug, diagnosis, and dosage and route may clarify what effects the drug will have. If the general effect is to block the parasympathetic system, then use the reflexive strokes and the mechanical strokes to achieve muscle relaxation and general relaxation. Recognize that the effects may take longer than usual because of the blocking effects of the drug. Rocking strokes may be helpful as well. If the systemic effect is stimulating the parasympathetic nervous system, then care must be taken not to overdo the relaxation effect by using more rapid effleurage, tapotement, deep compression, and shaking strokes that will counter the effects of the drug. Muscular relaxation can be achieved without the client being too sedated after the session.

Side Effects

Side effects will vary depending on the action of the drugs as discussed above. Many times the side effects the client is experiencing will be the biggest clue regarding how to proceed with a massage that will meet the client's needs. The most common side effects are low blood pressure, orthostatic hypotension, muscle cramping, and fasciculations. The first two require stimulating strokes at the end of the session and care in getting the client up from the table. The second two re-

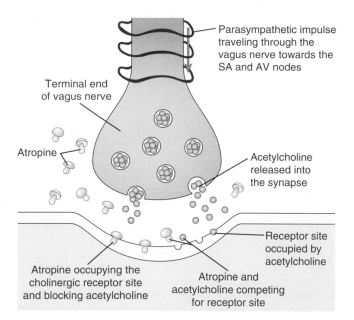

Parasympathetic impulse traveling through the vagus nerve towards the SA and AV nodes

Terminal end of vagus nerve

Atropine

Acetylcholine released into the synapse

Receptor site occupied by acetylcholine

Atropine occupying the cholinergic receptor site and blocking acetylcholine

Atropine and acetylcholine competing for receptor site

Figure 3-3 Increase in Heart Rate Caused by Atropine. To understand how atropine affects the heart, first consider how the heart's electrical conduction system functions. *Without the drug:* When the neurotransmitter acetylcholine is released, the vagus nerve stimulates the sinoatrial (SA) node (the heart's pacemaker) and the atrioventricular (AV) node, which controls conduction between the atria and the ventricles of the heart. This inhibits electrical conduction and causes the heart rate to slow. *With the drug:* When a patient receives atropine, a cholinergic blocking drug, the atropine competes with acetylcholine for binding with the cholinergic receptors on the SA and AV nodes. By blocking acetylcholine, atropine increases the heart rate.

Adverse Reactions to Cholinergic Blockers

Side Effects
- Dry mouth
- Decreased sweating
- Increased heart rate
- Constipation
- Anxiety
- Restlessness

Adverse Effects
- Blurred vision
- Arrhythmias
- Disorientation
- Hallucination
- Urinary retention
- Glaucoma
- Heatstroke

quire mechanical strokes and strokes that systemically relax the nervous system such as slow effleurage, pétrissage, and rocking or gentle shaking. Severe adverse effects are a contraindication and must be reported to the physician (see Sidebar: *Adverse Reactions to Cholinergic Blockers*).

Adrenergic Drugs

Adrenergic drugs are also called sympathomimetic drugs because they produce effects similar to those produced by the sympathetic nervous system. Adrenergic drugs are classified into two groups based on their chemical structure: catecholamines (both naturally occurring and synthetic) and noncatecholamines.

Adrenergic drugs are also divided by how they act. They can be direct-acting, in which case the drug acts directly on the organ or tissue innervated (supplied with nerves or nerve impulses) by the sympathetic nervous system. They can also be indirect-acting, in which case the drug triggers the release of a neurotransmitter, usually norepinephrine.

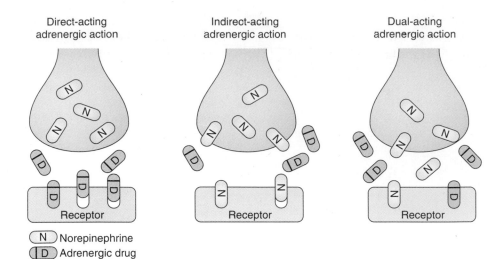

Figure 3-4 Understanding Adrenergic Drugs. Adrenergic drugs are distinguished by how they achieve their effect. The actions of direct-, indirect-, and dual-acting adrenergic drugs are shown. Direct-acting adrenergic drugs directly stimulate adrenergic receptors. Indirect-acting adrenergic drugs stimulate the release of norepinephrine from nerve endings into the synapse. Dual-acting adrenergic drugs stimulate both adrenergic receptor sites and the release of norepinephrine from nerve endings.

Finally, they can be dual-acting, in which case the drug has both direct and indirect actions (Fig. 3-4).

Therapeutic use of adrenergic drugs (catecholamines and noncatecholamines) depends on which receptors they stimulate and to what degree. Adrenergic drugs can affect alpha-adrenergic receptors, beta-adrenergic receptors, and dopamine receptors. Most of the adrenergic drugs produce their effects by stimulating alpha receptors and beta receptors. These drugs mimic the action of norepinephrine or epinephrine. Dopaminergic drugs act primarily on receptors in the sympathetic nervous system stimulated by dopamine.

Catecholamines

Common Drug Names

doputamine: Dobutrex

dopamine: Intropin

epinephrine: Adrenalin, AsthmaHaler (discontinued in the U.S.), Bronkaid Mist, EpiPen, Medihaler (discontinued in the U.S.), Primatene Mist, Sus-Phrine (discontinued in the U.S.)

isoproterenol: Isuprel, Medihaler-Iso (discontinued in the U.S.)

norepinephrine

Because of their common basic chemical structure, catecholamines share certain properties. They stimulate the nervous system, constrict peripheral blood vessels, increase heart rate, and dilate the bronchi. They can be manufactured in the body or in a laboratory.

Pharmacokinetics

Catecholamines cannot be taken orally because they are destroyed by digestive enzymes. When these drugs are given sublingually (under the tongue), they are rapidly absorbed through the mucous membranes. Any sublingual drug not completely absorbed is rapidly metabolized by swallowed saliva. SC injection absorption is slowed because these drugs cause the blood vessels around the injection site to constrict. IM absorption is more rapid because there is less constriction of local blood vessels.

Catecholamines are widely distributed in the body. They are metabolized and inactivated predominantly in the liver but can also be metabolized in the GI tract, lungs, kidneys, plasma, and other tissues. Catecholamines are excreted primarily in the urine; however, a small amount of isoproterenol is excreted in the feces, and some epinephrine is excreted in breast milk.

Pharmacodynamics

Catecholamines are primarily direct-acting. When catecholamines combine with alpha receptors or beta receptors, they cause either an excitatory or inhibitory effect. Typically, activation of alpha receptors generates an excitatory response except for intestinal relaxation. Activation of the beta receptors mostly produces an inhibitory response except in the cells of the heart, where norepinephrine produces excitatory effects.

The clinical effects of catecholamines depend on the dosage and on the route of administration. Catecholamines are potent inotropes (i.e., they make the heart contract more forcefully). As a result, the ventricles of the heart empty more completely with each heart beat, increasing the workload of the heart and the amount of oxygen it needs to do this harder work.

Catecholamines also produce a positive chronotropic effect, which means they cause the heart to beat faster. This is because the pacemaker cells in the sinoatrial (SA) node of the heart depolarize at a faster rate. As catecholamines cause blood vessels to constrict and blood pressure to rise, the heart rate can fall as the body tries to prevent an excessive rise in blood pressure.

Catecholamines can cause the Purkinje fibers (an intricate web of fibers that carry electrical impulses into the ventricles of the heart) to fire spontaneously, possibly producing abnormal heart rhythms (such as premature ventricular contractions and fibrillation). Epinephrine is more likely than norepinephrine to produce this spontaneous firing.

Pharmacotherapeutics

The therapeutic use of catecholamines depends on the particular receptor activity that is stimulated. Of the catecholamines, norepinephrine has the most nearly pure alpha activity. Dobutamine and isoproterenol have only beta-related therapeutic uses. Epinephrine stimulates alpha receptors and beta receptors. Dopamine primarily exhibits dopaminergic activity.

Catecholamines that stimulate alpha receptors are used to treat low blood pressure (hypotension). As a rule, catecholamines work best when used to treat hypotension caused by relaxation of the muscles of the blood vessels (also called a loss of vasomotor tone) and blood loss (such as from hemorrhage).

Catecholamines that stimulate $beta_1$ receptors are used to treat bradycardia, heart block (a delay or interruption in the conduction of electrical impulses between the atria and ventricles), low cardiac output, and paroxysmal atrial or nodal tachycardia (bursts of rapid heart rate). Catecholamines that exert $beta_2$ activity are used to treat acute and chronic bronchial asthma, emphysema, bronchitis, and acute hypersensitivity (allergic) reactions to drugs.

Because they are believed to make the heart more responsive to defibrillation (using an electrical current to terminate a deadly arrhythmia), $beta_1$-adrenergic drugs are used to treat ventricular fibrillation (quivering of the ventricles resulting in no pulse), asystole (no electrical activity in the heart), and cardiac arrest.

Dopamine, which stimulates the dopaminergic receptors, is used in low doses to improve blood flow to the kidneys because it dilates the renal blood vessels.

The effects of catecholamines produced by the body differ somewhat from the effects of manufactured catecholamines. Manufactured catecholamines have a short duration of action, which can limit their therapeutic usefulness.

Adverse Reactions to Adrenergic Catecholamines

Side Effects
- Restlessness
- Anxiety
- Dizziness
- Hypotension

Adverse Effects
- Headache
- Palpitations
- Cardiac arrhythmias
- Hypertension and hypertensive crisis
- Stroke
- Angina
- Increased blood glucose levels
- Tissue necrosis and sloughing (if any catecholamine given IV leaks into the surrounding tissue)

MASSAGE IMPLICATIONS AND ASSESSMENT

The adrenergic drugs stimulate the effects of the sympathetic nervous system. Sublingual and IM injections have effects on the entire body. Inhalation forms of these drugs work more specifically on the lungs; however, some systemic absorption occurs. Therefore, regular use of these inhalation forms also causes systemic effects. The effects of massage are blocked by these drugs. Strokes that work systemically to put the client into parasympathetic mode take longer to have an effect. Slow effleurage, rocking, and friction at the muscle–tendon juncture work best for systemic relaxation and bringing balance back to the body. This is especially important for someone receiving inhalation therapy. If the primary goal of the massage is muscle relaxation, then utilizing strokes with strong mechanical effects works best. Pétrissage, compression, more rapid effleurage, and even myofascial work bypass the systemic blocks and affect the local tissues. If the client is taking the drugs by injection, remember to avoid massage in the area of the injection site for at least several hours to prevent speeding the rate of absorption.

Side Effects

The side effects of adrenergic drugs are those of an activated sympathetic nervous system. In other words, the body shows signs of a stress reaction. Most common are restlessness, anxiety, dizziness, headache, and insomnia. The client may also exhibit weakness, tremors, and palpitations.

The goal of massage is often to help alleviate some of these effects. Slow rhythmic effleurage and rocking to entrain the body to a slower rhythm are the most beneficial. Because the effects of the drugs are very specific to target organs, performing massage to alleviate the general systemic effects does not interfere with drug treatment but helps the client to tolerate the drug regimen. In the case of EpiPen use (or injection of epinephrine, which is used for emergency situations such as bee sting or other severe allergic reactions), massage is contraindicated. More severe reactions, especially cardiac reactions, must be reported to a physician, and massage is contraindicated (see Sidebar: *Adverse Reactions to Adrenergic Catecholamines*).

Noncatecholamines

Common Drug Names

mephentermine: Wyamine Sulfate

metaraminol: Aramine

methoxamine

phenylephrine: AK-Nefrin Ophthalmic, Dionephrine, Mydfrin, Neo-Synephrine, Prefrin, Rhinall Nasal, Vicks Sinex Nasal

albuterol: Alti-Salbutamol, Apo-Salvent, Novo-Salmol, Proventil, Ventolin, Volmax

ephedrine: Pretz-D, Kondon's Nasal

isoetharine

terbutaline: Brethine, Bricanyl

ritodrine hydrochloride: Yutopar (discontinued in the U.S.)

metaproterenol: Alupent, Tanta Orciprenaline

levalbuterol: Xopenex

salmeterol: Serevent

formoterol: Foradil

Noncatecholamine adrenergic drugs have a variety of therapeutic uses because of the many effects these drugs can have on the body, including local or systemic constriction of blood vessels, nasal and eye decongestion, and dilation of the bronchioles smooth-muscle relaxation.

Pharmacokinetics

Although all these drugs are excreted in the urine, they are absorbed in different ways. Absorption of the noncatecholamine adrenergic drugs depends on the route of administration. Inhaled drugs, such as albuterol, are gradually absorbed from the bronchi of the lungs and result in lower drug levels in the body. Oral drugs are absorbed well from the GI tract and are distributed widely in the body fluids and tissues. Some noncatecholamine drugs (such as ephedrine) cross the blood–brain barrier and can be found in high concentrations in the brain and cerebrospinal fluid (fluid that moves through and protects the brain and spinal canal).

Metabolism and inactivation of noncatecholamines occur primarily in the liver but can also occur in the lungs, GI tract, and other tissues. Noncatecholamine drugs and their metabolites are excreted primarily in the urine. Some, such as inhaled albuterol, are excreted within 24 hours; others, such as oral albuterol, within 3 days. Acidic urine increases excretion of many noncatecholamines; alkaline urine slows excretion.

Pharmacodynamics

Noncatecholamines can be direct-acting, indirect-acting, or dual-acting (unlike catecholamines, which are primarily direct-acting). Direct-acting noncatecholamines that stimulate alpha activity include methoxamine and phenylephrine. Those that selectively exert beta$_2$ activity include albuterol, isoetharine, metaproterenol, ritodrine, and terbutaline. Indirect-acting noncatecholamines include phenylpropanolamine. Dual-acting noncatecholamines include ephedrine, mephentermine, and metaraminol. As with the catecholamines, these drugs are stimulating to the sympathetic nervous system. They may also have depressant effects, depending on the dose, route, and target organ.

Pharmacotherapeutics

Noncatecholamines stimulate the sympathetic nervous system and produce a variety of effects in the body. Metaraminol, for example, causes vasoconstriction and is used to treat hypotension in cases of severe shock. Ritodrine, in rare cases, is used to stop preterm labor. They are utilized much as the catecholamines are for hypotension, shock, bradycardia, heart block, arrhythmias, cardiac arrest, asthma, emphysema, bronchitis, and allergic reactions.

Adverse Reactions to Noncatecholamines

Side Effects
- Headache
- Restlessness
- Anxiety
- Irritability
- Trembling
- Drowsiness or insomnia
- Light-headedness

Adverse Effects
- Euphoria
- Incoherence
- Seizures
- Hypertension or hypotension
- Palpitations
- Bradycardia or tachycardia
- Irregular heart rhythm
- Cardiac arrest
- Cerebral hemorrhage
- Tingling or coldness in the arms or legs
- Angina
- Changes in heart rate and blood pressure in a pregnant woman and fetus

MASSAGE IMPLICATIONS AND ASSESSMENT

The noncatecholamine adrenergic drugs have all the same implications for massage as do the catecholamine adrenergics. Determining the desired action of the drug with the client, physician, and pharmacist, if needed, provides much information about the effects on the body. For the most part, a stimulatory effect on the sympathetic system requires use of systemic reflex strokes (such as effleurage and friction) and mechanical strokes (such as pétrissage). These will help achieve the desired effect of systemic relaxation and muscle release. They may need to be applied for longer times than normal to achieve optimal effect.

Side Effects

The side effects of concern to the massage therapist are caused by stimulation of the sympathetic system. They include nervousness, anxiety, insomnia, tremor, cramping, and sometimes hypotension. The strokes discussed above will help to overcome the systemic stimulation and bring balance back to the body. Rocking and rhythmic effleurage will entrain the body into a more relaxed state as well. Severe adverse reactions contraindicate massage (see Sidebar: *Adverse Reactions to Noncatecholamines*).

Adrenergic Blocking Drugs

Adrenergic blocking drugs, also called sympatholytic drugs, are used to disrupt sympathetic nervous system function. These drugs work by blocking impulse transmission (and thus sympathetic nervous system stimulation) at adrenergic neurons or adrenergic receptor sites. Their action at these sites can be exerted by interrupting the action of sympathomimetic (adrenergic) drugs, reducing available norepinephrine, and preventing the action of cholinergic drugs. Adrenergic blocking drugs are classified according to their site of action as alpha-adrenergic blockers or beta-adrenergic blockers.

Alpha-Adrenergic Blockers

Common Drug Names

doxazosin: Cardura

ergoid mesylates: dihydroergotamine, dihydroergotoxine, Hydergine, Migranal

ergotamine: Cafergot, Ergostat (discontinued in the U.S.), Ergomar (discontinued in the U.S.), Wigraine

phenoxybenzamine: Dibenzyline

phentolamine: Rogitine

prazosin: Alti-Prazosin, Apo-Prazosin, Minipress, Novo-Prazin, Nu-Prazo (prazosin and polythiazide: Minizide)

tamsulosin hydrochloride: Flomax

terazosin hydrochloride: Hytrin

Alpha-adrenergic blocking drugs work by interrupting the actions of the catecholamines epinephrine and norepinephrine at alpha receptors. This results in relaxation of the smooth muscle in the blood vessels, increased dilation of blood vessels, and decreased blood pressure.

Ergotamine is a mixed alpha agonist and antagonist. At high doses, it acts as an alpha blocker.

Pharmacokinetics

The action of alpha blockers in the body is not well understood. Most of these drugs are absorbed erratically when administered orally and more rapidly and completely when administered sublingually. The various alpha blockers vary considerably in their onset of action, peak concentration levels, and duration of action.

Pharmacodynamics

Alpha blockers work in one of two ways. First, they can interfere with or block the synthesis, storage, release, and reuptake of norepinephrine by neurons. Second, they can antagonize epinephrine, norepinephrine, or adrenergic (sympathomimetic) drugs at alpha receptor sites. Although alpha receptor sites are either $alpha_1$ or $alpha_2$ receptors, alpha blockers include drugs that block stimulation of $alpha_1$ receptors and that may block $alpha_2$ stimulation.

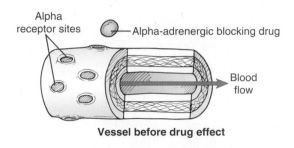

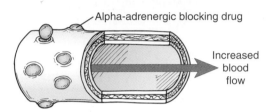

Figure 3-5 Alpha-Adrenergic Blocker Effects on Peripheral Blood Vessels. By occupying alpha receptor sites, alpha-adrenergic blocking drugs cause the blood vessel walls to relax. This leads to dilation of the blood vessels and reduced peripheral vascular resistance (the pressure that blood must overcome as it flows in a vessel). These effects can cause orthostatic hypotension, which is a drop in blood pressure that occurs when changing position from lying down to sitting or standing. Redistribution of blood to the dilated blood vessels of the legs causes hypotension.

Alpha blockers occupy alpha receptor sites on the smooth muscle of blood vessels (Fig. 3-5). This prevents catecholamines from occupying and stimulating the receptor sites. As a result, blood vessels dilate, increasing local blood flow to the skin and other organs. The decreased peripheral vascular resistance (resistance to blood flow) helps to decrease blood pressure.

The therapeutic effect of an alpha blocker depends on the sympathetic tone (the state of partial constriction of blood vessels) in the body before the drug is administered. For example, when the drug is given with the patient lying down, only a small change in blood pressure occurs. In this position, the sympathetic nerves release very little norepinephrine. Conversely, when a patient stands up, norepinephrine is released to constrict the veins and shoot blood back up to the heart. If the patient receives an alpha blocker, however, the veins cannot constrict and blood pools in the legs. Because blood return to the heart is reduced, blood pressure drops. This drop in blood pressure that occurs when a person stands up is called orthostatic hypotension.

Pharmacotherapeutics

Because alpha blockers cause smooth muscles to relax and blood vessels to dilate, they increase local blood flow to the skin and other organs as well as reduce blood pressure. As a result, they are used to treat hypertension and peripheral vascular disorders (disease of the blood vessels of the extremities), especially those in which spasm of the blood vessels causes poor local blood flow such as Raynaud's disease (intermittent pallor, cyanosis, or redness of fingers) and acrocyanosis (symmetric mottled cyanosis [bluish color] of the hands and feet). They are also used to treat frostbite, pheochromocytoma (a catecholamine-secreting tumor causing severe hypertension), and benign prostatic hypertrophy.

MASSAGE IMPLICATIONS AND ASSESSMENT

As always, the massage therapist needs to look at the action of the drug in the body. The alpha-adrenergic blockers stop the actions of epinephrine and norepinephrine (neurotransmitters made in the body). This stops stimulation of the sympathetic nervous system. The parasympathetic system is left in a normal state of activity but is not actually stimulated by the drugs. It is more a matter of the action of the sympathetic system not occurring to balance the body's reactions to changes. The client will experience parasympathetic relaxation very quickly with these drugs. The massage therapist needs to do less work to achieve relaxation both systemically and in the muscles. More stimulating strokes at the end of the session to allow the client to wake up may be needed. If the effect is strong, faster and more stimulating strokes may be needed throughout the massage.

Side Effects

The side effects of alpha-adrenergic blockers are orthostatic hypotension, lightheadedness, and sometimes flushing. The use of stimulating strokes such as rapid effleurage and tapotement is indicated. Shaking may also be used. This will help to prevent dizziness and a drop in blood pressure in many cases. Care still needs to be taken when clients are getting off the table. The therapist should stay and let the client sit on the side of the table until he or she is steady. Severe adverse reactions can occur. In such cases, the physician must be notified and massage withheld (see Sidebar: *Adverse Reactions to Alpha-Adrenergic Blocking Drugs*).

Adverse Reactions to Alpha-Adrenergic Blocking Drugs

Side Effects
- Hypotension
- Flushing
- Paresthesia
- Muscle weakness
- Fatigue
- Drowsiness

Adverse Effects
- Orthostatic hypotension or severe hypertension
- Bradycardia or tachycardia
- Edema
- Difficulty breathing
- Arrhythmias
- Angina
- Heart attack
- Cerebrovascular spasm
- Shocklike state
- Peptic ulcer
- Depression
- Confusion

Beta-Adrenergic Blockers

Common Drug Names: Nonselective

carvedilol: Coreg

labetalol: ibidomide, Normodyne, Trandate, Presolol

levobunolol: *l*-bunolol, Betagan, Novo-Levobunolol

nadolol: Alti-Nadolol, Apo-Nadolol, Corgard

penbutolol: Levatol

pindolol: Apo-Pindolol, Gen-Pindolol, Visken, Novo-Pindol, Syn-Pindolol

propranolol: Inderal, Apo-Propranolol, Detensol, Novopranol

sotalol: Alti-Sotalol, Apo-Sotalol, Betapace, Sorine, Sotacor

timolol: Apo-Timol, Apo-Timop, Betimol, Blocadren, Timoptic, Ocudose

---

Common Drug Names: Selective

acebutolol: Apo-Acebutolol, Gen-Acebutolol, Monitan, Rhotral, Sectral

atenolol: Apo-Atenolol, Gen-Atenolol, Tenormin, Tenolin

betaxolol: Betoptic, Kerlone

bisoprolol: Monocor, Zebeta

esmolol: Brevibloc

metoprolol: Apr-Metoprolol, Betaloc, Gen-Metoprolol, Lopressor, Nu-Metop, Topro-
   XL

Beta-adrenergic blockers, the most widely used adrenergic blockers, prevent stimulation of the sympathetic nervous system by inhibiting the action of catecholamines at beta-adrenergic receptors. These drugs are commonly referred to as "beta blockers."

Beta-adrenergic drugs are selective or nonselective. Nonselective beta-adrenergic drugs affect $beta_1$ receptor sites (located mainly in the heart) and $beta_2$ receptor sites (located in the bronchi, blood vessels, and uterus).

Pharmacokinetics

Beta-adrenergic blockers are usually absorbed rapidly and well from the GI tract and are protein-bound to some extent. Food does not inhibit their absorption and can enhance absorption of some drugs. Some beta-adrenergic blockers are absorbed more completely than others.

The onset of action of beta-adrenergic blockers is primarily dose-dependent and drug-dependent. The time it takes to reach peak concentration levels depends on the route of administration. Beta blockers given intravenously reach peak levels much more rapidly than when given by mouth.

Beta-adrenergic blockers are distributed widely in body tissues, with the highest concentrations found in the heart, liver, lungs, and saliva. With the exception of nadolol and atenolol, beta-adrenergic blockers are metabolized in the liver. They are excreted primarily in the urine as metabolites or in unchanged form, but can also be excreted in feces and bile with some secretion in breast milk.

Pharmacodynamics

Beta-adrenergic blockers have widespread effects in the body because they produce their blocking action not only at adrenergic nerve endings but also in the adrenal medulla. The following are some of the specific effects this can create.

Effects on the heart include increased peripheral vascular resistance, decreased blood pressure, decreased force of the contractions of the heart, decreased oxygen consumption by the heart, slowed conduction of impulses between the atria and ventricles of the heart, and decreased cardiac output (the amount of blood pumped by the heart each minute) (Fig. 3-6).

Some of the effects of beta-adrenergic blocking drugs depend on whether the drug is classified as selective or nonselective. Selective beta-adrenergic blockers, which preferentially block $beta_1$ receptor sites, reduce stimulation of the heart. They are often referred to as cardioselective beta-adrenergic blockers. Nonselective beta-adrenergic blockers, which block both $beta_1$ and $beta_2$ receptor sites, not only reduce stimulation of the heart but also

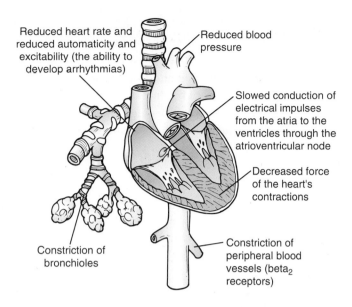

Reduced heart rate and reduced automaticity and excitability (the ability to develop arrhythmias)

Reduced blood pressure

Slowed conduction of electrical impulses from the atria to the ventricles through the atrioventricular node

Decreased force of the heart's contractions

Constriction of bronchioles

Constriction of peripheral blood vessels (beta$_2$ receptors)

Figure 3-6 Action of Beta-Adrenergic Blockers. By occupying beta receptor sites, beta-adrenergic blockers prevent catecholamines (norepinephrine and epinephrine) from occupying these sites and exerting their stimulating effects. The effects of beta-adrenergic blockers on the heart, lungs, and blood vessels are shown.

cause the bronchioles of the lungs to constrict. For example, nonselective beta-adrenergic blockers can cause bronchospasm in patients with chronic obstructive lung disorders. This adverse effect occurs less often when cardioselective drugs are given at lower doses.

Pharmacotherapeutics

Beta blockers are used to treat many conditions and are under investigation for use in many more. As mentioned previously, their clinical usefulness is based largely (but not exclusively) on how they affect the heart. Beta-adrenergic blockers can be prescribed after a heart attack to prevent another heart attack or to treat angina (chest pain), hypertension, hypertrophic cardiomyopathy (a disease of the heart muscle), and supraventricular arrhythmias (irregular heartbeats that originate in the atria, SA node, or atrioventricular node).

Beta-adrenergic blockers are also used to treat anxiety, cardiovascular symptoms associated with thyrotoxicosis (overproduction of thyroid hormones), essential tremor, migraine headaches, open-angle glaucoma, and pheochromocytoma.

MASSAGE IMPLICATIONS AND ASSESSMENT

Beta-adrenergic blockers are among the most commonly used drugs. The action of these drugs is to stop the sympathetic system effects on the body, especially the cardiovascular system and the lungs. The more selective drugs will have less systemic effects. The strokes utilized to relax the body and the muscles will all work more quickly with these drugs in the client's system. Oversedation during a massage may cause a client to have difficulty awakening. Using stimulating systemic

Adverse Reactions to Beta-Adrenergic Blockers

Side Effects
- Hypotension
- Flatulence
- Raynaud's syndrome

Adverse Effects
- Bradycardia
- Peripheral vascular insufficiency
- Atrioventricular block
- Heart failure
- Bronchospasm
- Diarrhea or constipation
- Nausea and vomiting
- Abdominal discomfort
- Anorexia
- Rash
- Fever with sore throat
- Spasm of the larynx
- Respiratory distress (allergic response)

reflexive and mechanical strokes either throughout the massage or just at the end will help prevent this and provide the muscle release and relaxation desired. Effleurage, pétrissage, friction, tapotement, deep tissue work, and shaking may all be used for this purpose. If the goal of the massage is to stimulate and warm up muscles, the mechanical, local strokes of effleurage and pétrissage work well. The systemic stimulation of the rapid effleurage and tapotement may take longer to have an effect.

Side Effects

The side effects of the beta-adrenergic blockers are similar to those of the alpha-adrenergics, although they may be less intense with the more selective cardiac drugs. Hypotension and orthostatic hypotension are the main areas of concern. Using stimulating strokes (as discussed above) at the end of the session helps with this problem. Again, the therapist should stay with clients as they sit up slowly. Clients should not be left alone until they are sure that they are not dizzy and that it is safe to get up. Some clients may have a side effect of Raynaud's syndrome. The blue or white color of the fingers, hands, or toes is due to a lack of circulation to the area. The cause is in the nervous system. At the time of the incident (which can come and go), no massage can be done to the locally affected area. Gentle warming holds only should be used so as not to damage the tissues that are deprived of oxygen. When the phenomenon is inactive, gentle massage of the area may be done. Other adverse reactions should be reported, and massage may need to be withheld until they are resolved (see Sidebar: *Adverse Reactions to Beta-Adrenergic Blockers*).

Quick Quiz

1. Your client is receiving Pilopine eye drops four times a day for glaucoma. What are the massage implications?

2. Your client is taking Aricept daily to treat early Alzheimer's disease. How should you alter your approach to massage with this client?

3. You are working on a cruise ship. Your client comes in with a transdermal skin patch and tells you it is Transderm Scōp for seasickness. How will this change your massage protocol?

4. Your client has asthma. She tells you she had to take her Primatine Mist about an hour ago, but is doing fine now. What do you need to consider when giving her a massage?

5. Your client is taking Lopressor daily for high blood pressure. Will this change your approach to the massage?

Neurologic and Neuromuscular Drugs

4

Skeletal Muscle Relaxants

Skeletal muscle relaxants relieve musculoskeletal pain or spasm and severe musculoskeletal spasticity (stiff, awkward movements). They are used to treat acute, painful musculoskeletal conditions and the muscle spasticity associated with multiple sclerosis (or MS, a progressive demyelination of the white matter of the brain and spinal cord, causing widespread neurologic dysfunction), cerebral palsy (a motor function disorder caused by neurologic damage), stroke (reduced oxygen supply to the brain resulting in neurologic deficits), and spinal cord injuries (injuries to the spinal cord that can result in paralysis or death).

This section discusses the two main classes of skeletal muscle relaxants: centrally acting and peripherally acting. It also discusses baclofen and diazepam, two drugs used to manage musculoskeletal disorders.

Exposure to severe cold, lack of blood flow to a muscle, or overexertion can send sensory impulses from the posterior sensory nerve fibers to the spinal cord and the higher levels of the central nervous system (CNS). These sensory impulses can cause a reflex (involuntary) muscle contraction or spasm from trauma, epilepsy, hypocalcemia (low calcium levels), or muscular disorders. The muscle contraction further stimulates the sensory receptors to a more intense contraction, establishing a cycle. Centrally acting muscle relaxants are believed to break this cycle by acting as CNS depressants.

Centrally Acting Skeletal Muscle Relaxants

Common Drug Names

carisoprodol: carisoprodate, isobamate, Soma

chlorzoxazone: Paraflex (discontinued in the U.S.), Parafon Forte, Remular-S, Strifon Forte *cyclobenzaprine:* Apo-Cyclobenzaprine, Flexeril, Flexitec, Novo-Cycloprine

metaxalone: Skelaxin

methocarbamol: Carbacot, Robaxin, Skelex, (with aspirin: Robaxisal)

orphenadrine: Banflex, Flexoject, Flexon, Myolin, Norflex, Orphenate, Rhoxal-orphen-drine

---

Centrally acting skeletal muscle relaxants, which act on the CNS, are used to treat acute spasms caused by such conditions as anxiety, inflammation, pain, and trauma. These drugs are not very effective in treating spasticity caused by a chronic neurologic disease such as cerebral palsy.

Pharmacokinetics (how drugs circulate)

There is still much we do not know about how centrally acting skeletal muscle relaxants circulate within the body. In general, these drugs are absorbed from the gastrointestinal (GI) tract, widely distributed in the body, metabolized in the liver, and excreted by the kidneys. When these drugs are administered orally, it can take from 30 to 60 minutes for effects to be achieved. Whereas the duration of action of most of these drugs varies from 4 to 6 hours, cyclobenzaprine has the longest duration of action at 12 to 25 hours.

Pharmacodynamics (how drugs act)

The centrally acting drugs do not relax skeletal muscles directly or depress neuron conduction, neuromuscular transmission, or muscle excitability. Although the precise mechanism of action of centrally acting drugs is unknown, these drugs are known to be CNS depressants. Skeletal muscle relaxant effects may be related to their sedative effects.

Pharmacotherapeutics (how drugs are used)

Patients receive centrally acting skeletal muscle relaxants to treat acute, painful musculoskeletal conditions. They are usually prescribed along with rest and physical therapy.

MASSAGE IMPLICATIONS AND ASSESSMENT

The main action of these drugs is depression of the CNS. Massage will not affect absorption because these drugs are taken orally. The types of strokes whose efficacy may be affected are the reflex strokes, both local and systemic. The effect of compression may be less effective since the reaction of the CNS to this stimulus will be slowed. The systemic reflex strokes, such as effleurage, may have increased and more rapid effects. The relaxation brought about by entrainment into the parasympathetic nervous system will be additive to the sedation already present due to the use of CNS depressant drugs. The most effective strokes in this situation are the local mechanical strokes (pétrissage, friction, and local effleurage) or gliding strokes. Myofascial work, which softens the local connective tissue, is also effective. Care must be taken to stimulate the client either during the entire massage or at the end of the massage with more rapid effleurage or tapotement. This helps to bring the client back to alertness.

Side Effects

The side effects of the centrally acting skeletal muscle relaxants are the result of CNS depression. They include drowsiness, dizziness, orthostatic hypotension, and constipation. The use of stimulating strokes either during or at the end of the massage, as discussed above, helps prevent problems with the client being too relaxed and ungrounded. It also helps prevent the drop in blood pressure that can occur with a change in position. It is advisable to assist the client to a sitting position before leaving the room. If constipation is a problem for the client, the use of effleurage on the abdomen and gliding strokes that follow the path of the large intestine may help alleviate this problem. Drinking extra fluids should also be suggested (see Sidebar: *Adverse Reactions to Centrally Acting Skeletal Muscle Relaxants*).

Peripherally Acting Skeletal Muscle Relaxants

Common Drug Names

dantrolene: Dantrium

Dantrolene is the most common peripherally acting skeletal muscle relaxant. Although dantrolene has a therapeutic effect similar to the centrally acting drugs, it works through a different mechanism of action. Because its major effect is on the muscle, dantrolene has a lower incidence of adverse CNS effects. High therapeutic doses, however, are toxic to the liver. Dantrolene seems most effective for spasticity of cerebral origin. Because it produces muscle weakness, dantrolene is of questionable benefit in patients with borderline strength.

Pharmacokinetics

Although the peak drug concentration of dantrolene occurs within approximately 5 hours after it is ingested, the patient may not note any therapeutic benefit for 1 week or more. Dantrolene is absorbed poorly from the GI tract. It is metabolized by the liver and excreted in the urine.

Pharmacodynamics

Dantrolene is chemically and pharmacologically unrelated to the other skeletal muscle relaxants. Dantrolene works by acting on the muscle itself. It interferes with calcium ion release from the sarcoplasmic reticulum and weakens the force of contractions. At therapeutic concentrations, dantrolene has little effect on cardiac or intestinal smooth muscle.

Pharmacotherapeutics

Dantrolene helps manage all types of spasticity but is most effective in patients with cerebral palsy, MS, spinal cord injury, and stroke. Dantrolene is also used to treat and prevent malignant hyperthermia. This rare but potentially fatal complication of anesthesia is

---

Adverse Reactions to Centrally Acting Skeletal Muscle Relaxants

Physical and psychological dependence can develop after long-term use of these drugs. Abruptly stopping any of these drugs can cause severe withdrawal symptoms. Other adverse reactions can also occur.

Side Effects
- Dizziness
- Drowsiness
- Constipation

Adverse Effects
- Abdominal distress
- Ataxia
- Diarrhea
- Heartburn
- Nausea and vomiting

characterized by skeletal muscle rigidity and high fever (see Sidebar: *Dantrolene and Muscle Rigidity Reduction*).

MASSAGE IMPLICATIONS AND ASSESSMENT

Dantrolene acts directly on the muscle by making it less responsive to the impulses of the CNS. It follows, therefore, that massage strokes that rely on the feedback reflex mechanisms for the muscles (local reflexes) would be less effective. These include compression, friction, and deep tissue. It is better to use mechanical strokes and the more systemic strokes, such as pétrissage and effleurage, in clients taking dantrolene. Because persons taking this drug are often struggling with problems of chronic spasticity of muscles, the use of rhythmic effleurage and rocking is helpful in entraining the body to a more relaxed state overall.

Side Effects

The side effects of this drug are similar to the centrally acting relaxants. The sedating effects are not as strong, but care must be taken to bring the client to full awareness with stimulating strokes at the end of the massage if necessary. Effleurage of the abdomen is helpful if constipation is a problem (see Sidebar: *Adverse Reactions to Peripherally Acting Skeletal Muscle Relaxants*).

Other Skeletal Muscle Relaxants

Common Drug Names

baclofen: Clofen

diazepam: Valium

tizanidine: Lioresal

Valium is primarily an antianxiety drug. It is a CNS depressant and is rarely used for muscle relaxation anymore. This section discusses baclofen and tizanidine only.

Pharmacokinetics

Both drugs are absorbed rapidly from the GI tract. They are distributed widely, undergo minimal liver metabolism, and are excreted primarily unchanged in the urine. It can take from hours to weeks before the patient notes any beneficial effects of baclofen. Abrupt withdrawal of the drug can cause hallucinations, seizures, and worsening of spasticity.

Pharmacodynamics

The exact mechanisms of action of baclofen and tizanidine are not known. The drugs are chemically similar to the neurotransmitter gamma-aminobutyric acid and probably act in the spinal cord. It seems that the drugs lessen neuron activity, decreasing the number and severity of muscle spasms, and reduce associated pain. Because baclofen and tizanidine produce less sedation than diazepam and less peripheral muscle weakness than dantrolene, they are the drugs of choice to treat spasticity.

Pharmacotherapeutics

The major clinical use is for paraplegic or quadriplegic patients with spinal cord lesions, most commonly caused by MS or trauma. For these patients, the drugs significantly reduce the number and severity of painful flexor spasms. Aside from these benefits, however, they do not improve stiff gait, manual dexterity, or residual muscle function.

MASSAGE IMPLICATIONS AND ASSESSMENT

In the case of diazepam or Valium, the massage practitioner must consider this drug in the same way as the centrally acting skeletal muscle relaxants discussed above. Because baclofen seems to act in the spinal cord, it would affect the local reflexes in the muscles. Deep tissue, compression, and friction are less effective in this case. Using mechanical strokes (myofascial, effleurage, pétrissage) and systemic reflex strokes to entrain the body to relaxation and balance is most effective.

Side Effects

The side effects of baclofen are much less than those of the other skeletal muscle relaxants. Some drowsiness may occur. Being sure that the client is fully awake at the end of the massage is important (see Sidebar: *Adverse Reactions to Other Skeletal Muscle Relaxants*).

> ### Adverse Reactions to Other Skeletal Muscle Relaxants
>
> **Side Effects**
> - Drowsiness
> - Dizziness
>
> **Adverse Effects**
> - Nausea
> - Hypotonia
> - Muscle weakness
> - Depression
> - Headache

Neuromuscular Blocking Drugs

Neuromuscular blocking drugs relax skeletal muscles by disrupting the transmission of nerve impulses at the motor end plate (the branching terminals of a motor nerve axon) (Fig. 4-1). Neuromuscular blockers have three major clinical indications: to relax skeletal muscles during surgery, to reduce the intensity of muscle spasms in drug or electrically induced seizures, and to manage patients who are fighting the use of a ventilator to help with breathing.

There are two main classes of natural and synthetic drugs used as neuromuscular blockers: nondepolarizing and depolarizing. Nondepolarizing blockers compete with acetylcholine at the cholinergic receptor sites of the skeletal muscle membrane. This blocks the neurotransmitter action of acetylcholine, preventing the muscle from contracting. The effect can be counteracted by anticholinesterase drugs, such as neostigmine or pyridostigmine, which inhibit the action of acetylcholinesterase, the enzyme that destroys acetylcholine.

The initial muscle weakness produced by these drugs quickly changes to a flaccid (loss of muscle tone) paralysis that affects the muscles in a specific sequence. The first muscles to exhibit flaccid paralysis are those of the eyes, face, and neck. Next, the limbs, abdomen, and trunk muscles become flaccid. Finally, the intercostal muscles (between the ribs) and diaphragm (the breathing muscle) are paralyzed. Recovery from paralysis usually occurs in the reverse order.

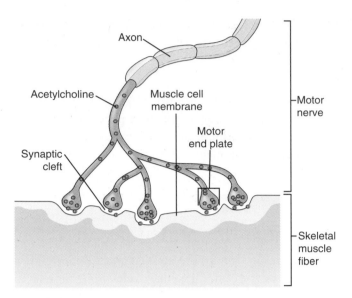

Figure 4-1 Motor End Plate. The motor nerve axon divides to form branching terminals called motor end plates. These are enfolded in muscle fibers but are separated from the fibers by the synaptic cleft. A stimulus to the nerve causes the release of acetylcholine into the synaptic cleft. There, acetylcholine occupies receptor sites on the muscle cell membrane, depolarizing the membrane and causing muscle contraction. Neuromuscular blocking agents act at the motor end plate by competing with acetylcholine for the receptor sites or by blocking depolarization.

Nondepolarizing blockers are used for intermediate or prolonged muscle relaxation to ease the passage of an endotracheal (ET) tube (a tube placed in the trachea), to decrease the amount of anesthetic required during surgery, and to facilitate realigning broken bones and dislocated joints. They are also used to paralyze patients who need ventilatory support but who fight the ET tube and ventilation, and to prevent muscle injury during electroconvulsive therapy (ECT) (passing an electric current through the brain to treat depression) by reducing the intensity of muscle spasms.

Of the depolarizing blocking drugs, succinylcholine is the only therapeutic drug. Although it is similar to the nondepolarizing blockers in its therapeutic effect, its mechanism of action differs. Succinylcholine acts like acetylcholine but is not inactivated by cholinesterase. It is the drug of choice when short-term muscle relaxation is needed. Succinylcholine is also the drug of choice for short-term muscle relaxation, such as during intubation and ECT.

MASSAGE IMPLICATIONS AND ASSESSMENT

Because these drugs paralyze the client, they are in most cases a complete contraindication for massage. They are used very specifically in procedures during which massage is inappropriate in any case. In rare cases, a client on long-term ventilator support who struggles against the action of the respirator may be given low doses of one of these drugs. In these cases, massage that is extremely gentle, effleurage mostly, could be used with permission of the physician.

Anti-Parkinson Drugs

Drug therapy is an important part of treatment of Parkinson's disease, which is a progressive neurologic disorder characterized by four cardinal features: muscle rigidity (inflexibility), akinesia (loss of muscle movement), tremors at rest, and disturbances of posture and balance. Parkinson's disease affects the extrapyramidal system, which influences movement. The extrapyramidal system includes the corpus striatum, globus pallidus, and substantia nigra of the brain.

In Parkinson's disease, a dopamine deficiency occurs in the basal ganglia, the dopamine-releasing pathway that connects the substantia nigra to the corpus striatum. Reduction of dopamine in the corpus striatum upsets the normal balance between two neurotransmitters, acetylcholine and dopamine. This results in increased cholinergic activity. The excessive excitation caused by cholinergic activity creates the movement disorders of Parkinson's disease. Parkinsonism can also result from drugs, encephalitis, neurotoxins, trauma, arteriosclerosis, or other neurologic disorders and environmental factors.

The goals of drug intervention are twofold: promote the secretion of dopamine (with dopaminergic drugs) and inhibit cholinergic effects (with anticholinergic drugs).

Anticholinergic Anti-Parkinson Drugs

Common Drug Names: Synthetic Tertiary Amines

benztropine: Apo-Benztropine, Cogentin

biperiden hydrochloride: Akineton, biperiden lactate

procyclidine: Kemadrin, Procyclid

trihexyphenidyl: Apo-Trihex, Artane, Trihexane, Trihexy-2, Trihexy-5

Common Drug Names: Antihistamines

diphenhydramine: Aler-Dryl, Banophen, Benadryl, Benylin,

orphenadrine: Banflex, Flexoject, Flexon, Myolin, Norflex, Orphenate

Anticholinergic drugs are sometimes called parasympatholytic drugs because they inhibit the action of acetylcholine at special receptors in the parasympathetic nervous system. Anticholinergics used to treat Parkinsonism are classified into two chemical categories according to their chemical structure. First are the synthetic tertiary amines, such as benztropine, biperiden hydrochloride, biperiden lactate, procyclidine, and trihexyphenidyl. Second are the antihistamines, such as diphenhydramine and orphenadrine.

Pharmacokinetics

Typically, anticholinergic drugs are well absorbed from the GI tract and cross to their action site in the brain. Most are metabolized in the liver, at least partially, and are excreted by the kidneys as metabolites and unchanged drug. The exact distribution of these drugs is unknown.

Benztropine is a long-acting drug, with a duration of action of up to 24 hours in some patients. For most anticholinergics, half-life is undetermined. In addition to the oral route, some anticholinergics can be given intramuscularly or intravenously.

Pharmacodynamics

High acetylcholine levels produce an excitatory effect on the CNS, which can cause Parkinsonian tremor. Patients with Parkinson's disease take anticholinergic drugs to inhibit the action of acetylcholine at receptor sites in the CNS and autonomic nervous system, thus reducing tremor.

Pharmacotherapeutics

Anticholinergics are used to treat all forms of Parkinsonism. They are used most commonly in the early stages of Parkinson's disease when symptoms are mild and do not have a major impact on the patient's lifestyle. These drugs effectively control sialorrhea (excessive flow of saliva) and are approximately 20% effective in reducing the incidence and severity of akinesia and rigidity. Anticholinergics can be used alone or with amantadine in the early stages of Parkinson's disease. These drugs can also be given with levodopa during the later stages to further relieve symptoms.

Adverse Reactions to Anticholinergics

Mild, dose-related adverse reactions to anticholinergics are seen in 30% to 50% of patients. Dry mouth may be a dose-related reaction to trihexyphenidyl.

Side Effects
- Restlessness
- Agitation and excitement
- Drowsiness or insomnia
- Constipation

Adverse Effects
- Confusion
- Tachycardia or palpitations
- Nausea and vomiting
- Urinary retention
- Increased intraocular pressure, blurred vision, pupil dilation, and photophobia
- Hives
- Allergic rashes

MASSAGE IMPLICATIONS AND ASSESSMENT

Anticholinergic drugs are also discussed in Chapter 3 under "Cholinergic Blocking Drugs." Their main action is to inhibit acetylcholine. In Parkinson's disease, this produces a decrease in CNS stimulation and in the rigidity and tremor characteristic of the disorder. The normal contraction and relaxation of muscle cells, and therefore muscle tone, are impaired in this disease. The muscles will not react normally to the local reflex strokes and sometimes not even to the mechanical strokes of massage. The acetylcholine excess leads to lack of muscle relaxation. The massage strokes that are most helpful to the client and that will work with the drug are the systemic reflex strokes of effleurage and rocking. When paired with some mechanical strokes, the parasympathetic nervous system is brought into play and can help relax the client and the muscles.

Side Effects

The main side effects are usually restlessness, agitation, constipation, and insomnia. The above use of massage helps to ameliorate all these symptoms. Drowsiness also occurs in some cases, and care in getting the client up from the table and alert after the massage must be taken (see Sidebar: *Adverse Reactions to Anticholinergics*).

Dopaminergics

Common Drug Names

amantadine: Antadine, Endantadine, Symmetrel, Symadine

bromocriptine: Apo-Bromocriptine, Parlodel

carbidopa-levodopa: Apo-Levocarb, Nu-Levocarb, Sinemet

entacapone: Comtan

levodopa: Dopar, Larodopa, Lidopa

pergolide: Permax

pramipexole: Mirapex

ropinirole: ReQuip

selegiline: Carbex, Eldepryl

tolcapone: Tasmar

Dopaminergics include drugs that are chemically unrelated:

- amantadine, an antiviral drug
- bromocriptine, a semisynthetic ergot alkaloid
- carbidopa-levodopa, a combination drug composed of carbidopa and levodopa
- levodopa, the metabolic precursor to dopamine
- pergolide and pramipexole, two dopamine agonists
- selegiline, a type B monoamine oxidase inhibitor (MAOI)

Pharmacokinetics

Like anticholinergic drugs, dopaminergic drugs are absorbed from the GI tract into the bloodstream and are delivered to their action site in the brain. Dopaminergic drugs are metabolized extensively in various areas of the body and eliminated by the liver, the kidneys, or both.

Pharmacodynamics

Dopaminergic drugs act in the brain to improve motor function in one of two ways: by increasing the dopamine concentration or by enhancing neurotransmission of dopamine.

Pharmacotherapeutics

Usually, dopaminergic drugs are used to treat patients with severe Parkinsonism or those who do not respond to anticholinergics alone. Levodopa is the most effective drug used to treat Parkinson's disease; however, it loses its effectiveness after 3 to 5 years. When carbidopa is given with levodopa, the dosage of levodopa can be reduced, decreasing the risk of GI and cardiovascular adverse effects.

Some dopaminergic drugs, such as amantadine, pramipexole, and bromocriptine, must be gradually tapered to avoid precipitating Parkinsonian crisis (sudden significant clinical deterioration) and possible life-threatening complications.

In some patients, levodopa can produce a significant interaction with foods. Dietary amino acids can decrease the effectiveness of levodopa by competing with it for absorption from the intestine and slowing its transport to the brain.

MASSAGE IMPLICATIONS AND ASSESSMENT

The dopaminergic drugs act on the neurotransmitter dopamine and act to decrease the rigidity of the muscles. The same implications for massage hold true here as for the anticholinergic drugs discussed above. Mechanical strokes mixed with systemic reflex strokes can help restore balance to the body of the client with Parkinson's disease.

Side Effects

The side effect common to almost all dopaminergic drugs is that of orthostatic hypotension. The massage practitioner needs to be aware of this and stay with clients as they sit up after the massage to ensure they are steady and safe. In more severe cases of Parkinson's disease, it may be necessary to assist the client with dressing (see Sidebar: *Adverse Reactions to Dopaminergics*).

Adverse Reactions to Dopaminergics

Side Effects

- Orthostatic hypotension
- Constipation
- Dizziness

Adverse Effects

Levodopa

- Nausea and vomiting
- Anorexia
- Neuroleptic malignant syndrome
- Arrhythmias
- Irritability
- Confusion

Bromocriptine

- Persistent orthostatic hypotension
- Ventricular tachycardia
- Bradycardia
- Worsening angina

Pergolide

- Confusion
- Dyskinesia
- Hallucinations
- Nausea

Pramipexole

- Confusion
- Insomnia

Anticonvulsant Drugs

Anticonvulsant drugs inhibit neuromuscular transmission. These agents are prescribed for long-term management of chronic epilepsy (recurrent seizures) and for short-term management of acute isolated seizures not caused by epilepsy, such as after trauma or brain surgery. In addition, some anticonvulsants are used in the emergency treatment of status epilepticus (a continuous seizure state). Anticonvulsants fall into five major classes: hydantoins and sodium channel blockers, barbiturates and those with gamma-aminobutyric acid (GABA) receptor effects, iminostilbenes, benzodiazepines, and other.

Hydantoins and Sodium Channel Blockers

Common Drug Names

ethosuximide: Zarontin

ethotoin: Peganone

fosphenytoin: Cerebyx

lamotrigine: Lamictal

mephenytoin

phenytoin: Dilantin, phenytoin sodium, Phenytek

topiramate: Topamax

zonisamide: Zonegran

The two most commonly prescribed anticonvulsant drugs (phenytoin and phenytoin sodium) belong to the hydantoin class. Less commonly used hydantoins include fosphenytoin, mephenytoin, and ethotoin.

Pharmacokinetics

The pharmacokinetics of hydantoins vary from drug to drug. Phenytoin is absorbed slowly after both oral and intramuscular administration. It is distributed rapidly to all tissues. Phenytoin is metabolized in the liver. Inactive metabolites are excreted in bile and then reabsorbed from the GI tract. Eventually, however, they are excreted in the urine.

Mephenytoin is absorbed rapidly after oral administration. It is metabolized by the liver to an active metabolite believed to possess the therapeutic and toxic effects attributed to mephenytoin. Excretion occurs via the urine.

Ethotoin is metabolized by the liver and is excreted in the urine.

Fosphenytoin is indicated for short-term intramuscular or intravenous administration. It is widely distributed throughout the body. Fosphenytoin is metabolized by the liver and is excreted in the urine.

Pharmacodynamics

In most cases, these anticonvulsants stabilize nerve cells to keep them from getting overexcited by blocking sodium transport. They appear to work in the motor cortex of the brain, where they stop the spread of seizure activity. The pharmacodynamics of fosphenytoin, mephenytoin, ethotoin, and the other "anticonvulsant" drugs are thought to mimic those of phenytoin. Phenytoin is also used as an antiarrhythmic drug to control irregular heart rhythms, with properties similar to those of quinidine or procainamide.

Pharmacotherapeutics

Because of its effectiveness and relatively low toxicity, phenytoin is the most commonly prescribed anticonvulsant. It is one of the drugs of choice to treat complex partial seizures (also called psychomotor or temporal lobe seizures) and tonic-clonic seizures.

Health care providers sometimes prescribe mephenytoin and ethotoin in combination with other anticonvulsants for partial and tonic-clonic seizures in patients whose conditions are resistant to or intolerant of other anticonvulsants.

MASSAGE IMPLICATIONS AND ASSESSMENT

Since the hydantoins work in the motor cortex of the CNS and decrease the sensitivity and excitability of the neuron cell membrane, they may alter the effectiveness of the local reflex strokes and the systemic reflex strokes. The use of mechanical strokes such as effleurage, pétrissage, myofascial techniques, and some friction can be used if this is the case. The effect will often depend on the dosage the client needs to control seizure activity. If low, the effect on massage may be small.

Adverse Reactions to Hydantoins

Side Effects
- Drowsiness
- Irritability
- Restlessness
- Dizziness
- Headache

Adverse Effects
- Ataxia
- Nystagmus
- Dysarthria
- Nausea and vomiting
- Abdominal pain
- Anorexia
- Depressed atrial and ventricular conduction
- Ventricular fibrillation (in toxic states)
- Bradycardia, hypotension, and cardiac arrest (with intravenous administration)
- Hypersensitivity reactions

Side Effects

The side effects of the hydantoins are drowsiness, irritability, restlessness, and dizziness. Massage can assist in easing these effects. Care again must be taken at the end of the massage to bring the client to full alertness before leaving the room (see Sidebar: *Adverse Reactions to Hydantoins*).

Barbiturates and GABA Receptor Drugs

Common Drug Names

gabapentin: Neurontin

mephobarbital

phenobarbital: Ancalixir, Barbita (discontinued in the U.S.), Luminal, Solfoton, phenobarbitone

primidone: Apo-Primidone, Mysoline, PMS Primidone, Sertan

tiagabine: Gabitril

The long-acting barbiturate phenobarbital was formerly one of the most widely used anticonvulsants. It is now used less frequently because of its sedative effects. Phenobarbital is sometimes used for long-term treatment of epilepsy and is prescribed selectively for acute treatment of status epilepticus. Mephobarbital, also a long-acting barbiturate, is sometimes used as an anticonvulsant. Primidone, which is closely related chemically to the barbiturates, is also used in the chronic treatment of epilepsy.

Pharmacokinetics

Each barbiturate has a slightly different set of pharmacokinetic properties. Phenobarbital is absorbed slowly but well from the GI tract. Phenobarbital is metabolized by the liver and is excreted in the urine.

Almost half of a mephobarbital dose is absorbed from the GI tract and well distributed in body tissues. Mephobarbital undergoes extensive metabolism by the liver and is excreted in the urine.

Primidone is absorbed from the GI tract and distributed evenly among body tissues. It is metabolized in the liver and excreted in the urine. It is also excreted in breast milk.

Pharmacodynamics

Barbiturates exhibit anticonvulsant action at doses lower than drugs that produce hypnotic effects. For this reason, barbiturates usually do not produce dependency when used to treat epilepsy. Their action is unknown but may be by decreasing neural activity or increasing GABA (an inhibitory neurotransmitter) effects.

Pharmacotherapeutics

The barbiturate anticonvulsants are effective in treating partial seizures, tonic-clonic seizures, and febrile seizures. Barbiturates can be used alone or with other anticonvulsants. Intravenous phenobarbital is also used to treat status epilepticus. The major disadvantage of using phenobarbital for status epilepticus is that it has a delayed onset of action when an immediate response is needed. Barbiturate anticonvulsants are ineffective in treating absence seizures. Mephobarbital has no advantage over phenobarbital and is used when patients cannot tolerate the adverse effects of phenobarbital. Primidone is used primarily with other anticonvulsants.

MASSAGE IMPLICATIONS AND ASSESSMENT

Although the action of barbiturates in unclear, it is believed to be that of CNS depression, specifically in decreasing the transmission of impulses to the motor cortex of the brain. As with the hydantoins, the effect of systemic and local reflex strokes may be slowed and/or reduced. The use of mechanical strokes is more effective in this case. In addition, more time may be required for reflex strokes to be effective.

Side Effects

The common side effects of barbiturates are drowsiness, dizziness, hypotension, and hair loss. Massage practitioners again need to be aware of safety in ending the session. In addition, scalp massage may be contraindicated if hair loss is an issue (see Sidebar: *Adverse Reactions to Barbiturates*).

Adverse Reactions to Barbiturates

Side Effects
- Drowsiness, lethargy, and dizziness
- Hair loss

Adverse Effects
- Nystagmus, confusion, and ataxia (with large doses)
- Laryngospasm, respiratory depression, and hypotension (when administered intravenously)
- Primidone can cause the same CNS and GI adverse reactions as phenobarbital; primidone can also cause acute psychoses, hair loss, impotence, and osteomalacia
- All three barbiturate anticonvulsants can produce a hypersensitivity rash, other rashes, lupus erythematosus–like syndrome (an inflammatory disorder), and enlarged lymph nodes

---

Iminostilbenes

Common Drug Names

carbamazepine: Apo-Carbamazepine, Atretol, Carbatrol, Epitol, Novo-Carbamaz, Tegretol, Teril

oxcarbazepine: Trileptal

Carbamazepine is the most commonly used iminostilbene anticonvulsant. It effectively treats partial and generalized tonic-clonic seizures and mixed seizure types.

Pharmacokinetics

Carbamazepine is absorbed slowly and erratically from the GI tract. Metabolism occurs in the liver, and carbamazepine is excreted in the urine. A small amount crosses the placenta, and some is secreted in breast milk.

Pharmacodynamics

Carbamazepine's anticonvulsant effect is similar to that of phenytoin. The drug's anticonvulsant action can occur because of its ability to inhibit the spread of seizure activity or neuromuscular transmission in general.

Pharmacotherapeutics

Carbamazepine is the drug of choice, in adults and children, for treating generalized tonic-clonic seizures as well as simple and complex partial seizures. Carbamazepine also relieves pain when used to treat trigeminal neuralgia (tic douloureux, characterized by excruciating facial pain along the trigeminal nerve).

<table>
<tr><td>

Adverse Reactions to Iminostilbenes

Side Effects
- Dizziness
- Drowsiness
- Fatigue
- Hypotension
- Dry mouth
- Sweating

Adverse Effects
- Ataxia
- Increased seizures
- Heart failure
- Nystagmus
- Diplopia
- Nausea/vomiting
- Abdominal pain
- Stomatitis/glossitis
- Urinary problems
- Impotence
- Increased blood urea nitrogen (BUN) levels
- Aplastic anemia
- Hepatitis
- Rash
- Stevens-Johnson syndrome in children

</td><td>

MASSAGE IMPLICATIONS AND ASSESSMENT

The decrease in transmission of impulses in the motor neurons of the CNS is similar to that of the hydantoins, and massage is approached in the same way. If the reflex strokes are slow in effectiveness, the use of mechanical strokes is effective on the muscles. Again, this effect may be dose-related.

Side Effects

The side effects of the iminostilbenes are drowsiness, dizziness, fatigue, hypotension, dry mouth, and increased sweating. Care for safety at the end of the massage is an important consideration. Having drinking water available during the massage may also add to the client's comfort (see Sidebar: *Adverse Reactions to Iminostilbenes*).

</td></tr>
</table>

Benzodiazepines

Common Drug Names

diazepam: Apo-Diazepam, Diastat, Diazemuls, Novo-Dipam, Valium, Vivol
clonazepam: Klonopin, Rivotril
clorazepate: Tranxene, Apo-Chlorazepate, Gen-XENE, Novo-Clopate, Clorazecaps

All of the above drugs provide anticonvulsant effects. Only clonazepam is recommended for long-term treatment of epilepsy. Diazepam is restricted to acute treatment of status epilepticus. Clorazepate is prescribed as an adjunct in treating partial seizures.

Pharmacokinetics

Patients can receive benzodiazepines orally or parenterally. Benzodiazepines are absorbed rapidly and almost completely from the GI tract but are distributed at different rates. Benzodiazepines are metabolized in the liver to multiple metabolites and are then excreted in the urine. These agents readily cross the placenta and are excreted in breast milk.

Pharmacodynamics

Benzodiazepines act as anticonvulsants, antianxiety agents, sedative-hypnotics, and muscle relaxants. Their mechanism of action is poorly understood. They may act on neural activity or GABA receptors.

Pharmacotherapeutics

Each of the benzodiazepines can be used in slightly different ways. Clonazepam is used to treat the following types of seizures: absence (petit mal), atypical absence (Lennox-Gastaut syndrome), atonic, and myoclonic.

Diazepam is not recommended for long-term treatment because of its potential for addiction and the high serum concentrations required to control seizures. Intravenous diazepam is used to control status epilepticus. Because diazepam provides only short-term effects of less than 1 hour, the patient must also be given a long-acting anticonvulsant, such as phenytoin or phenobarbital, during diazepam therapy.

Clorazepate is used with other drugs to treat partial seizures.

MASSAGE IMPLICATIONS AND ASSESSMENT

The action of benzodiazepines is unclear. It is believed they increase the action of GABA, a neurotransmitter that has an inhibitory effect on transmission of neural impulses in the brain. In essence, they seem to be CNS depressants. Therefore, systemic and local reflex strokes might be affected, in that their effectiveness might be slowed. The use of mechanical strokes is indicated if this is the case.

Side Effects

The side effects are those of dizziness and drowsiness and sometimes hypotension. The effect of this on safety is clear. The use of stimulatory strokes at the end or even during the massage helps to alleviate too much drowsiness (see Sidebar: *Adverse Reactions to Benzodiazepines*).

Adverse Reactions to Benzodiazepines

Side Effects
- Drowsiness
- Dizziness
- Headache
- Tremor

Adverse Effects
- Confusion
- Ataxia
- Weakness
- Nystagmus
- Fainting
- Dysarthria
- Glassy-eyed appearance
- Depression of the heart and breathing (with high doses and with intravenous diazepam)
- Rash and acute hypersensitivity reactions

Other Anticonvulsants

Common Drug Names

acetazolamide: Diamox

divalproex: Depakote, Epival

levetiracetam: Keppra

valproic acid: Depacon, Depakene, Myproic Acid

Valproic acid is unrelated structurally to the other anticonvulsants. The two major drugs in the valproic acid class are valproate and divalproex. Miscellaneous drugs include acetazolamide and levetiracetam.

Pharmacokinetics

Valproate is converted rapidly to valproic acid in the stomach. Divalproex is a precursor of valproic acid and separates into valproic acid in the GI tract. Valproic acid is absorbed well, is strongly protein-bound, and is metabolized in the liver. Metabolites and unchanged drug are excreted in urine. Valproic acid readily crosses the placental barrier and also appears in breast milk.

Pharmacodynamics

The mechanism of action for valproic acid remains unknown. It is thought to increase GABA levels. Diamox and Keppra also have unclear actions.

Pharmacotherapeutics

These drugs are prescribed for long-term treatment of absence seizures, myoclonic seizures, and tonic-clonic seizures. Valproic acid is administered rectally for status epilepticus that does not respond to other anticonvulsants. Valproic acid must be used cautiously in a young child or in a patient receiving multiple anticonvulsants. With these patients, valproic acid carries a risk of potentially fatal liver toxicity. This risk limits the use of valproic acid as a drug of choice for seizure disorders.

Adverse Reactions to Valproic Acid

Side Effects
- Sedation
- Dizziness
- Constipation
- Headache
- Indigestion
- Easy bruising

Adverse Effects

Rare but deadly liver toxicity has occurred with this drug. For this reason, the drug is not routinely prescribed. Most other adverse reactions to valproic acid are tolerable and dose-related. These include:
- Nausea and vomiting
- Diarrhea
- Ataxia
- Muscle weakness

MASSAGE IMPLICATIONS AND ASSESSMENT

With the knowledge that valproic acid may increase GABA and inhibit motor neuron transmission, the use of mechanical strokes in massage is indicated. Reflex strokes may take longer to be effective if used.

Side Effects

This drug class has the same side effects as many of the other anticonvulsants. Safety and the use of stimulation at the end of the massage are indicated. All drugs that affect the CNS require caution when using deep tissue massage because reaction to depth and perception of depth may be altered (see Sidebar: *Adverse Reactions to Valproic Acid*).

Quick Quiz

1. A 15-year-old patient has a tonic-clonic seizure disorder and is prescribed phenytoin. He describes his side effects as those of sleepiness and dizziness when moving too quickly. He is still experiencing seizures regularly, and his physician is trying to regulate dosages of the medication. His mother wants you to massage the patient for relaxation. What should you do?

2. A client has myoclonic seizures. She has trouble sleeping at times and wants massage for relaxation and to work out the knots in her shoulders. Her condition is well regulated with medication, and she has had no seizure activity for 5 years. She is taking Depakene. What are the indications for massage?

3. A 48-year-old patient has been prescribed Artane for Parkinson's disease. She has mild tremors and some rigidity but is independent and still working. What are some side effects she may have, and what massage strokes might be helpful?

Pain Medications

5

Drugs used to control pain range from mild, over-the-counter (OTC) preparations, such as acetaminophen (Tylenol), to potent general anesthetics.

Nonnarcotic Analgesics, Antipyretics, and Nonsteroidal Anti-Inflammatory Drugs

Nonnarcotic analgesics, antipyretics, and nonsteroidal anti-inflammatory drugs (NSAIDs) are a broad group of pain medications. They are discussed together because, in addition to pain control, they also produce antipyretic (fever control) and anti-inflammatory effects. The drug classes included in this group are salicylates (especially aspirin), which are widely used; the para-aminophenol derivative acetaminophen (Tylenol); NSAIDs; and the urinary tract analgesic phenazopyridine hydrochloride.

Salicylates

Common Drug Names

acetylsalicylic acid: Apo-ASA, aspirin, ASA, Bayer, Ecotrin, Empirin, Novorin

choline magnesium trisalicylate: Tricosal, Trilisate

choline salicylate: Arthropan, Teejel

diflunisal: Dolobid, Apo-Diflunisal, Novo-Diflunisal

magnesium salicylate: Doan's, Mobidin

salsalate: Amigesic, Argesic, Mono-Gesic

sodium thiosalicylate: Rexolate

Salicylates are among the most commonly used pain medications. They are used regularly to control pain and reduce fever and inflammation. These agents usually cost less than other analgesics and are readily available without a prescription. Aspirin, the most commonly used salicylate, remains the cornerstone of anti-inflammatory drug therapy.

Pharmacokinetics (how drugs circulate)

Taken orally, salicylates are absorbed partly in the stomach but primarily in the upper part of the small intestine. The pure and buffered forms of aspirin are absorbed readily, but sustained-release and enteric-coated salicylate preparations or food or antacids in the stomach delay absorption. Salicylates given rectally have a slower, more erratic absorption. Salicylates are distributed widely throughout body tissues and fluids, including breast milk. In addition, they easily cross the placenta. The liver metabolizes salicylates extensively into several metabolites. The kidneys excrete the metabolites and some unchanged drug.

Pharmacodynamics (how drugs act)

The different effects of salicylates stem from their separate mechanisms of action. They relieve pain primarily by inhibiting the synthesis of prostaglandin. (Recall that prostaglandin is a chemical mediator that sensitizes nerve cells to pain.) In addition, they may also reduce inflammation by inhibiting the prostaglandin synthesis and release that occurs during inflammation. Salicylates reduce fever by stimulating the hypothalamus, producing dilation of the peripheral blood vessels and increased sweating. This promotes heat loss through the skin and cooling by evaporation. Also, because prostaglandin E increases body temperature, inhibiting its production lowers a fever.

One salicylate, aspirin, inhibits platelet aggregation (the clumping of platelets to form a blood clot) by interfering with the production of a substance called thromboxane A_2, which is necessary for platelet aggregation. As a result, aspirin can be used to enhance blood flow during myocardial infarction.

Pharmacotherapeutics (how drugs are used)

Salicylates are used primarily to relieve pain and reduce fever. However, they do not effectively relieve visceral pain (pain from the organs and smooth muscle) or severe pain from trauma. Salicylates will not reduce a normal body temperature. They can reduce an elevated body temperature and will relieve headache and muscle ache at the same time. Salicylates can provide considerable relief in 24 hours when they are used to reduce inflammation in rheumatic fever and rheumatoid arthritis.

No matter what the clinical indication, the main guideline of salicylate therapy is to use the lowest dose that provides relief. This reduces the likelihood of side effects or adverse reactions.

MASSAGE IMPLICATIONS AND ASSESSMENT

The action of this class of drugs is primarily that of decreasing prostaglandin synthesis. This leads to decreased sensitivity to pain, reduced inflammation, and reduced fever. Also, dilation of peripheral blood vessels and increased sweating are actions of these drugs. Aspirin alone will decrease platelet clumping and improve blood flow.

When looking at the individual massage strokes, decreased sensitivity to pain always means that caution must be used with depth/pressure exerted with all strokes. All massage strokes, especially effleurage, pétrissage, and friction, dilate peripheral blood vessels. Because this is an action of this drug, care needs to be taken that the effect is not compounded, leading to a drop in blood pressure. This is especially needed in the elderly or in anyone with low blood pressure. Simply utilizing the above strokes differently toward the end of the massage (increased speed to stimulate sympathetic nervous system) or using a stimulating stroke, such as tapotement, is sufficient.

Side Effects

The only side effect of salicylates that would be of concern is dizziness related to peripheral blood vessel dilation. The above actions, plus care when sitting the client up after a massage, are all that is needed. Adverse reactions are more serious and should be referred to a physician (see Sidebar: *Adverse Reactions to Salicylates*).

> ### Adverse Reactions to Salicylates
>
> **Side Effects**
> • Gastric distress
> • Dizziness
>
> **Adverse Effects**
> • Hearing loss (when taken for prolonged periods)
> • Diarrhea, thirst, sweating, tinnitus, confusion, nausea, vomiting, impaired vision, and hyperventilation (rapid breathing)
> • Reye's syndrome (when given to children with chickenpox or with flulike symptoms)

Acetaminophen

Common Drug Names

acetaminophen: Anacin, APAP, Atasol, Panadol, paracetamol, Robigesic, Tylenol

Although the class of para-aminophenol derivatives includes two drugs—phenacetin and acetaminophen—only acetaminophen is available in the United States. Acetaminophen (Tylenol) is an OTC drug that produces analgesic and antipyretic effects. It appears in many products designed to relieve pain and symptoms associated with colds and influenza.

Pharmacokinetics

Acetaminophen is absorbed rapidly and completely from the gastrointestinal (GI) tract. It is also absorbed well from the mucous membranes of the rectum. Acetaminophen is distributed widely in body fluids and readily crosses the placenta. After acetaminophen is metabolized by the liver, it is excreted by the kidneys and, in small amounts, in breast milk.

Pharmacodynamics

Acetaminophen reduces pain and fever, but unlike salicylates, it does not affect inflammation or platelet function. The pain-control effects of acetaminophen are not well understood. It may work in the central nervous system (CNS) by inhibiting prostaglandin synthesis and in the peripheral nervous system in some unknown way. It reduces fever by acting directly on the heat-regulating center in the hypothalamus.

Pharmacotherapeutics

Acetaminophen is used to reduce fever and relieve headache, muscle ache, and general pain. Acetaminophen is the drug of choice to treat fever and flulike symptoms in children. Recently, the American Arthritis Association has indicated that acetaminophen is an effective pain reliever for some types of arthritis.

Adverse Reactions to Acetaminophen

Side Effects

Most patients tolerate acetaminophen well. Unlike the salicylates, acetaminophen rarely causes gastric irritation or bleeding tendencies.

Adverse Effects

- Hemolytic anemia
- Jaundice
- Liver damage
- Rash
- Hypoglycemia

MASSAGE IMPLICATIONS AND ASSESSMENT

Because the actions of this drug in the body are poorly understood, the effects are all that can be assessed in the context of how the drug might affect massage. As always, reduction of sensitivity to pain requires caution in the depth and pressure applied with all massage strokes.

Side Effects

There are no side effects of this drug that influence massage. There are, however, some serious adverse effects that should be reported to a physician (see Sidebar: *Adverse Reactions to Acetaminophen*).

NSAIDs

Common Drug Names

carprofen: Rimadyl

celecoxib: Celebrex

diclofenac: Cataflam

etodolac: Lodine

etoricoxib: Arcoxia

flurbiprofen: Ansaid

ibuprofen: Advil, Amersol, Excedrin IB (discontinued in the U.S.), Motrin, Novo-Profen, Nuprin

indomethacin: Indocid, Indocin, Novo-Methacin

ketoprofen: Actron, Apo-Keto, Orudis, Rhodis

mefenamic acid: Ponstan, Ponstel

meloxicam: Mobic

nabumetone: Relafen

naproxen sodium: Aleve, Anaprox, Naprosyn, Synflex

oxaprozin: Daypro

piroxicam: Apo-Piroxicam, Feldene, Novo-Pirocam

rofecoxib: Vioxx

sulindac: Clinoril, Novo-Sundac

tolmetin: Tolectin

valdecoxib: Bextra, Voltaren

As their name suggests, NSAIDs are often used to combat inflammation, and their anti-inflammatory action equals that of aspirin. They also have analgesic and antipyretic effects but are seldom prescribed for fever. Drugs in this class include indomethacin (Indocin), ibuprofen (Advil), mefenamic acid (Ponstel), celecoxib (Celebrex), piroxicam (Feldene), and sulindac (Clinoril).

Pharmacokinetics

All NSAIDs are absorbed in the GI tract. They are mostly metabolized in the liver and excreted primarily by the kidneys.

Pharmacodynamics

Researchers believe that NSAIDs produce their effects by inhibiting prostaglandin synthesis. For example, a new class of NSAIDs, called cyclooxygenase-2 (Cox-2) inhibitors, inhibit Cox-2, an enzyme responsible for prostaglandin synthesis. Another type of NSAIDs, fenamates, may compete with prostaglandins at receptor-binding sites. As with aspirin, decreased prostaglandin production means less sensitivity to pain and less inflammation.

Pharmacotherapeutics

NSAIDs are used primarily to decrease inflammation. They are secondarily used to relieve pain but are seldom prescribed to reduce fever (except in children, in whom they are used extensively as anti-pyretics). The following conditions respond favorably to treatment with NSAIDs: ankylosing spondylitis (an inflammatory joint disease that first affects the spine); moderate to severe rheumatoid arthritis (an inflammatory disease of peripheral joints); osteoarthritis (a degenerative joint disease) in the hip, shoulder, or other large joints; osteoarthritis accompanied by inflammation; acute gouty arthritis (urate deposits in the joints); and dysmenorrhea (painful menstruation).

MASSAGE IMPLICATIONS AND ASSESSMENT

As with the salicylates, the main action of NSAIDs is on prostaglandins. With these drugs, prostaglandins are either decreased or interfered with. Thus, pain and inflammation are decreased. Decreased pain sensation requires extra caution in the depth and pressure of any massage stroke used.

Side Effects

The main side effects of these drugs that may increase or decrease the effects of massage are drowsiness and dizziness. A simple use of more rapid strokes or more stimulating strokes at the end of the session is indicated here. Special care should be taken with elderly patients, who tend to have more problems with dizziness because of a slower response of the nervous system to changes of position. Other adverse effects should be reported to a physician (see Sidebar: *Adverse Reactions to NSAIDs*).

Adverse Reactions to NSAIDs

Side Effects
- Drowsiness
- Dizziness
- Headache

Adverse Effects
- Abdominal pain
- Bleeding
- Anorexia
- Diarrhea
- Nausea
- Ulcers
- Liver toxicity
- Jaundice
- Confusion
- Tinnitus
- Vertigo
- Depression
- Bladder infection
- Blood in the urine
- Kidney necrosis

Phenazopyridine Hydrochloride

Common Drug Names

phenazopyridine hydrochloride: Azo-Dine, Phenazo, Phenazodine, Pyridiate, Urodine, Pyridium

Phenazopyridine hydrochloride (Pyridium), an azo dye used in commercial coloring, produces a local analgesic effect on the urinary tract, usually within 24 to 48 hours after therapy begins. It relieves the pain, burning, urgency, and frequency that occur with urinary tract infections. When taken orally, phenazopyridine is 35% metabolized in the liver, with the remainder excreted unchanged in the urine, which may take on an orange or red color. If the drug is accumulating, the skin and sclera of the eye may take on a yellow tinge and the phenazopyridine may need to be stopped.

> **Adverse Reactions to Phenazopyridine**
>
> **Side Effects**
> - Dark urine
> - Nausea
>
> **Adverse Effects**
> - Headache
> - Hemolytic anemia
> - Rash

MASSAGE IMPLICATIONS AND ASSESSMENT

Because the action of this drug is localized to the internal genitourinary tract, there are no implications for massage or changes in application of massage necessary (see Sidebar: *Adverse Reactions to Phenazopyridine*).

Narcotic Agonist and Antagonist Drugs

The word narcotic refers to any derivative of the opium plant or any synthetic drug that imitates natural narcotics. Narcotic agonists (also called narcotic analgesics) include opium derivatives and synthetic drugs with similar properties. They are used to relieve or decrease pain without causing the person to lose consciousness. Some narcotic agonists may also have antitussive and antidiarrheal effects.

Narcotic antagonists are not pain medications; they block the effects of narcotic agonists and are used to reverse adverse drug reactions, such as respiratory and CNS depression, produced by those drugs. Unfortunately, by reversing the analgesic effect, they also cause pain to recur.

Some narcotic analgesics, called mixed narcotic agonist-antagonists, have both agonist and antagonist properties. The agonist component relieves pain, and the antagonist component decreases the risk of toxicity and drug dependence. These mixed narcotic agonist-antagonists reduce the risk of respiratory depression and drug abuse.

Narcotic Agonists

Common Drug Names

codeine: Paveral

fentanyl citrate: Duragesic, Sublimaze

hydromorphone hydrochloride: Dilaudid, Hydromorph Contin

levorphanol tartrate: Levo-Dromoran

meperidine hydrochloride: Demerol

methadone hydrochloride: Dolophine, Methadose

morphine sulfate (including morphine sulfate sustained-release tablets and intensified oral solution): Morphitec, MS Contin, Roxanol

Morphine sulfate is the standard against which the effectiveness and adverse reactions of other pain medications are measured.

Pharmacokinetics

A person may receive narcotic agonists by any administration route, although inhalation administration is uncommon. Oral doses are absorbed readily from the GI tract. Narcotic agonists administered intravenously provide the most rapid (almost immediate) and reliable pain relief. The subcutaneous and intramuscular routes may result in delayed absorption, especially in patients with poor circulation.

Narcotic agonists are distributed widely throughout body tissues and are metabolized extensively in the liver. Metabolites are excreted by the kidneys. A small amount is excreted in stool through the biliary tract.

Pharmacodynamics

Narcotic agonists reduce pain by binding to opiate receptor sites in the peripheral nervous system and the CNS. When these drugs stimulate the opiate receptors, they mimic the effects of endorphins (naturally occurring opiates that are part of the body's pain relief system). This receptor-site binding produces the therapeutic effects of analgesia and cough suppression as well as adverse reactions, such as respiratory depression and constipation (Fig. 5-1).

Narcotic agonists, especially morphine, affect the smooth muscle of the GI and genitourinary tracts (the organs of the reproductive and urinary systems). This causes contraction of the bladder and ureters and slowed intestinal peristalsis (rhythmic contractions that move food along the digestive tract).

These drugs also cause blood vessels to dilate, especially in the face, head, and neck. In addition, they suppress the cough center in the brain, producing antitussive effects and causing constriction of the bronchial muscles. Any of these effects can become adverse reactions if they are produced in excess. For example, if the blood vessels dilate too much, hypotension can occur.

Pharmacotherapeutics

Narcotic agonists are prescribed to relieve severe pain in acute, chronic, and terminal illnesses. They also reduce anxiety before a patient receives anesthesia and are sometimes prescribed to control diarrhea and suppress coughing.

Morphine is also used to relieve shortness of breath in patients with pulmonary edema (fluid in the lungs) and left-sided heart failure (inability of the heart to pump enough blood to meet the needs of the body).

MASSAGE IMPLICATIONS AND ASSESSMENT

The main action of this class of drugs is that of binding to opiate receptors and decreasing the response to stimuli, especially pain. Because binding to these receptors slows all responses, care must be taken with the amount of depth and pressure

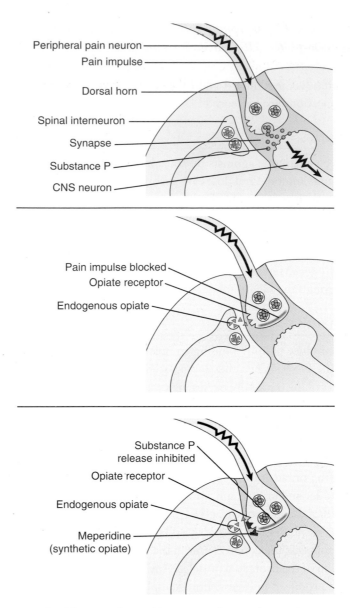

Figure 5-1 Pain Control With Narcotic Agonists. Narcotic agonists, such as meperidine, inhibit pain transmission by mimicking the body's natural pain control mechanisms. In the dorsal horn of the spinal cord, peripheral pain neurons meet central nervous system (CNS) neurons. At the synapse, the pain neuron releases a pain neurotransmitter (substance P). This agent helps transfer pain impulses to the CNS neurons that carry the impulse to the brain. In theory, the spinal interneurons respond to stimulation from the descending neurons of the CNS by releasing endogenous opiates. These opiates bind to the peripheral pain neuron to inhibit release of substance P and to retard the transmission of pain impulses. Synthetic opiates supplement this pain-blocking effect by binding with free opiate receptors to inhibit the release of substance P. Opiates also alter consciousness of pain, but how this mechanism works remains unknown.

with all massage strokes. In addition, response to somatic reflex arcs may be slowed as well, making strokes such as compression, friction, and stretching/movement less effective. Because these drugs also act like the body's own endorphins, the normal response of relaxation and euphoria brought on by general massage may be increased significantly. To counter this and to keep the body in balance, the therapist must alter the systemic reflexive strokes of effleurage and pétrissage by making them more rapidly applied. Use of tapotement and rapid extended friction at the end of a session is also indicated. If the drugs are given parenterally, either intramuscular or subcutaneous injection sites should be avoided to prevent increasing the rate of absorption. Usually, subcutaneous doses take longer to absorb (up to 4 hours). Doses given intramuscularly take 1 to 2 hours to absorb, based on onset and peak effect times.

Side Effects

The side effects of these powerful drugs are many. The main side effects come from the drug action on the nervous system. Drowsiness, hypotension from dilation of blood vessels, and euphoria are the most common. The modifications described above help prevent the massage from exacerbating these symptoms. Other side effects slow the GI tract and can lead to constipation. In this case, effleurage on the abdomen (in the direction that follows the flow of the colon) is a helpful addition to massage. Severe problems with any of the above side effects or any other adverse effects must be reported to the physician and the massage postponed (see Sidebar: *Adverse Reactions to Narcotic Agonists*).

> ### *Adverse Reactions to Narcotic Agonists*
>
> **Side Effects**
> - Orthostatic hypotension
> - Flushing
> - Pupil constriction
> - Dizziness
> - Constipation
> - Drowsiness
>
> **Adverse Effects**
> - Decreased respirations
> - Asthma attacks
> - Tremors
> - Palpitations
> - Delirium
> - Euphoria
> - Urine retention

Combination Narcotic Pain Relievers

Both narcotic agonist and mixed narcotic angonist-antagonists are frequently combined with other pain-relieving drugs, most commonly with acetaminophen, aspirin, and NSAIDs. In these situations, look at the action and side effects of both drugs through the Drug Regimen Assessment Process (see Chapter 1) to see how massage will be affected (see Sidebar: *Drug Combinations for Pain*).

Mixed Narcotic Agonist-Antagonists

Common Drug Names

buprenorphine hydrochloride: Buprenex, Temgesic

buprenorphine with naloxone: Suboxone

butorphanol tartrate: Stadol

hydrocodone: (used in combination only; related to morphine)

nalbuphine hydrochloride: Nubain

oxycodone hydrochloride: OxyContin, Roxicodone, Supeudol

pentazocine hydrochloride: Fortral, Talwin

propoxyphene hydrochloride: Darvon, Novo-Propoxyn

Mixed narcotic agonist-antagonists attempt to relieve pain while reducing toxic effects and dependency.

> ### *Drug Combinations for Pain*
>
> - Acetaminophen and codeine: Empracet, Tylenol #1, Tylenol #2, Tylenol #3, Tylenol #4
> - Propoxyphene hydrochloride and acetaminophen: Darvocet
> - Propoxyphene hydrochloride, acetaminophen, and caffeine: Darvon Compound
> - Oxycodone and aspirin: Endocin, Oxycodan, Percodan
> - Oxycodone and acetaminophen: Endocet, Oxycocet, Percocet, Roxicet
> - Hydrocodone and acetaminophen: Vicodin

Originally, mixed narcotic agonist-antagonists appeared to have less abuse potential than the pure narcotic agonists. However, butorphanol and pentazocine have reportedly caused dependence.

Pharmacokinetics

Absorption of mixed narcotic agonist-antagonists occurs rapidly from parenteral sites. These drugs are distributed to most body tissues and also cross the placenta. They are metabolized in the liver and excreted primarily by the kidneys, although more than 10% of a butorphanol dose and a small amount of dezocine and pentazocine doses are excreted in stool.

Pharmacodynamics

The exact mechanism of action of the mixed narcotic agonist-antagonists is not known. Buprenorphine binds with receptors in the CNS, altering both perception of and emotional response to pain through an unknown mechanism. It seems to release slowly from binding sites, producing a longer duration of action than the other drugs in this class.

The site of action of butorphanol may be opiate receptors in the limbic system (part of the brain involved in emotion). Like pentazocine, butorphanol also acts on pulmonary circulation, increasing pulmonary vascular resistance (the resistance in the blood vessels of the lungs that the right ventricle must pump against). Both drugs also increase blood pressure and the workload of the heart.

Pharmacotherapeutics

Mixed narcotic agonist-antagonists are prescribed primarily for relief of moderate to severe pain and as preoperative medication to reduce anxiety and pain. They are also used as analgesia during childbirth. Mixed narcotic agonist-antagonists are sometimes prescribed in place of narcotic agonists because they have a lower risk of drug dependence. Mixed narcotic agonist-antagonists also are less likely to cause respiratory depression, although they can produce some adverse reactions. Patients with a history of narcotic abuse should not receive any of the mixed narcotic agonist-antagonists because they can cause symptoms of withdrawal.

MASSAGE IMPLICATIONS AND ASSESSMENT

These drugs act directly on the receptors in the CNS to decrease pain perception. The depth and pressure of all strokes must be modified. In addition, the therapist must recognize that the somatic reflex reactions to strokes such as compression, petrissage, friction, and stretching/movement may be slowed. As with narcotic agonists, injection sites need to be avoided to prevent increasing the rate of absorption of the drug (usually 1 to 2 hours based on onset and peak effect times for the drug).

Side Effects

The side effects of this class of drugs include dizziness, euphoria, and sedation. Because the CNS is acted on, these side effects may be significant. Massage effects of relaxation are greatly increased in clients taking these drugs. Using rapid stimulating strokes is indicated throughout most of the massage. Tapotement and rapid and prolonged friction are also useful.

These drugs may often be used during childbirth or before invasive procedures. The sedative effect is the desired outcome in these cases, and therefore no stimulating strokes should be used. Rather, stay with gentle effleurage and pétrissage. Any serious adverse reactions should be reported to the physician (see Sidebar: *Adverse Reactions to Narcotic Agonist-Antagonists*).

Narcotic Antagonists

Common Drug Names

nalmefene: Revex

naloxone hydrochloride: Narcan

naltrexone hydrochloride: Depade, ReVia

> ### Adverse Reactions to Narcotic Agonist-Antagonists
>
> **Side Effects**
> - Light-headedness
> - Sedation
> - Euphoria
>
> **Adverse Effects**
> - Nausea
> - Vomiting
> - Delirium
> - Withdrawal symptoms
>
> Patients with a history of narcotic abuse should not receive mixed narcotic agonist-antagonists because withdrawal symptoms may result.

Narcotic antagonists attach to opiate receptors but do not stimulate them. Narcotic antagonists have a greater attraction for opiate receptors than do narcotics. As a result, they prevent narcotic drugs, enkephalins, and endorphins from producing their effects.

Pharmacokinetics

Naloxone and Nalmefene are administered intramuscularly, subcutaneously, or intravenously. Naltrexone is administered orally in tablet or liquid form. These drugs are metabolized by the liver and excreted by the kidneys.

Pharmacodynamics

Narcotic antagonists block the effects of narcotics by occupying the opiate receptor sites, displacing any narcotics attached to opiate receptors, and blocking further narcotic binding at these sites. The process by which they work is known as competitive inhibition.

Pharmacotherapeutics

Naloxone and Nalmefene are the drugs of choice for managing a narcotic overdose. They reverse respiratory depression and sedation and help stabilize the patient's vital signs within seconds after administration. Because naloxone also reverses the analgesic effects of narcotic drugs, a patient who was given a narcotic drug for pain relief may complain of pain or even experience withdrawal symptoms.

Naltrexone is used along with psychotherapy or counseling to treat drug abuse. However, it is only given to patients who have gone through a detoxification program to remove all narcotics from the body. That is because a patient who still has narcotics in the body may experience acute withdrawal symptoms if he or she receives naltrexone.

Adverse Reactions to Narcotic Antagonists

Side Effects
- Palpitations
- Anxiety
- Insomnia
- Dizziness
- Shortness of breath
- Headache

Adverse Effects
- Hypertension
- Tachycardia
- Hyperventilation
- Tremors
- Edema
- Disorientation
- Nausea
- Vomiting
- Urinary frequency
- Diarrhea
- Anorexia
- Liver toxicity
- Jaundice

MASSAGE IMPLICATIONS AND ASSESSMENT

Because these drugs are used in narcotic overdose and reverse the effects of narcotics by opening and freeing the opiate receptors, they can produce violent side effects and should only be administered in the presence of trained physicians. Massage done at this time (if any) would be under close supervision of a physician and should be aimed at stimulation to assist in the work of the drugs. Simple rapid effleurage and friction could be used. A physician may prefer that no massage be done until the crisis is over.

Side Effects

Clients who are taking this drug as part of a drug rehabilitation program may experience many side effects. Headache, nervousness, insomnia, anxiety, and high blood pressure are just a few. Massage with this client must be done under the close supervision of a physician. Strokes soothing to the nervous system are best. Rocking and gentle, rhythmic effleurage use the systemic reflex and entrain the body to a calmer state. Extra sensitivity to pain precludes the use of deep tissue work. Severe reactions must be reported to the physician immediately and the massage postponed (see Sidebar: *Adverse Reactions to Narcotic Antagonists*).

Anesthetic Drugs

Anesthetic drugs are divided into three groups: general anesthetics, local anesthetics, and topical anesthetics. General anesthetic drugs are further subdivided into two main types, those given by inhalation and those given by injection.

Inhalation and Injection Anesthetics

General anesthetics that are given by injection or inhalation are only used during surgery or surgical procedures. Massage is contraindicated during these times.

MASSAGE IMPLICATIONS AND ASSESSMENT

After a surgical procedure, these drugs take a long time to be metabolized by the liver and kidney and excreted from the body. With physician approval, use of some gentle effleurage (for its systemic effect on increasing circulation through the body) helps with this elimination. Caution is called for, however; limit the amount and time of the effleurage so as not to move fluids too fast and overwhelm the liver and kidney. If massage is being used to help with pain relief, use the systemic reflexive strokes that increase endorphin production, such as friction at the attachment site of muscles, tendons, and ligaments.

Injection anesthetics are a type of general anesthesia usually used when anesthesia is needed for only a short period, such as in outpatient surgery. These drugs are also used to promote rapid induction of anesthesia or to supplement inhalation anesthetics. Massage is contraindicated during these times.

Local Anesthetics

Common Drug Names

amides: bupivacaine, ropivacaine, etidocaine, lidocaine, mepivacaine, prilocaine

esters: chloroprocaine, procaine, tetracaine

Local anesthetics are administered to prevent or relieve pain in a specific area of the body. In addition, these drugs are often used as an alternative to general anesthesia for elderly or debilitated patients. Local anesthetics are "amide" drugs (with nitrogen in the molecular chain) and "ester" drugs (with oxygen in the molecular chain). These are all the "-caine" drugs, the most common of which is lidocaine.

Pharmacokinetics

Absorption of local anesthetics varies widely, but distribution occurs throughout the body. Esters and amides undergo different types of metabolism, but both yield metabolites that are excreted in the urine.

Pharmacodynamics

Local anesthetics block nerve impulses at the point of contact in all kinds of nerves. They accumulate and cause the nerve cell membrane to expand. As the membrane expands, the cell loses its ability to depolarize, which is necessary for impulse transmission.

Pharmacotherapeutics

Local anesthetics are used to prevent and relieve pain from medical procedures, disease, or injury. Local anesthetics are used for severe pain that topical anesthetics or analgesics cannot relieve. Local anesthetics are usually preferred to general anesthetics for surgery in an elderly or debilitated patient or in a patient with a disorder that affects respiratory function, such as chronic obstructive pulmonary disease and myasthenia gravis. For some procedures, a local anesthetic is combined with a drug such as epinephrine that constricts blood vessels. Vasoconstriction helps control local bleeding and reduces absorption of the anesthetic. Reduced absorption prolongs the anesthetic's action at the site and limits its distribution and CNS effects.

MASSAGE IMPLICATIONS AND ASSESSMENT

Local anesthetics used for surgical procedures are a contraindication to massage. In some cases of chronic pain, anesthetics are injected locally into a nerve to block the pain sensation. Massage therapists need to be aware that all sensation to the local area is blocked, not just pain. No deep work is done in that area. Gentle local mechanical strokes such as effleurage are appropriate.

Topical Anesthetics

Common Drug Names

benzocaine and resorcinol: Vagicaine, Vagisil

capsaicin: Capsin, Zostrix

lidocaine hydrochloride: Xylocaine

procaine hydrochloride: Novocain

Biofreeze, Mineral Ice, Tiger Balm, Icy Hot, and other similar topical anesthetics have combinations of products that use thermal properties to temporarily overwhelm peripheral sensors and decrease sensation to an area. They are not as strong as many other topical anesthetics but can be quite effective.

Topical anesthetics are applied directly to the skin or mucous membranes. All topical anesthetics are used to prevent or relieve minor pain. Some injectable local anesthetics, such as lidocaine and tetracaine, also are effective topically. In addition, some topical anesthetics are combined in products.

Pharmacokinetics

Topical anesthetics produce little systemic absorption, except for the application of cocaine to mucous membranes. However, systemic absorption may occur if the patient receives frequent or high-dose applications to the eye or large areas of burned or injured skin. Tetracaine and other esters are metabolized extensively in the blood and to a lesser extent in the liver. Dibucaine, lidocaine, and other amides are metabolized primarily in the liver. Both types of topical anesthetics are excreted in the urine.

Pharmacodynamics

Benzocaine, butacaine, butamben, cocaine, dyclonine, and pramoxine produce topical anesthesia by blocking nerve impulse transmission. They accumulate in the nerve cell membrane, causing it to expand and lose its ability to depolarize; thus, impulse transmission is blocked. Dibucaine, lidocaine, and tetracaine may block impulse transmission across the nerve cell membranes.

The aromatic compounds, such as benzyl alcohol and clove oil, appear to stimulate nerve endings. This stimulation causes counterirritation that interferes with pain perception.

Ethyl chloride superficially freezes the tissue, stimulating the cold sensation receptors and blocking the nerve endings in the frozen area. Menthol selectively stimulates the sensory nerve endings for cold, causing a cool sensation and some local pain relief.

Pharmacotherapeutics

Topical anesthetics are used to relieve or prevent pain, especially minor burn pain; relieve itching and irritation; anesthetize an area before an injection is given; numb mucosal surfaces before a tube, such as a urinary catheter, is inserted; and alleviate sore throat or mouth pain when used in a spray or solution.

MASSAGE IMPLICATIONS AND ASSESSMENT

Care needs to be taken with topical anesthetics when it comes to the site of application. Obviously, some massage is used to apply the drug to the local surface. However, prolonged massage to the area increases the absorption rate of the drug and must be avoided. The numbing effects of the topical anesthetic are not as strong as those of the local injectable. The same issues do exist, in that all sensation to the area is altered and deep tissue work in the area needs to be avoided. Many massage therapists work with OTC types of topical anesthetics (i.e., Biofreeze) and must be aware of the above cautions. The use of ice during massage also has the same effects.

Quick Quiz

1. A client is taking ibuprofen (800 mg three times a day) for pain related to systemic lupus erythamatosis. She has very tight neck and shoulders and wants to decrease her pain and increase her range of motion. How will her medication and disease affect massage?

2. A client comes in with a strain of the lower back. He is taking Tylenol #3 every 4 hours for pain. His low back is very tight and he also states that his upper back and neck are tight. He wants the muscles to "let go" and is requesting deep work all over the back and neck. What is your response?

Cardiovascular Drugs

6

The heart, arteries, veins, and lymphatics make up the cardiovascular system. These structures transport life-supporting oxygen and nutrients to cells, remove metabolic waste products, and carry hormones from one part of the body to another. Because this system performs such vital functions, any problem with the heart or blood vessels can seriously affect a person's health.

Types of drugs used to improve cardiovascular function include digitalis glycosides and phosphodiesterase (PDE) inhibitors, antiarrhythmic drugs, antianginal drugs, antihypertensive drugs, diuretic drugs, and antilipemic drugs.

Digitalis Glycosides and PDE Inhibitors

Digitalis glycosides and PDE inhibitors increase the force of the heart's contractions. Increasing the force of contractions is known as a positive inotropic effect, so these drugs are also called inotropic drugs. (Inotropic means affecting the force or energy of muscular contractions.) Digitalis glycosides also slow the heart rate (called a negative chronotropic effect) and slow electrical impulse conduction through the atrioventricular (AV) node (called a negative dromotropic effect).

Digitalis Glycosides

Common Drug Names

digitalis: Digitek, digoxin, Lanoxicaps, Lanoxin

Digitalis glycosides are a group of drugs derived from digitalis, a substance that occurs naturally in foxglove plants and certain toads. The most frequently used digitalis glycoside is digoxin. Another digitalis glycoside, digitoxin, is no longer available in the United States.

Pharmacokinetics (how drugs circulate)

The intestinal absorption of digoxin varies greatly; the capsules are absorbed most efficiently, followed by the elixir form, and then tablets. Digoxin is distributed widely throughout the body. In most patients, digoxin is metabolized in the liver and gut by bacteria. This effect varies and may be substantial in some people. Most of the drug is excreted by the kidneys as unchanged drug.

Pharmacodynamics (how drugs act)

Digoxin is used to treat heart failure because it strengthens the contraction of the ventricles. It does this by boosting intracellular calcium at the cell membrane, enabling stronger heart contractions. Digoxin also may enhance the movement of calcium into the myocardial cells and stimulate the release, or block the reuptake, of norepinephrine at the adrenergic nerve terminal. Digoxin acts on the central nervous system (CNS) to slow the heart rate, thus making it useful for treating supraventricular arrhythmias (an abnormal heart rhythm that originates above the bundle branches of the heart's conduction system), such as atrial fibrillation and atrial flutter. It also increases the refractory period (the period when the cells of the conduction system cannot conduct an impulse).

Pharmacotherapeutics (how drugs are used)

In addition to treating heart failure and supraventricular arrhythmias, digoxin is used to treat paroxysmal atrial tachycardia (an arrhythmia marked by brief periods of tachycardia that alternate with brief periods of sinus rhythm).

Adverse Reactions to Digitalis Glycosides

Side Effects
- Fatigue
- Muscle weakness
- Dizziness
- Hypotension

Adverse Effects
- Agitation
- Hallucinations
- Arrhythmias
- Heart failure
- Seeing yellow-green halos around objects
- Blurred vision
- Photophobia
- Diplopia

Because digitalis glycosides have a narrow therapeutic index (margin of safety), they may produce digitalis toxicity. To prevent digitalis toxicity, the dosage should be individualized based on the patient's serum digitalis concentration.

MASSAGE IMPLICATIONS AND ASSESSMENT

There are no concerns with massage increasing the absorption rate of this drug. Its actions are mostly on the heart muscle itself, with secondary actions in the CNS that are poorly understood. The action slows the heart rate while increasing strength of contractions and efficiency of the heart's pumping action. There are no strokes that are directly impacted by this action. All strokes are effective. Choice of strokes is based on the individual's condition and needs.

Side Effects

There are a few side effects that may be of concern to the massage practitioner. Dizziness and hypotension must be addressed by exerting care when getting the client off the table. Stimulating strokes may help; however, the use of more rapid effleurage (which moves blood and fluid systemically) is prohibited if the client has severe cardiac failure (see Sidebar: *Adverse Reactions to Digitalis Glycosides*).

PDE Inhibitors

Common Drug Names

inamrinone lactate milrinone: Primacor

PDE inhibitors are typically used for short-term management of heart failure or long-term management of patients awaiting heart transplant surgery. In the United States, two PDE inhibitors, inamrinone lactate and milrinone (Primacor), have been approved for use.

Pharmacokinetics

Inamrinone is administered intravenously, distributed rapidly, metabolized by the liver, and excreted by the kidneys. Milrinone is also administered intravenously, distributed rapidly, and excreted by the kidneys, primarily as unchanged drug.

Pharmacodynamics

PDE inhibitors improve cardiac output by strengthening contractions. These drugs are believed to help move calcium into the cardiac cell or to increase calcium storage in the sarcoplasmic reticulum. By directly relaxing vascular smooth muscle, they also decrease peripheral vascular resistance (afterload) and the amount of blood returning to the heart (preload).

Pharmacotherapeutics

Inamrinone and milrinone are used for the management of heart failure in patients whose conditions have not responded adequately to treatment with digitalis glycosides, diuretics, or vasodilators. Prolonged use of these drugs may increase the risk of complications and death.

MASSAGE IMPLICATIONS AND ASSESSMENT

These drugs are used short term for severe cases of heart failure. In such situations, massage may be contraindicated by the client's condition. If massage is performed, the medication's action does not affect any of the actions of the strokes. Strokes are chosen based on the client's condition.

Antiarrhythmic Drugs

Antiarrhythmic drugs are used to treat arrhythmias, disturbances of the normal heart rhythm. Unfortunately, many antiarrhythmic drugs are also capable of worsening or causing the very arrhythmias they are supposed to treat. The benefits need to be weighed against the risks of antiarrhythmic therapy. Antiarrhythmics are categorized into four classes: I (which includes class IA, IB, and IC), II, III, and IV.

Class I antiarrhythmics consist of sodium channel blockers. This is the largest group of antiarrhythmic drugs. Class I agents are frequently subdivided into Class IA, IB, and IC. One drug, adenosine, does not fall into any of these classes.

The mechanisms of action of antiarrhythmic drugs vary widely, and a few drugs exhibit properties common to more than one class.

Class IA Antiarrhythmics

Common Drug Names

disopyramide phosphate: Norpace, Rythmodan,

procainamide hydrochloride: Procainamide Durules, Procan, Promine, Pronestyl

quinidine gluconate: Dura-Tabs, Quinalan, Quinate

quinidine polygalacturonate: Cardioquin

quinidine sulfate: Apo-Quinidine, Cin-Quin, Novoquinidin, Quinaglute, Quinidex, Quinora

---

The above Class IA antiarrhythmics are used to treat a wide variety of atrial and ventricular arrhythmias.

Pharmacokinetics

When administered orally, class IA drugs are rapidly absorbed and metabolized. Because they work so quickly, sustained-release forms of these drugs were developed to help maintain therapeutic levels. These drugs are distributed through all body tissues. Quinidine, however, is the only one that crosses the blood–brain barrier. All class IA antiarrhythmics are metabolized in the liver and are excreted unchanged by the kidneys. Acidic urine increases the excretion of quinidine.

Pharmacodynamics

Class IA antiarrhythmics control arrhythmias by altering the myocardial cell membrane and interfering with autonomic nervous system control of pacemaker cells. These agents also block parasympathetic stimulation of the sinoatrial (SA) and AV nodes. Because stimulation of the parasympathetic nervous system causes the heart rate to slow, drugs that block the parasympathetic nervous system increase the conduction rate of the AV node. This increase in the conduction rate can produce dangerous increases in the ventricular heart rate if rapid atrial activity is present, as in a patient with atrial fibrillation. In turn, the increased ventricular heart rate can offset the ability of the antiarrhythmics to convert atrial arrhythmias to a regular rhythm.

Pharmacotherapeutics

Class IA antiarrhythmics are prescribed to treat such arrhythmias as premature ventricular contractions, ventricular tachycardia, atrial fibrillation, atrial flutter, and paroxysmal atrial tachycardia.

MASSAGE IMPLICATIONS AND ASSESSMENT

Oral administration of these medications means that absorption is not an issue for the massage therapist. The action of this class of antiarrhythmics is very specific to the myocardial muscle cell and to the electrical conduction system of the heart. There is little or no change in the effectiveness of the various massage strokes related to the medication.

Side Effects

Dizziness is a side effect of these drugs. Care for the patient's safety in changing positions is appropriate. Other adverse effects are reasons to stop the massage and contact a physician (see Sidebar: *Adverse Reactions to Class IA Antiarrhythmics*).

> **Adverse Reactions to Class IA Antiarrhythmics**
>
> **Side Effects**
> - Dizziness
> - Headache
> - Increased salivation
>
> **Adverse Effects**
> - Confusion
> - Tachycardia
> - Arrhythmias
> - Heart failure
> - Nausea/vomiting
> - Hematologic changes
> - Liver toxicity
> - Acute asthma
> - Heart block

Class IB Antiarrhythmics

Common Drug Names

lidocaine hydrochloride: LidoPen, Xylocaine, Xylocard

mexiletine hydrochloride: Mexitil

tocainide hydrochloride: Tonocard

Lidocaine hydrochloride, a class IB antiarrhythmic, is one of the antiarrhythmics most widely used for treating acute ventricular arrhythmias. Other class IB antiarrhythmics include mexiletine hydrochloride and tocainide hydrochloride.

Pharmacokinetics

With the exception of lidocaine, which is typically administered intravenously, all class IB antiarrhythmics are absorbed well from the GI tract after oral administration.

Lidocaine is distributed widely throughout the body, including the brain. Lidocaine and mexiletine are moderately bound to plasma proteins. (Remember, only that portion of a drug that is unbound can produce a response.) Tocainide is mostly unbound.

Class IB antiarrhythmics are metabolized in the liver and excreted in the urine. Mexiletine also is excreted in breast milk.

Pharmacodynamics

Class IB drugs work by blocking the rapid influx of sodium ions during the depolarization phase of the heart's depolarization-repolarization cycle, resulting in a decreased refractory period, which reduces the risk of arrhythmia.

Because class IB antiarrhythmics especially affect the Purkinje fibers (fibers in the conducting system of the heart) and myocardial cells in the ventricles, they are used only to treat ventricular arrhythmias.

Pharmacotherapeutics

Class IB antiarrhythmics are used to treat ventricular ectopic beats, ventricular tachycardia, and ventricular fibrillation. Because class IB antiarrhythmics usually do not produce serious adverse reactions, they are the drugs of choice in acute care.

Adverse Reactions to Class IB Antiarrhythmics

Side Effects
- Drowsiness
- Dizziness
- Hypotension

Adverse Effects
- Bradycardia
- Paresthesias
- Sensory disturbances
- Seizures
- Respiratory arrest
- Heart block
- Confusion
- Ataxia

MASSAGE IMPLICATIONS AND ASSESSMENT

Class IB drugs are used for life-threatening ventricular arrhythmias. In these cases, anything that could stimulate the nervous system or the cardiovascular system (including massage) may be contraindicated. In these patients, massage must be approved by a physician and is limited by the condition of the patient (see Sidebar: *Adverse Reactions to Class IB Antiarrhythmics*).

Class IC Antiarrhythmics

Common Drug Names

flecainide acetate: Tambocor

moricizine: Ethmozine

propafenone hydrochloride: Rythmol

Class IC antiarrhythmics are used to treat certain severe, refractory (resistant) ventricular arrhythmias. Class IC antiarrhythmics include flecainide acetate, moricizine, and propafenone hydrochloride.

Pharmacokinetics

After oral administration, class IC antiarrhythmics are absorbed well, distributed in varying degrees, and probably metabolized by the liver. They are excreted primarily by the kidneys, except for propafenone, which is excreted primarily in stool.

Pharmacodynamics

Class IC antiarrhythmics primarily slow conduction along the heart's conduction system. Moricizine decreases the fast inward current of sodium ions of the action potential, depressing the depolarization rate and effective refractory period.

Pharmacotherapeutics

Like class IB antiarrhythmics, class IC antiarrhythmic drugs are used to treat life-threatening ventricular arrhythmias. They are also used to treat supraventricular arrhythmias (abnormal heart rhythms that originate above the bundle branches of the heart's conduction system). Flecainide also may be used to prevent paroxysmal supraventricular tachycardia (PSVT) in patients without structural heart disease. Moricizine is used to manage life-threatening ventricular arrhythmias such as sustained ventricular tachycardia.

MASSAGE IMPLICATIONS AND ASSESSMENT

As with the other class I antiarrhythmics, the action of these drugs is specific to the heart conduction system and does not change the effect of massage strokes. The client's condition guides the choice of strokes used. A physician's approval for massage is required for patients with these serious cardiac conditions (see Sidebar: *Adverse Reactions to Class IC Antiarrhythmics*).

Adverse Reactions to Class IC Antiarrhythmics

Side Effects
- Anxiety
- Drowsiness
- Dizziness
- Fatigue
- Insomnia
- Weakness
- Tremor
- Dry mouth
- Constipation

Adverse Effects
- Atrial fibrillation
- Heart block
- Angina
- Edema
- Ventricular tachycardia
- Dyspnea
- Bronchospasm
- Cardiac arrest

Class II Antiarrhythmics

Common Drug Names

acebutolol: Monitan, Sectral

esmolol: Brevibloc

propranolol: Apo-Propranolol, Detensol, Inderal, Novopranol

Class II antiarrhythmics are composed of beta-adrenergic antagonists, or beta blockers. Beta blockers used as antiarrhythmics include acebutolol hydrochloride, esmolol hydrochloride, and propranolol hydrochloride.

Pharmacokinetics

Acebutolol and propranolol are absorbed almost entirely from the GI tract after an oral dose. Esmolol, which can only be given intravenously, is immediately available throughout the body. Acebutolol and propranolol undergo significant first-pass effect, leaving only a small portion of these drugs available to reach the circulation to be distributed to the body. Approximately 35% of an acebutolol dose is excreted in the urine and 55% in stool. Most of an esmolol dose is metabolized to an inactive metabolite, which is excreted in the urine. Propranolol's metabolites are excreted in the urine as well.

Pharmacodynamics

Class II antiarrhythmics block beta-adrenergic receptor sites in the conduction system of the heart. As a result, the ability of the SA node to fire spontaneously (automaticity) is slowed. The ability of the AV node and other cells to receive and conduct an electrical impulse to nearby cells (conductivity) is also reduced. Class II antiarrhythmics also reduce the strength of the heart's contractions. When the heart beats less forcefully, it does not require as much oxygen to do its work.

Pharmacotherapeutics

Class II antiarrhythmics slow ventricular rates in patients with atrial flutter, atrial fibrillation, and paroxysmal atrial tachycardia.

MASSAGE IMPLICATIONS AND ASSESSMENT

The action of these drugs is quite specific to the heart conduction system and does not affect the efficacy of the various massage strokes. The patient's condition dictates the types of massage to be used. Physician approval is appropriate.

Side Effects

The side effects of concern to the massage practitioner are lethargy and hypotension. Because stimulation of the nervous system or cardiovascular system may be contraindicated in severe arrhythmias, the therapist would be unable to do tapotement or rapid effleurage. Staying with clients until they are seated on the side of the table and are not experiencing any dizziness is the safest way to handle these possible side effects (see Sidebar: *Adverse Reactions to Class II Antiarrhythmics*).

Class III Antiarrhythmics

Common Drug Names

amiodarone: Aratac, Cordarone

bretylium tosylate: Bretylate

Class III antiarrhythmics are used to treat ventricular arrhythmias. The two drugs in this class are amiodarone hydrochloride and bretylium tosylate.

Pharmacokinetics

The absorption of these two antiarrhythmics varies widely. After oral administration, amiodarone is absorbed slowly at widely varying rates. The drug is distributed extensively and accumulates in many sites, especially in organs with a rich blood supply and fatty tissue. Because GI absorption is so erratic, bretylium is given intravenously. Bretylium is distributed widely throughout the body and is excreted unchanged by the kidneys.

Pharmacodynamics

Although the exact mechanism of action is not known, class III antiarrhythmics are believed to suppress arrhythmias. They have little or no effect on depolarization.

Pharmacotherapeutics

Because of their adverse effects, class III antiarrhythmics are not the drugs of choice for antiarrhythmic therapy. They are used for life-threatening arrhythmias that are resistant to other antiarrhythmic treatment.

MASSAGE IMPLICATIONS AND ASSESSMENT

Because this class of drugs is used only in life-threatening arrhythmias, massage is more than likely contraindicated. The action of the drugs themselves does affect not the action of the massage strokes, but the client's condition dictates contraindication or great caution. The side effects of the drugs are many and increase the instability of the client condition's (see Sidebar: *Adverse Reactions to Class III Antiarrhythmics*).

Adverse Reactions to Class III Antiarrhythmics

Side Effects
- Hypotension
- Peripheral neuropathy
- Headache
- Fatigue
- Constipation

Adverse Effects
- Extrapyramidal symptoms
- Arrhythmias
- Heart block
- Heart failure
- Hepatic dysfunction
- Thyroid dysfunction
- Blue-gray skin
- Gynecomastia
- Pulmonary toxicity

Class IV Antiarrhythmics

Class IV antiarrhythmics are composed of calcium channel blockers. Calcium channel blockers used to treat arrhythmias include verapamil and diltiazem. Verapamil and diltiazem are used to treat supraventricular arrhythmias with rapid ventricular response rates (rapid heart rate in which the rhythm originates above the ventricles). For a thorough discussion of calcium channel blockers and how they work, see the section on calcium channel blockers under "Antianginal Drugs" in this chapter.

Adenosine

Adenosine is an injectable antiarrhythmic drug indicated for acute treatment of paroxysmal supraventricular tachycardia (PSVT). Because this is an unstable, life-threatening condition, massage is contraindicated in many cases and is dictated by the client's condition and not the medications.

Antianginal Drugs

Although angina's cardinal symptom is chest pain, the drugs used to treat angina are not typically analgesics. Instead, antianginal drugs treat angina by reducing myocardial oxygen demand (reducing the amount of oxygen the heart needs to do its work), by increasing the supply of oxygen to the heart, or both (Fig. 6-1). The three classes of antianginal drugs discussed in this section include nitrates (for treating acute angina), beta blockers (for long-term prevention of angina), and calcium channel blockers (for use when other drugs fail to prevent angina).

Nitrates

Common Drug Names

isosorbide dinitrate: Apo-ISDN, Cedocard, Coronex, Isordil, Isotrate, Sorbitrate

isosorbide mononitrate: IMDUR, Monoket,

nitroglycerin: Nitrodisc, Nitro-Bid, Nitro-Dur, Nitrogard, Nitrol, Nitrostat, NTG, Transderm-Nitro, Tridil

---

Nitrates are the drugs of choice for relieving acute angina.

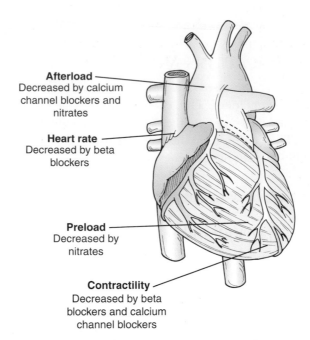

Afterload
Decreased by calcium
channel blockers and
nitrates

Heart rate
Decreased by beta
blockers

Preload
Decreased by
nitrates

Contractility
Decreased by beta
blockers and calcium
channel blockers

Figure 6-1 Antianginal Drug Effects on the Cardiovascular System. Angina occurs when the coronary arteries, the heart's primary source of oxygen, supply insufficient oxygen to the myocardium. This increases the heart's workload, which increases heart rate, preload (blood volume in the ventricle at the end of diastole), afterload (pressure in the arteries leading from the ventricle), and force of myocardial contractility. The antianginal drugs (nitrates, beta blockers, and calcium channel blockers) relieve angina by decreasing one or more of these four factors.

Pharmacokinetics

Nitrates can be administered in a variety of ways. Nitrates given sublingually (under the tongue), buccally (in the pocket of the cheek), as chewable tablets, or as lingual aerosols (sprayed onto or under the tongue) are absorbed almost completely. That is because the mucous membranes of the mouth have a rich blood supply.

Swallowed nitrate capsules are absorbed through the mucous membranes of the GI tract, and only about half the dose enters circulation. Transdermal nitrates (a patch or ointment placed on the skin) are absorbed slowly and in varying amounts, depending on the quantity of drug applied, the location where the patch is applied, the surface area of skin used, and the circulation to the skin. Intravenous nitroglycerin, which does not need to be absorbed, goes directly into the circulation.

Pharmacodynamics

Nitrates cause the smooth muscle of the veins and, to a lesser extent, the arteries to relax and dilate. When the veins dilate, less blood returns to the heart. This, in turn, reduces the amount of blood in the ventricles at the end of diastole, when the ventricles are full. (This blood volume in the ventricles just before contraction is called preload.) By reducing preload, nitrates reduce ventricular size and ventricular wall tension (the left ventricle does not have to stretch as much to pump blood). This, in turn, reduces the oxygen requirements of the heart.

The arterioles provide the most resistance to the blood pumped by the left ventricle (called peripheral vascular resistance). Nitrates decrease afterload by dilating the arterioles, reducing resistance, easing the heart's workload, and easing the demand for oxygen.

Pharmacotherapeutics

Nitrates are used to relieve and prevent angina. The rapidly absorbed nitrates, such as nitroglycerin, are the drugs of choice for relief of acute angina because they have a rapid onset of action, they are easy to take, and they are inexpensive. Longer-acting nitrates, such as the daily nitroglycerin transdermal patch, are convenient and can be used to prevent chronic angina. Oral nitrates are also used because they seldom produce serious adverse reactions.

MASSAGE IMPLICATIONS AND ASSESSMENT

The method of administration of nitrates needs to be addressed by the massage therapist in the case of transdermal patches or ointments applied to the skin. Effects and absorption continue for up to 8 hours for ointments and for 24 hours for transdermal patches. Massage over the site of administration is contraindicated in both cases, and massage of the adjacent tissues (i.e., the entire upper arm if the patch is on the deltoid muscle) must be limited so as not to increase the rate of absorption.

The action of these drugs is to relax the smooth muscle of both veins and arteries. This does not affect the action of reflex strokes. The mechanical strokes and the body system effects of effleurage are potentiated by these medications. Although they may still be used, caution is indicated. Decreasing the amount of time effleurage and pétrissage are used could help prevent a drop in blood pressure and feelings of weakness. Tapotement is a good choice at the end of the massage to stimulate the client.

Side Effects

There are many side effects related to the action of these drugs that concern the massage therapist. Flushing, orthostatic hypotension, dizziness, and weakness are the most common. The above alterations in the application of massage help. Also, the therapist must stay with clients as they sit up after a massage and until they feel steady (see Sidebar: *Adverse Reactions to Nitrates*).

Adverse Reactions to Nitrates

Side Effects
- Headache
- Dizziness
- Weakness
- Orthostatic hypotension
- Flushing

Adverse Effects
- Tachycardia
- Edema
- Severe hypotension

Beta-Adrenergic Antianginals

Common Drug Names

atenolol: Apo-Atenol, Noten, Nu-Atenol, Tenormin

metoprolol: Apo-Metoprolol, Betaloc, Lopressor, Toprol XL

nadolol: Corgard, Syn-Nadolol

propranolol: Apo-Propranolol, Detensol, Inderal, Novopranol

Beta-adrenergic antagonists (also called beta blockers) are used for long-term prevention of angina and are one of the main types of drugs used to treat hypertension.

Pharmacokinetics

Metoprolol and propranolol are absorbed almost entirely from the GI tract, whereas less than half the dose of atenolol or nadolol is absorbed. These beta blockers are distributed widely.

Propranolol and metoprolol are metabolized in the liver, and their metabolites are excreted in the urine. Atenolol and nadolol are not metabolized and are excreted unchanged in the urine and stool.

Pharmacodynamics

Beta blockers decrease blood pressure and block beta-adrenergic receptor sites in the heart muscle and conduction system, decreasing heart rate and reducing the force of the heart's contractions. This results in lower demand for oxygen.

Pharmacotherapeutics

Beta blockers are indicated for long-term prevention of angina. Because of their longer onset, they are not used to provide immediate relief of an angina attack or to prevent an imminent one. Because of their ability to reduce blood pressure, beta blockers are also first-line therapy for treating hypertension.

Adverse Reactions to Beta Blockers

Side Effects
- Fatigue
- Lethargy
- Hypotension

Adverse Effects
- Bradycardia
- Angina
- Fainting
- Fluid retention
- Peripheral edema
- Shock
- Heart failure
- Arrhythmias, especially atrioventricular block
- Nausea and vomiting
- Diarrhea
- Significant constriction of the bronchioles
- Acute myocardial infarction

MASSAGE IMPLICATIONS AND ASSESSMENT

Adrenergic blockers stop the stimulation of the sympathetic nervous system. Whereas beta-adrenergic blockers are more heart-specific than others, there is still the effect systemically of making it a little harder to wake up and a little easier to go into parasympathetic nervous system activity. Because massage generally puts the client into parasympathetic activity, the use of more rapid and stimulatory strokes during and/or at the end of the massage may be needed to prevent lethargy.

Side Effects

Common side effects to these drugs are due to their actions in blocking the awakening of the sympathetic nervous system. Fatigue, hypotension, lethargy, and dizziness are a few. The modifications to massage application discussed above help balance these effects. Staying with clients may also be needed while they are changing positions if these side effects are present (see Sidebar: *Adverse Reactions to Beta Blockers*).

Calcium Channel Blockers

Common Drug Names

amlodipine besylate: Norvasc

diltiazem hydrochloride: Cardizem, Dilacor XR, Tiamate, Tiazac *nicardipine:* Cardene

nifedipine hydrochloride: Adalat (discontinued in the U.S.), Procardia, Nu-Nifed

verapamil hydrochloride: Calan, Isoptin, Apo-Verap, Novo-Veramil, Nu-Verap

Calcium channel blockers are commonly used to prevent angina that does not respond to drugs in either of the other antianginal classes. As mentioned previously, several of the calcium channel blockers are also used as antiarrhythmics.

Pharmacokinetics

When administered orally, calcium channel blockers are absorbed quickly and almost completely. Because of the first-pass effect, however, the bioavailability of these drugs is much lower. All calcium channel blockers are metabolized rapidly and almost completely in the liver.

Pharmacodynamics

Calcium channel blockers prevent the passage of calcium ions across the myocardial cell membrane and vascular smooth muscle cells. This causes dilation of the coronary and peripheral arteries, which decreases the force of the heart's contractions and reduces the workload of the heart (Fig. 6-2). By preventing arterioles from constricting, calcium channel blockers also reduce afterload. Decreasing afterload also decreases the oxygen demands of the heart. Calcium channel blockers also reduce the heart rate by slowing conduction through the SA and AV nodes. A slower heart rate reduces the heart's need for additional oxygen.

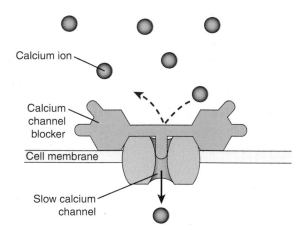

Figure 6-2 Effects of Calcium Channel Blockers.
Calcium channel blockers increase the myocardial oxygen supply and slow the heart rate. Apparently the drugs produce these effects by blocking the slow calcium channel. This action inhibits the influx of extracellular calcium ions across both myocardial and vascular smooth muscle cell membranes. Calcium channel blockers achieve this blockade without changing serum calcium concentrations. This calcium blockade causes the coronary arteries (and, to a lesser extent, the peripheral arteries and arterioles) to dilate, decreasing afterload and increasing myocardial oxygen supply. The blockade also slows sinoatrial and atrioventricular node conduction, slightly reducing heart rate.

Pharmacotherapeutics

Calcium channel blockers are used only for long-term prevention of angina, not for short-term relief of chest pain. Calcium channel blockers are particularly effective for preventing Prinzmetal's angina.

Adverse Reactions to Calcium Channel Blockers

Side Effects
- Orthostatic hypotension
- Dizziness
- Headache
- Flushing

Adverse Effects
- Edema
- Heart failure
- Arrhythmias
- Heart block

MASSAGE IMPLICATIONS AND ASSESSMENT

The action of the calcium channel blockers is on the heart muscle and the smooth muscle of the arteries, causing dilation. The effects of the various massage strokes on the skeletal muscle are not affected. The action of mechanical massage strokes is increased because dilation of blood vessels occurs with these strokes. Application of these strokes (effleurage and pétrissage especially) should be slightly more rapid and stimulatory during or at the end of the massage to balance this effect. Tapotement may also be used.

Side Effects

The side effects of these drugs are similar to other antianginals. Flushing, hypotension, and dizziness are most common. The above changes in application to massage will prevent problems with these effects (see Sidebar: *Adverse Reactions to Calcium Channel Blockers*).

Antihypertensive Drugs

Antihypertensive drugs, which act to reduce blood pressure, are used to treat hypertension. Hypertension is a disorder characterized by elevation in systolic blood pressure, diastolic blood pressure, or both. Treatment of hypertension begins with beta blockers and diuretics. If those drugs are not effective, treatment continues with sympatholytic drugs (other than beta blockers), vasodilators, angiotensin-converting enzyme (ACE) inhibitors, or a combination of drugs.

Sympatholytic Drugs

Common Drug Names

clonidine hydrochloride: Catapres, Dixarit, Duraclon

doxazosin mesylate: Cardura

guanabenz acetate: Wytensin (discontinued in the U.S.)

guanadrel sulfate: Hylorel

guanethidine monosulfate: Ismelin

guanfacine: Tenex

labetalol: Normodyne, Presolol, Trandate,

methyldopa: Aldomet, Apo-Methyldopa, Dopamet, Hydopa, Novo-Medopa, Nu-Medopa

phentolamine: Regitine (discontinued in the U.S.), Rogitine *prazosin hydrochloride:* Minipress

terazosin: Hytrin

Sympatholytic drugs include several different types of drugs, but all reduce blood pressure by inhibiting or blocking the sympathetic nervous system. They are classified by their site or mechanism of action and include:

- Central-acting sympathetic nervous system inhibitors (clonidine hydrochloride, guanabenz acetate, guanfacine, and methyldopa)
- Alpha blockers (doxazosin mesylate, phentolamine, prazosin hydrochloride, and terazosin)
- Mixed alpha and beta blockers (labetalol)
- Norepinephrine depletors (guanadrel sulfate, guanethidine monosulfate, and reserpine)

Pharmacokinetics

Most sympatholytic drugs are absorbed well from the GI tract, distributed widely, metabolized in the liver, and excreted primarily in the urine.

Pharmacodynamics

All sympatholytic drugs inhibit stimulation of the sympathetic nervous system. This causes dilation of the peripheral blood vessels or decreased cardiac output, thereby reducing blood pressure.

Pharmacotherapeutics

Beta blockers (along with diuretics) are the initial drugs for treating hypertension. If blood pressure fails to be controlled, an alpha blocker (such as prazosin) or an alpha-beta blocker (such as labetalol) may be used. If the patient's condition fails to respond (i.e., the desired blood pressure is not achieved), the physician may add a drug from a different class, substitute a drug in the same class, or increase the drug dosage.

MASSAGE IMPLICATIONS AND ASSESSMENT

The sympatholytic drugs stop the action of the sympathetic nervous system. Because massage also works to decrease sympathetic stimulation and put the client into parasympathetic system, massage effects may be increased by these drugs. The use of slightly more rapid and stimulating strokes helps the client to feel relaxed (rather than lethargic), yet more balanced at the end of the massage.

Side Effects

The above modifications to massage assist with the most common of the side effects experienced by those taking sympatholytic drugs. These side effects are hypotension, drowsiness, and fatigue. Some clients will also experience numbness and tingling. If so, deep tissue should be used with great caution (see Sidebar: *Adverse Reactions to Sympatholytics*).

Adverse Reactions to Sympatholytics

Side Effects
- Hypotension
- Drowsiness
- Depression
- Numbness and tingling
- Dizziness
- Weight gain

Adverse Effects
- Edema
- Liver dysfunction
- Bronchoconstriction
- Arrhythmias
- Angina

Vasodilating Drugs

Common Drug Names

diazoxide: Hyperstat, Proglycem
hydralazine hydrochloride: Apo-Hydralazine, Apresoline, Novo-Hylazin, Nu-Hydral
minoxidil: Apo-Gain, Loniten, Minox, Rogaine
nitroprusside sodium: Nipride, Nitropress

There are two types of vasodilating drugs: direct vasodilators and calcium channel blockers. Both types decrease systolic and diastolic blood pressure. All of the above listed drugs are direct vasodilators. These agents act on arteries, veins, or both.

Hydralazine and minoxidil are usually used to treat resistant or refractory hypertension (a rare use for minoxidil, more often used for hair loss). Diazoxide and nitroprusside are reserved for use in hypertensive crisis.

Calcium channel blockers produce arteriolar relaxation by preventing the entry of calcium into the cells. This prevents the contraction of vascular smooth muscle. For a more in-depth discussion, see the section on calcium channel blockers under "Antianginal Drugs" in this chapter.

Pharmacokinetics

Most of these drugs are absorbed rapidly and distributed well. They all are metabolized in the liver, and most are excreted by the kidneys.

Pharmacodynamics

The direct vasodilators relax peripheral vascular smooth muscles, causing the blood vessels to dilate. This lowers blood pressure by increasing the diameter of the blood vessels, reducing total peripheral resistance.

Pharmacotherapeutics

Vasodilating drugs are rarely used alone to treat hypertension. Instead, they are usually used in combination with other drugs to treat the patient with moderate to severe hypertension (hypertensive crisis). Calcium channel blockers are occasionally used alone to treat mild to moderate hypertension.

MASSAGE IMPLICATIONS AND ASSESSMENT

The action of the various strokes on muscles is not affected by vasodilating drugs. The action of the mechanical strokes of massage in dilating blood vessels is increased. Again, slightly increasing the rate of these strokes (effleurage and pétrissage) during the massage and using tapotement at the end of the massage gives the client less chance of feeling dizzy or weak from dilation of blood vessels.

Side Effects

Hypotension is the main side effect of these drugs. The needed changes to massage are addressed above. Another side effect may be that of breast tenderness in both men and women. Sensitivity to this when working the chest may be needed (see Sidebar: *Adverse Reactions to Vasodilators*).

Adverse Reactions to Vasodilators

Side Effects
- Fatigue
- Headache
- Breast tenderness
- Hypotension

Adverse Effects
- Palpitations
- Angina
- Edema
- Rash
- Severe pericardial effusion

Angiotensin-Converting Enzyme Inhibitors

Common Drug Names

benazepril hydrochloride: Lotensin

captopril: Alti-Captopril, Apo-Capto, Capoten (with hydrochlorothiazide: Capozide)

enalapril: Vasotec

fosinopril: Monopril

lisinopril: Prinivil, Zestril

quinapril hydrochloride: Accupril

ramipril: Altace

Angiotensin-converting enzyme (ACE) inhibitors reduce blood pressure by interrupting the renin-angiotensin-aldosterone system.

Pharmacokinetics

ACE inhibitors are absorbed from the GI tract, distributed to most body tissues, metabolized somewhat in the liver, and excreted by the kidneys. Ramipril also is excreted in stool.

Pharmacodynamics

ACE inhibitors act by interfering with the renin-angiotensin-aldosterone system. Normally, the kidneys maintain blood pressure by releasing the hormone renin. Renin acts on the plasma protein angiotensinogen to form angiotensin I. Angiotensin I is then converted to angiotensin II. Angiotensin II, a potent vasoconstrictor, increases peripheral resistance and promotes the excretion of aldosterone. Aldosterone, in turn, promotes the retention of sodium and water, increasing the volume of blood the heart needs to pump.

ACE inhibitors work by preventing the conversion of angiotensin I to angiotensin II. As angiotensin II is reduced, arterioles dilate, reducing peripheral vascular resistance. By reducing aldosterone secretion, ACE inhibitors promote the excretion of sodium and water, reducing the amount of blood the heart needs to pump and resulting in decreased blood pressure.

Pharmacotherapeutics

ACE inhibitors may be used alone or in combination with another drug, such as a thiazide diuretic, to treat hypertension. They are commonly used when beta blockers or diuretics are ineffective. They are also used to manage heart failure.

Adverse Reactions to ACE Inhibitors

Side Effects
- Headache and fatigue
- Dry, nonproductive, persistent cough
- Hypotension

Adverse Effects
- Angioedema
- GI reactions
- Increased serum potassium concentrations
- Transient elevations of blood urea nitrogen and serum creatinine levels (indicators of kidney function)

MASSAGE IMPLICATIONS AND ASSESSMENT

The ACE inhibitors dilate the vessels; therefore, the effects of mechanical massage strokes on the blood vessels may be enhanced. Slightly increasing the rate of application and the use of tapotement may ease any problems that could arise, such as weakness or dizziness and fatigue. Because ACE inhibitors also affect the rate of excretion of sodium and water from the body, the use of systemic strokes that increase circulation (i.e., effleurage) is limited in duration.

Side Effects

Hypotension is the main side effect of the ACE inhibitors that concerns the massage therapist. The above modifications help to prevent problems. Staying with clients while they sit up after a massage is indicated if this is an issue (see Sidebar: *Adverse Reactions to ACE Inhibitors*).

Diuretics

Diuretics are used to promote the excretion of water and electrolytes by the kidneys. By doing so, diuretics play a major role in the treatment of hypertension and other cardiovascular conditions. The major diuretics used as cardiovascular drugs include thiazide and thiazide-like diuretics, loop diuretics, and potassium-sparing diuretics.

Thiazide and Thiazide-Like Diuretics

Common Drug Names

bendroflumethiazide: Naturetin

chlorthalidone: Apo-Chlorthalidone, Thalitone

hydrochlorothiazide: Apo-Hydro, Ezide, HCTZ, HydroDIURIL, Microzide (with triamterene: Dyazide)

indapamide: Apo-Indapamide, Lozide, Lozol

methyclothiazide: Aquatensen, Enduron

polythiazide: Renese

trichlormethiazide: Aquacot, Metatensin, Naqua, Trichlorex

Thiazide and thiazide-like diuretics are sulfonamide derivatives. Thiazide diuretics include:

- bendroflumethiazide
- benzthiazide
- chlorothiazide
- hydrochlorothiazide

- hydroflumethiazide
- methyclothiazide
- polythiazide
- trichlormethiazide

Thiazide-like diuretics include:

- chlorthalidone
- indapamide

Pharmacokinetics

Thiazide diuretics are absorbed rapidly but incompletely from the GI tract after oral administration. Thiazide diuretics cross the placenta and are secreted in breast milk. These drugs differ in how well they are metabolized. They are excreted primarily in the urine.

Thiazide-like diuretics are absorbed from the GI tract. Indapamide is distributed widely into body tissues and metabolized in the liver. These drugs are excreted primarily in the urine.

Pharmacodynamics

Thiazide and thiazide-like diuretics work by preventing sodium from being reabsorbed in the kidney. As sodium is excreted, it pulls water along with it. Thiazide and thiazide-like diuretics also increase the excretion of chloride, potassium, and bicarbonate, which can result in electrolyte imbalances.

Initially, these drugs decrease circulating blood volume, leading to a reduced cardiac output. However, if therapy is maintained, cardiac output stabilizes but plasma fluid volume decreases.

Pharmacotherapeutics

Thiazides are used as long-term treatment of hypertension and are also used to treat edema caused by mild or moderate heart failure, liver disease, kidney disease, and corticosteroid and estrogen therapy. Because these drugs decrease the level of calcium in the urine, they are also used alone or with other drugs to prevent the development and recurrence of calcium kidney stones.

Diabetes insipidus is a disorder characterized by excessively large amounts of urine and excessive thirst, caused by reduced secretion of antidiuretic hormone by the pituitary gland. This condition is not related to diabetes mellitus, in which insulin and blood sugar are affected. In patients with diabetes insipidus, thiazides paradoxically decrease urine volume, possibly through sodium depletion and plasma volume reduction.

MASSAGE IMPLICATIONS AND ASSESSMENT

The action of these drugs is to increase secretion of sodium and water. The mechanical strokes that affect circulation (effleurage) have an increased action by speeding blood to the kidneys and increasing excretion further. It is appropriate in these clients to limit the use of effleurage to prevent this.

Side Effects

Orthostatic hypotension can be a problem in massage, especially in clients taking diuretics. Because effleurage must be limited, more rapid pétrissage, friction, and tapotement are used to help alleviate some of the problems associated with orthostatic hypotension. In addition, the loss of sodium, potassium, and other electrolytes may lead to cramping of muscles. Massage can help alleviate an isolated case, but a referral to a physician is required to evaluate if cramping is caused by an electrolyte imbalance (see Sidebar: *Adverse Reactions to Thiazide and Thiazide-Like Diuretics*).

Loop Diuretics

Common Drug Names

bumetanide: Bumex, Burinex

ethacrynate sodium: Edecril, Edecrin, ethacrynic acid

furosemide: Apo-Furosemide, Furocot, Lasix

torsemide: Demadex

Pharmacokinetics

Loop diuretics usually are absorbed well and distributed rapidly. For the most part, these agents undergo partial or complete metabolism in the liver, except for furosemide, which is excreted primarily unchanged. Loop diuretics are excreted primarily by the kidneys.

Pharmacodynamics

Loop diuretics are the most potent diuretics available, producing the greatest volume of diuresis (urine production). They also have a high potential for causing severe adverse reactions. Bumetanide is the shortest-acting diuretic. It is 40 times more potent than furosemide.

Loop diuretics receive their name because they act primarily on the thick ascending loop of Henle (the part of the nephron responsible for concentrating urine) to increase the secretion of sodium, chloride, and water. These drugs also may inhibit sodium, chloride, and water reabsorption.

Pharmacotherapeutics

Loop diuretics are used to treat edema associated with heart failure as well as hypertension (usually with a potassium-sparing diuretic or a potassium supplement to prevent hypokalemia). Loop diuretics are also used to treat edema associated with liver disease or nephrotic syndrome (kidney disease).

MASSAGE IMPLICATIONS AND ASSESSMENT

As with other diuretics, use of effleurage should be limited so as not to increase the action of the drug. Because these diuretics may also be used in edematous conditions, such as heart failure and liver disease, consultation with a physician on the condition of the client may also be indicated.

Side Effects

Orthostatic hypotension and muscle cramping are the most common side effects of loop diuretics. Taking care when the client is changing positions and notifying a physician if cramping is a problem are appropriate actions to take (see Sidebar: *Adverse Reactions to Loop Diuretics*).

> ### Adverse Reactions to Loop Diuretics
>
> **Side Effects**
> - Orthostatic hypotension
> - Muscle cramps
>
> **Adverse Effects**
> - Shock
> - Dehydration
> - Altered electrolytes
> - Confusion
> - Arrhythmias

Potassium-Sparing Diuretics

Common Drug Names

amiloride: Kaluril, Midamor

eplerenome: Inspra

spironolactone: Aldactone, Novo-Spiroton, Spiractin

triamterene: Dyrenium

Potassium-sparing diuretics have weaker diuretic and antihypertensive effects than other diuretics. However, they have the advantage of conserving potassium.

Pharmacokinetics

Potassium-sparing diuretics are only available orally and are absorbed in the GI tract. They are metabolized in the liver (except for amiloride, which is not metabolized) and excreted primarily in the urine and bile.

Pharmacodynamics

The direct action of potassium-sparing diuretics on the distal tubule of the kidneys produces the following effects: (1) urinary excretion of sodium and water increases, as does excretion of chloride and calcium ions, and (2) excretion of potassium and hydrogen ions decreases. These effects lead to reduced blood pressure and increased serum potassium levels.

Spironolactone, one of the main potassium-sparing diuretics, is structurally similar to aldosterone and acts as an aldosterone antagonist. Recall that aldosterone promotes the retention of sodium and water and loss of potassium. Spironolactone counteracts these effects by competing with aldosterone for receptor sites. As a result, sodium, chloride, and water are excreted and potassium is retained.

Pharmacotherapeutics

Potassium-sparing diuretics are used to treat edema, diuretic-induced hypokalemia in patients with heart failure, cirrhosis, nephrotic syndrome (abnormal condition of the kidneys), and hypertension. Spironolactone, in particular, is also used to treat hyperaldosteronism (excessive secretion of aldosterone) and hirsutism (excessive hair growth), including hirsutism associated with Stein-Leventhal (polycystic ovary) syndrome. Potassium-sparing diuretics are commonly used with other diuretics to potentiate their action or counteract their potassium-wasting effects.

Adverse Reactions to Potassium-Sparing Diuretics

Side Effects
- Muscle cramps
- Headache
- Drowsiness
- Breast soreness

Adverse Effects
- Hyperkalemia
- Arrhythmias
- Peptic ulcer
- Dehydration
- Rash
- Gynecomastia

MASSAGE IMPLICATIONS AND ASSESSMENT

Regarding excretion of sodium and water, potassium-sparing diuretics have a weaker effect on their own than when combined with other drugs. Effleurage may be used, but with caution, so as not to increase circulation to the kidneys and excretion. When potassium-sparing diuretics are used in combination, their effects can be potentiated. In such cases, limiting or eliminating the use of effleurage may be indicated. In edema caused by heart failure, kidney disease, or liver disease, approval of a physician is necessary for massage to take place.

Side Effects

There is less chance of hypotension and cramping with the potassium-sparing diuretics when they are used alone. These side effects, when present, are treated in the same manner as when they are caused by other diuretics. Breast soreness can be a side effect of these drugs, so care must be taken with the depth of chest massage (see Sidebar: *Adverse Reactions to Potassium-Sparing Diuretics*).

Antilipemic Drugs

Antilipemic drugs are used to lower abnormally high blood levels of lipids, such as cholesterol, triglycerides, and phospholipids. The risk of developing coronary artery disease increases when serum lipid levels are elevated. Drugs are used when lifestyle changes, such as proper diet, weight loss, and exercise, and treatment of an underlying disorder causing the lipid abnormality fail to lower lipid levels. Antilipemic drug classes include bile-sequestering drugs (cholestyramine and colestipol hydrochloride), fibric acid derivatives (clofibrate and gemfibrozil), and cholesterol synthesis inhibitors (lovastatin, pravastatin sodium, and simvastatin).

Bile-Sequestering Drugs

Common Drug Names

cholestyramine: LoCHOLEST, Novo-Cholamine, Prevalite, Questran
colestipol hydrochloride: Colestid

The two bile-sequestering drugs are cholestyramine and colestipol hydrochloride. These two drugs are resins that remove excess bile acids from the fat depots under the skin.

Pharmacokinetics

Bile-sequestering drugs are not absorbed from the GI tract. Instead, they remain in the intestine, where they combine with bile acids for approximately 5 hours. Eventually, they are excreted in stool.

Pharmacodynamics

These drugs combine with bile acids in the intestines to form an insoluble compound that is then excreted in stool. The decreasing level of bile acid in the gallbladder triggers the liver to synthesize more bile acids from their precursor, cholesterol. As cholesterol leaves the bloodstream and other storage areas to replace the lost bile acids, blood cholesterol levels decrease.

Pharmacotherapeutics

Bile-sequestering drugs are the drugs of choice for treating type IIa hyperlipoproteinemia (familial hypercholesterolemia) in the patient whose low-density lipoprotein (LDL) cholesterol levels have not been lowered through dietary changes. A patient whose blood cholesterol levels indicate a severe risk of coronary artery disease is most likely to require one of these drugs to supplement his or her diet.

MASSAGE IMPLICATIONS AND ASSESSMENT

The actions of this drug class take place in the intestines and do not affect the action of the various massage strokes.

Side Effects

One of the most common side effects of the bile-sequestering agents is constipation. The massage therapist can help with this problem by performing abdominal massage. If the client complains of abdominal pain and tenderness and has not had a bowel movement in several days, massage *cannot* be performed. The client must be evaluated for a bowel obstruction immediately by a physician or urgent care center (see Sidebar: *Adverse Reactions to Bile-Sequestering Drugs*).

> **Adverse Reactions to Bile-Sequestering Drugs**
>
> **Side Effects**
> - Constipation
> - Nausea
>
> **Adverse Effects**
> - Fecal impaction
> - Diarrhea
> - Peptic ulcers and bleeding
> - Gallstones

Fibric Acid Derivatives

Common Drug Names

clofibrate: Atromid-S, Claripex

fenofibrate: Tricor

gemfibrozil: Apo-Gemfibrozil, Lopid

Fibric acid is produced by several fungi. Two derivatives of this acid are clofibrate and gemfibrozil. These drugs are used to reduce high triglyceride levels and, to a lesser extent, high LDL levels.

Pharmacokinetics

Clofibrate and gemfibrozil are absorbed readily from the GI tract and are highly protein bound. Clofibrate is hydrolyzed and gemfibrozil undergoes extensive metabolism in the liver before both drugs are excreted in the urine.

Pharmacodynamics

Although the exact mechanism of action for these drugs is not known, researchers believe that fibric acid derivatives may reduce cholesterol production early in its formation, mobilize cholesterol from the tissues, increase cholesterol excretion, decrease synthesis and secretion of lipoproteins, and decrease synthesis of triglycerides. Gemfibrozil produces two other effects. It increases high-density lipoprotein levels in the blood (remember, this is "good" cholesterol), and it increases the serum's capacity to dissolve additional cholesterol.

Pharmacotherapeutics

Fibric acid drugs are used primarily to reduce triglyceride levels, especially very-low-density triglycerides, and secondarily to reduce blood cholesterol levels. Because of their ability to reduce triglyceride levels, fibric acid derivatives are useful in treating patients with types II, III, IV, and mild-type V hyperlipoproteinemia.

Adverse Reactions to Fibric Acid Derivatives

Side Effects
- Dyspepsia
- Flatulence
- Fatigue
- Constipation

Adverse Effects
- Arrhythmias
- Diarrhea
- Impotence
- Acute renal failure
- Gallstones
- Altered liver function
- Anemia
- Arthralgia

MASSAGE IMPLICATIONS AND ASSESSMENT

As with bile-sequestering drugs, the fibric acid drugs do not affect the efficacy of the various massage strokes.

Side Effects

Because fibric acid drugs can also lead to constipation, abdominal massage is indicated (see Sidebar: *Adverse Reactions to Fibric Acid Derivatives*).

Cholesterol Synthesis Inhibitors

Common Drug Names

atorvastatin: Lipitor

ezetimibe: Zetia

fluvastatin: Lescol

lovastatin: Altocor, Apo-Lovastatin, Mevacor

pravastatin: Lin-Pravastatin, Pravachol

simvastatin: Lipex, Zocor

As their name implies, cholesterol synthesis inhibitors (also known as the "statins") lower lipid levels by interfering with cholesterol synthesis. These drugs include lovastatin, pravastatin sodium, and simvastatin.

Pharmacokinetics

These drugs each have slightly different pharmacokinetic properties. After oral administration, lovastatin is absorbed incompletely, and much of the drug dose is lost because of the extensive first-pass metabolism in the liver. Food may increase the drug's systemic absorption. Pravastatin is absorbed rapidly but incompletely after being taken orally. Pravastatin also undergoes extensive first-pass metabolism in the liver. Simvastatin is absorbed incompletely and also undergoes extensive first-pass metabolism in the liver.

Pharmacodynamics

Cholesterol synthesis inhibitors reduce cholesterol levels by inhibiting enzyme activity. This interferes with an early step of cholesterol synthesis, thereby reducing the synthesis of LDL and enhancing LDL breakdown.

Pharmacotherapeutics

Cholesterol synthesis inhibitors are used to treat elevated total cholesterol and LDL levels in patients with primary hypercholesterolemia (types IIa and IIb). By lowering cholesterol levels, the cholesterol synthesis inhibitors reduce the risk of coronary artery disease.

MASSAGE IMPLICATIONS AND ASSESSMENT

The actions of these drugs do not affect the actions of any of the massage strokes.

Side Effects

GI disturbances, such as nausea and heartburn, are the most common side effects. The massage therapist should elevate a client's head if these are present (see Sidebar: *Adverse Reactions to Cholesterol Synthesis Inhibitors*).

Adverse Reactions to Cholesterol Synthesis Inhibitors

Side Effects
- Nausea
- Headache

Adverse Effects
- Liver toxicity
- Chest pain
- Renal failure
- Myalgia

Quick Quiz

1. Your long-term client, a 72-year-old woman with a history of coronary artery disease with angina, is taking Isordil. She tells you she gets very flushed and red-faced in the morning after taking her medicine. What does this mean?

2. Your client is taking Catapres, a sympatholytic antihypertensive, and HydroDIURIL, a thiazide diuretic. You give her a Swedish massage for relaxation and after the session, she states she is feeling nauseated and dizzy. You take her blood pressure and it is 90/60 mm Hg. Her blood pressure is usually 140/80 mm Hg. What could you have done to prevent this? What should you do now?

Hematologic Drugs

7

The hematologic system includes plasma (the liquid component of blood) and blood cells, such as red blood cells (RBCs), white blood cells (WBCs), and platelets. Types of drugs used to treat disorders of the hematologic system include hematinic drugs, anticoagulant drugs, and thrombolytic drugs.

Hematinic Drugs

Hematinic drugs provide essential building blocks for RBC production. They do so by increasing hemoglobin, the necessary element for oxygen transportation. This section discusses hematinic drugs used to treat microcytic and macrocytic anemia—iron, vitamin B_{12}, and folic acid. It also describes the use of epoetin alfa to treat normocytic anemia.

Iron

Common Drug Names

iron

ferrous fumarate: Femiron, Feostat, Fumerin, Neo-Fer, Palafer

ferrous gluconate: Fergon, Fertinic, Novoferogluc

ferrous sulfate: Slow-Fe, Ferralyn, Feosol, Fer-In-Sol, Fer-Iron

iron dextran: DexFerrum, Dexiron, INFeD

Iron preparations are used to treat the most common form of anemia, iron deficiency anemia.

Pharmacokinetics (how drugs circulate)

Iron is absorbed primarily from the duodenum and upper jejunum of the intestine. The amount of iron absorbed depends partially on the body stores of iron. When body stores are low or RBC production is accelerated, iron absorption may increase by 20% to 30%. Conversely, when total iron stores are large, only approximately 5% to 10% of iron is absorbed. Enteric-coated preparations decrease iron absorption because in that form iron is not released until after it leaves the duodenum. The lymphatic system absorbs the parenteral form after intramuscular (IM) injections.

Iron is transported by the blood and bound to transferrin, its carrier plasma protein. Approximately one-third of the iron is stored primarily as hemosiderin or ferritin in the reticuloendothelial cells of the liver, spleen, and bone marrow. Approximately two-thirds of the total body iron is contained in hemoglobin. Iron is excreted in urine, stool, sweat, and through intestinal cell sloughing and is secreted in breast milk.

Pharmacodynamics (how drugs act)

Although iron has other roles, its most important role is the production of hemoglobin. Approximately 80% of iron in the plasma goes to the bone marrow, where it is used for erythropoiesis (production of RBCs).

Pharmacotherapeutics (how drugs are used)

Oral iron therapy is used to prevent or treat iron deficiency anemia. It is also used to prevent anemias in children age 6 months to 2 years because this is a period of rapid growth and development. Pregnant women may need iron supplements to replace the iron used by the developing fetus. Treatment of iron deficiency anemia usually lasts for 6 months.

Parenteral iron therapy is used for patients who cannot absorb oral preparations, are not compliant with oral therapy, or have bowel disorders (such as ulcerative colitis). The only currently available parenteral form is iron dextran, which builds up iron stores more rapidly than the oral drugs but does not correct anemia any faster.

Adverse Reactions to Iron

Side Effects
- Bruising
- Constipation
- Black stools

Adverse Effects
- Gastric upset
- GI bleeding

MASSAGE IMPLICATIONS AND ASSESSMENT

The only concern for massage increasing the absorption of iron is with the parenteral IM injection. If this is the form used, massage is locally contraindicated for the area of the injection for up to 3 days. Even after this time, intramuscular iron may remain in the tissues and continue to be absorbed over the next 3 weeks. The area must be avoided completely for 3 days and massage limited during intramuscular iron therapy. In addition, intramuscular iron is very painful, often causing bruising and discoloration of the skin. This is another reason for local contraindication for the first days after injection. Because the action of the drug is that of replacement of a needed nutritional agent, no effect on the efficacy of massage strokes is present.

Side Effects

The side effect of iron therapy that is of concern for a massage therapist is constipation. The therapist should encourage increased fluid intake and perform abdominal work to encourage the movement of stool (see Sidebar: *Adverse Reactions to Iron*).

Vitamin B$_{12}$

Common Drug Names

cyanocobalamin: Anacobin, Bedoz, Crystamine, Crysti 1000, Cyomin (discontinued in the U.S.), LA-12

hydroxocobalamin: Hydro Cobex (discontinued in the U.S.)

Vitamin B$_{12}$ preparations are used to treat pernicious anemia.

Pharmacokinetics

Vitamin B$_{12}$ is available in both oral and injectable forms. A substance called intrinsic factor, secreted by the gastric mucosa, is needed for vitamin B$_{12}$ absorption. People who have a deficiency of intrinsic factor develop a special type of anemia known as vitamin B$_{12}$-deficiency pernicious anemia. Because people with this disorder cannot absorb vitamin B$_{12}$, an injectable form of the drug is used.

When cyanocobalamin is injected by the intramuscular or subcutaneous route, it is absorbed and binds to transcobalamin II for transport to the tissues. It is then transported in the bloodstream to the liver, where 90% of the body's supply of vitamin B$_{12}$ is stored.

Although hydroxocobalamin is absorbed more slowly from the injection site, its uptake in the liver may be greater than that of cyanocobalamin. With either drug, the liver slowly releases vitamin B$_{12}$ as needed by the body. It is secreted in breast milk. About 3 to 8 µg of vitamin B$_{12}$ is excreted in bile each day and then reabsorbed in the ileum.

Pharmacodynamics

When vitamin B$_{12}$ is administered, it replaces the vitamin B$_{12}$ that the body normally would absorb from the diet. This vitamin is essential for cell growth and replication as well as for the maintenance of myelin (nerve coverings) throughout the nervous system. Vitamin B$_{12}$ also may be involved in lipid and carbohydrate metabolism.

Pharmacotherapeutics

Cyanocobalamin and hydroxocobalamin are used to treat pernicious anemia, a megaloblastic anemia characterized by decreased gastric production of hydrochloric acid and the deficiency of intrinsic factor. Intrinsic factor is a substance normally secreted by the parietal cells of the gastric mucosa that is essential for vitamin B$_{12}$ absorption.

MASSAGE IMPLICATIONS AND ASSESSMENT

The only implication for massage therapy is that of avoiding the injection site for approximately 1 hour after an injection. In most cases of pernicious anemia, the drug is given as an IM injection once a month. It is a replacement drug, and its action has no effect on the use of massage strokes or their efficacy.

Adverse Reactions to Vitamin B₁₂

No dose-related adverse reactions occur with vitamin B_{12} therapy. However, some rare reactions may occur when vitamin B_{12} is administered parenterally.

Parenteral Problems
Adverse reactions to parenteral administration include hypersensitivity reactions that could result in anaphylaxis and death, pulmonary edema, heart failure, peripheral vascular thrombosis, polycythemia vera, hypokalemia, and itching.

Side Effects
Other than occasional bruising at the injection site, vitamin B_{12} does not have any side effects that concern massage therapists. Rare adverse reactions are emergency situations (see Sidebar: *Adverse Reactions to Vitamin B_{12}*).

Folic Acid

Common Drug Names

folic acid: Apo-Folic, folate, Folvite, Novo-Folacid
leucovorin calcium: citrovorum factor, folinic acid, Wellcovorin

Folic acid is given to treat folic acid deficiency. It is typically known simply as folic acid, although a preparation called leucovorin calcium is also used.

Pharmacokinetics

Folic acid is absorbed rapidly in the first third of the small intestine and distributed into all body tissues. Folic acid is metabolized in the liver. Excess folate is excreted unchanged in the urine, and small amounts of folic acid are excreted in stool. Folates are excreted in urine and stool and secreted in breast milk.

Pharmacodynamics

Folic acid is an essential component for normal RBC production and growth. A deficiency in folic acid results in pernicious anemia as well as low serum and RBC folate levels.

Pharmacotherapeutics

Folic acid is used to treat folic acid deficiency. Patients who are pregnant or who are undergoing treatment of liver disease, hemolytic anemia, alcohol abuse, skin disease, or renal failure typically need preventive folic acid therapy.

Adverse Reactions to Folic Acid

There are no side effects of folic acid.

Adverse Reactions
- Erythema
- Itching
- Rash

MASSAGE IMPLICATIONS AND ASSESSMENT
Folic acid is given orally; therefore, absorption is not a consideration in massage therapy. The drug therapy itself does not affect the applications of massage strokes because folic acid is also a replacement therapy.

Side Effects
There are no common side effects of folic acid therapy that are of concern to the massage therapist. Adverse effects must be reported to a physician. If severe, massage is contraindicated. (see Sidebar: *Adverse Reactions to Folic Acid*).

Special Note: Although drug therapy with hematinic drugs itself does not require a change in massage techniques, the condition of the client must be considered. In severe anemia, clients may have massage cautions and contraindications owing to their conditions.

Red and White Blood Cell-Stimulating Drugs

Common Drug Names: Red Blood Cell Stimulators

darbepoetin alfa: Aranesp
epoetin alfa: Epogen, Eprex, Procrit

Common Drug Names: White Blood Cell Stimulators

filgrastim: Neupogen
pegfilgrastim: Neulasta
sargramostim: Leukine, Prokine

This section discusses drugs that stimulate RBC production and those that stimulate WBC production.

Pharmacokinetics

Epoetin alfa may be given subcutaneously or intravenously. After subcutaneous administration, peak serum levels occur within 5 to 24 hours. Distribution, metabolism, and excretion are still unknown. Darbepoetin is also given by injection. It is a long-acting version given every 2 weeks instead of every week as with epoetin. Drugs that stimulate WBC production are also injectables with unknown distribution, metabolism, and excretion.

Pharmacodynamics

Epoetin alfa and darbepoetin boost the production of erythropoietin, thus stimulating RBC production in bone marrow. Normally, erythropoietin is formed in the kidneys in response to hypoxia (reduced oxygen) and anemia. Patients with conditions that decrease production of erythropoietin develop chronic normocytic anemia, necessitating administration of these drugs.

Drugs that stimulate WBC production are synthetic versions (recombinant DNA) of naturally occurring chemical proteins in the body called cytokines. They stimulate the bone marrow to increase production of WBCs.

Pharmacotherapeutics

Epoetin alfa and darbepoetin are used to treat patients with normocytic anemia (characterized by a decrease in hemoglobin content, packed RBC volume, and the number of RBCs per cubic millimeter of blood) caused by chronic renal failure. These agents are also used to treat anemia associated with zidovudine therapy in patients with human immunodeficiency virus infection. Finally, these drugs decrease the need for transfusions in patients with certain types of leukemia.

Special Note: These drugs have been used illegally as performance-enhancing drugs by athletes.

White blood cell-stimulating drugs are used to increase WBCs in patients with bone marrow suppression from chemotherapy and bone marrow transplant.

MASSAGE IMPLICATIONS AND ASSESSMENT

Because these drugs are given by injection, massage is contraindicated in the local area where the injection was given. The drug's absorption may last as long as 24 hours, so massage in the area is withheld for at least that amount of time. The action of the drug is directly on the kidneys or the bone marrow and does not affect the application of massage strokes. Physician approval must be obtained before performing massage and the absorption times at the injection sites (local contraindication time) verified.

Side Effects

The side effects of blood cell stimulators that may be of concern to a massage practitioner are fatigue, weakness, dizziness, and muscle pain Shorter sessions may be indicated if the client is fatigued. Also, care must be taken in getting the client off the table to ensure safety. Other adverse effects must be reported to a physician and contraindicate massage (see Sidebar: *Adverse Reactions to Epoetin Alfa*). Clients receiving this drug are often very ill and/or are receiving chemotherapy. The implications for modifying massage techniques come from the client's condition or illness rather than from the drug therapy.

Anticoagulant Drugs

Anticoagulant drugs are used to reduce the ability of the blood to clot. Major categories of anticoagulants include heparin, oral anticoagulants, and antiplatelet drugs.

Heparin

Common Drug Names

heparin sodium: Hepalean, Heparin Leo, Liquaemin Sodium, Uniparin,
dalteparin sodium: Fragmin
enoxaparin sodium: Lovenox

Heparin, prepared commercially from animal tissue, is used to prevent clot formation. Because it does not affect the synthesis of clotting factors, heparin cannot dissolve already formed clots.

Low molecular-weight heparins, such as dalteparin sodium and enoxaparin sodium, have been developed to prevent deep vein thrombosis (a blood clot in the deep veins, usually of the legs) in surgical patients.

Pharmacokinetics

Because heparin is not absorbed well from the gastrointestinal (GI) tract, it must be administered parenterally. Distribution is immediate after intravenous administration, but it is not as predictable with subcutaneous injection. Heparin is not given intramuscularly because of the risk of local bleeding. Heparin is metabolized in the liver, and its metabolites are excreted in urine.

Pharmacodynamics

Heparin prevents the formation of new thrombi in the following way. Heparin inhibits the formation of thrombin and fibrin by activating antithrombin III. Antithrombin III then inactivates factors IXa, Xa, XIa, and XIIa in the intrinsic and common pathways. The end result is prevention of a stable fibrin clot. In low doses, heparin increases the activity of antithrombin III against factor Xa and thrombin and inhibits clot formation. Much larger doses are necessary to inhibit fibrin formation after a clot has been formed. This relationship between dose and effect is the rationale for using low-dose heparin to prevent clotting.

Pharmacotherapeutics

Heparin may be used in a number of clinical situations to prevent the formation of new clots or the extension of existing clots. These situations include:

- Preventing or treating venous thromboemboli, characterized by inappropriate or excessive intravascular activation of blood clotting
- Treating disseminated intravascular coagulation, a complication of other diseases, resulting in accelerated clotting
- Treating arterial clotting and preventing embolus formation in patients with atrial fibrillation, an arrhythmia in which ineffective atrial contractions cause blood to pool in the atria, increasing the risk of clot formation
- Preventing thrombus formation and promoting cardiac circulation in an acute myocardial infarction (MI) by preventing further clot formation at the site of the already formed clot

Heparin can be used to prevent clotting whenever the patient's blood must circulate outside the body through a machine, such as the cardiopulmonary bypass machine or hemodialysis machine. Heparin is also useful for preventing clotting during orthopedic surgery. (This type of surgery, in many cases, activates the coagulation mechanisms excessively.) In fact, heparin is the drug of choice for orthopedic surgery.

MASSAGE IMPLICATIONS AND ASSESSMENT

Heparin is only given parenterally. The local site of injection of subcutaneous heparin should not be massaged for 4 to 5 hours after administration. This prevents increasing the absorption rate. The action of heparin in slowing clot formation itself does not change how the body will react to the massage strokes. However, because heparin is used in conditions for which there is a very high risk of clotting or there is already a clot present, massage is totally contraindicated except for simple touch holds and energetic modalities in which no manipulation of soft tissue occurs. In cases in which heparin is used in small doses to keep venous access devices (such as those used for dialysis or chemotherapy) open, some massage may be given with physician consent. Deep tissue work is contraindicated because of the risk of bruising, and systemic strokes that move fluids and blood are limited. The client's condition may require further modifications in massage application.

Side Effects
The most common side effect of heparin therapy is easy bruising. As stated above, deep tissue work is therefore contraindicated (see Sidebar: *Adverse Reactions to Heparin*).

Oral Anticoagulants

Common Drug Names
dicumarol: bishydroxycoumarin
warfarin sodium: Coumadin, Warfilone Sodium

The major oral anticoagulants used in the United States are the coumarin compounds warfarin sodium and dicumarol.

Pharmacokinetics
Warfarin is absorbed rapidly and almost completely when it is taken orally. Dicumarol is absorbed more slowly and erratically. Warfarin and dicumarol are both metabolized in the liver and excreted in urine.

Pharmacodynamics
Oral anticoagulants alter the ability of the liver to synthesize vitamin K-dependent clotting factors, including prothrombin and factors VII, IX, and X. However, clotting factors already in the bloodstream continue to coagulate blood until they become depleted; thus, anticoagulation does not begin immediately.

Pharmacotherapeutics
Oral anticoagulants are prescribed to treat thromboembolism and, in this situation, are started while the patient is still receiving heparin. Warfarin, however, may be started without heparin in outpatients at high risk for thromboembolism.

Oral anticoagulants also are the drugs of choice to prevent deep vein thrombosis and for patients with prosthetic heart valves or diseased mitral valves. They sometimes are combined with an antiplatelet drug, such as dipyridamole, to decrease the risk of arterial clotting.

MASSAGE IMPLICATIONS AND ASSESSMENT

Oral anticoagulants do not pose any problem of increased absorption rates with massage. The action of the drugs is to prevent synthesis of certain clotting factors, thus decreasing clot formation rate and speed. This action does not affect the efficacy of any of the massage strokes. The conditions for the use of these drugs are of concern, however. Massage must not be done if blood clots are present. If the drugs are being used in the long term for preventive therapy, massage may be given if the physician believes that the client's condition is stable and gives approval. No deep tissue work and minimizing strokes that affect the circulation of blood and fluid systemically (effleurage and tapotement, especially) are appropriate.

Side Effects

The side effects of the drugs for anticoagulation do concern the massage practitioner. Most common is the side effect of easy bruising. This means contraindication for deep tissue massage. Other adverse effects must be reported to a physician and are a contraindication for massage (see Sidebar: *Adverse Reactions to Oral Anticoagulants*).

Adverse Reactions to Oral Anticoagulants

Side Effects
• Bruising

Adverse Effects
• Bleeding

Antiplatelet Drugs

Common Drug Names

aspirin: acetylsalicylic acid, Ancasal, ASA, Ecotrin, Empirin

cilostazol: Pletal

clopidogrel: Plavix

dipyridamole: Apo-Dipyridamole, Novo-Dipiradol, Persantin, Persantine

pentoxifylline: Trental

sulfinpyrazone: Anturan, Anturane

ticlopidine: Alti-Ticlopidine, Ticlid

Antiplatelet drugs are used to prevent arterial thromboembolism, particularly in patients at risk for MI, stroke, arteriosclerosis (hardening of the arteries), and atherosclerosis.

Pharmacokinetics

All antiplatelet drugs are taken orally, absorbed very quickly, and reach peak concentration between 1 and 2 hours after administration. Aspirin maintains its antiplatelet effect for approximately 10 days, or as long as platelets normally survive. Sulfinpyrazone may require several days of administration.

Pharmacodynamics

Antiplatelet drugs interfere with platelet activity in different drug-specific and dose-related ways. Low dosages of aspirin (50 to 325 mg/day) appear to inhibit clot formation by blocking the synthesis of prostaglandin, which in turn prevents formation of the platelet-aggregating substance thromboxane A_2. Dipyridamole may inhibit platelet aggregation.

Sulfinpyrazone appears to inhibit several platelet functions. At dosages of 400 to 800 mg/day, it lengthens platelet survival; dosages of more than 600 mg/day prolong the patency of arteriovenous shunts used for hemodialysis. A single dose rapidly inhibits platelet aggregation.

Ticlopidine and clopidogrel inhibit the binding of fibrinogen to platelets during the first stage of the clotting cascade. Dipyridamole decreases fibrinogen concentrations, and cilostazol decreases platelet aggregation.

Pharmacotherapeutics

Antiplatelet drugs have many different uses. Aspirin is used in patients with a previous MI or in unstable angina to reduce the risk of death and in men to reduce the risk of transient ischemic attacks (TIAs) (temporary reduction in circulation to the brain). After an MI, sulfinpyrazone may be used to decrease the risk of sudden cardiac death. In patients with mitral stenosis (a narrowed mitral valve) caused by rheumatic fever, it may decrease the risk of systemic embolism.

Dipyridamole is used with a coumarin compound to prevent thrombus formation after cardiac valve replacement. Dipyridamole with aspirin has been used to prevent thromboembolic disorders in patients with aortocoronary bypass grafts (bypass surgery) or prosthetic (artificial) heart valves. Ticlopidine is used to reduce the risk of thrombotic stroke in high-risk patients (including those with a history of frequent TIAs) and in patients who have already had a thrombotic stroke.

Other uses include treatment of ischemic strokes, angina, intermittent claudication, and peripheral vascular disease.

Adverse Reactions to Antiplatelet Drugs

Side Effects
- Stomach upset
- Heartburn
- Nausea
- Constipation
- Flushing
- Dizziness
- Weakness
- Headache

Adverse Effects
- Blood in stool
- GI bleeding
- Rash
- Liver impairment
- Neutropenia
- Anaphylactic shock

MASSAGE IMPLICATIONS AND ASSESSMENT

There are no concerns about the route of administration for antiplatelet drugs. The action of the drugs is on the blood clotting factors and does not change the effect of any of the massage strokes. The condition of the client may require modification of massage; a physician must be consulted.

Side Effects

The massage therapist is concerned with the side effects of heartburn, constipation, and possible easy bruising. Although these drugs are not as strong as anticoagulants, care should be taken with deep tissue work to avoid bruising the client. If heartburn is a problem, the client may not be able to lie flat or on the stomach for long periods. Constipation is an indication for abdominal massage (see Sidebar: *Adverse Reactions to Antiplatelet Drugs*).

Thrombolytic Drugs

Common Drug Names

alteplase: Actilyse, Activase

anistreplase: Eminase

streptokinase: Kabikinase, Streptase

Thrombolytic drugs are used to dissolve a preexisting clot or thrombus, often in an acute or emergency situation.

Pharmacokinetics

After intravenous or intracoronary administration, thrombolytic drugs are distributed immediately throughout the circulation, quickly activating plasminogen (a precursor to plasmin, which dissolves fibrin clots). Alteplase is cleared rapidly from circulating plasma, primarily by the liver. Anistreplase is metabolized in the plasma. Streptokinase is removed rapidly from the circulation by antibodies and the reticuloendothelial system (a body system involved in defending against infection and disposing products of cell breakdown). It does not appear to cross the placenta.

Pharmacodynamics

Thrombolytic drugs convert plasminogen to plasmin, which lyses (dissolves) thrombi, fibrinogen, and other plasma proteins.

Pharmacotherapeutics

Thrombolytic drugs have a number of uses. They are used to treat certain thromboembolic disorders and are also used to dissolve thrombi in arteriovenous cannulas (used in dialysis) and intravenous catheters to reestablish blood flow. Thrombolytic drugs are the drugs of choice to break down newly formed thrombi. They seem most effective when administered immediately after thrombosis, although they can be used for up to 6 hours after the onset of symptoms.

In addition, each drug has specific uses. Alteplase is used to treat acute MI, pulmonary embolism, and acute ischemic stroke. Anistreplase is also used in acute MI. Streptokinase is used to treat acute MI, pulmonary embolus, deep vein thrombosis, arterial thrombosis, and arterial embolism as well as to clear an occluded arteriovenous cannula.

MASSAGE IMPLICATIONS AND ASSESSMENT

Because these drugs are only used in emergency situations and in the presence of blood clots, massage is totally contraindicated.

Quick Quiz

1. A client comes in for a massage. He is taking Warfarin. When you ask why, he tells you that he recently had a deep vein thrombosis. What should you do?

2. Your client tells you that she has been taking Ticlid for about 5 years to help her circulation. What implications does this have for massage?

Respiratory Drugs

8

The respiratory system, extending from the nose to the pulmonary capillaries, performs the essential function of gas exchange between the body and its environment. In other words, it takes in oxygen and expels carbon dioxide. Drugs used to improve respiratory function include methylxanthines, expectorants, antitussives, mucolytics, and decongestants.

Methylxanthines

Methylxanthines, also called xanthines, are used to treat breathing disorders.

Types of Methylxanthines

Common Drug Names

aminophylline: Phyllocontin

anhydrous theophylline: Accurbron, Aquaphyllin (discontinued in the U.S.), Asmalix, Bronkodyl, Elixophyllin, Slo-bid (discontinued in the U.S.) , Slo-Phyllin, Theo-Dur, Theobid (discontinued in the U.S.)

oxtriphylline: Choledyl SA

theophylline sodium glycinate

Methylxanthines include anhydrous theophylline and its derivative salts aminophylline, oxtriphylline, and theophylline sodium glycinate.

Pharmacokinetics (how drugs circulate)

The pharmacokinetics of methylxanthines vary according to which drug the patient is receiving, the dosage form, and the route of administration.

When theophylline is given as an oral solution or a rapid-release tablet, it is absorbed rapidly and completely. Absorption of some of theophylline's slow-release forms depends on gastric pH. Food can alter absorption. Theophylline is metabolized primarily in the liver. In adults and children, approximately 10% of a dose is excreted unchanged in the urine. Because infants have immature livers with reduced metabolic functioning, as much as half a dose may be excreted unchanged in their urine.

Pharmacodynamics (how drugs act)

Methylxanthines act in a number of ways. Methylxanthines decrease airway reactivity and relieve bronchospasm by relaxing bronchial smooth muscle. Their specific mechanism of action in reversible obstructive airway diseases, such as asthma, is not completely understood.

In nonreversible obstructive airway diseases (chronic bronchitis, emphysema, and apnea), methylxanthines appear to increase the sensitivity of the brain's respiratory center to carbon dioxide and to stimulate the respiratory drive. In chronic bronchitis and emphysema, these drugs decrease fatigue of the diaphragm, the respiratory muscle that separates the abdomen from the thoracic cavity. They also improve ventricular function and, therefore, the heart's pumping action.

Pharmacotherapeutics (how drugs are used)

Theophylline and its salts are used to treat asthma (as second- or third-line drugs), chronic bronchitis, and emphysema. Whereas investigation by the Food and Drug Administration is still ongoing, theophylline has been used in clinical trials to treat neonatal apnea (periods of not breathing in the newborn).

Adverse Reactions to Methylxanthines

Side Effects
- Irritability
- Restlessness
- Anxiety
- Insomnia
- Dizziness

Adverse Effects
- Nausea
- Vomiting
- Abdominal cramping
- Anorexia
- Diarrhea
- Tachycardia
- Palpitations
- Arrhythmias

Smoking increases the elimination of theophylline, which reduces its effectiveness.

MASSAGE IMPLICATIONS AND ASSESSMENT

Methylxanthines are given by several different routes of administration. Most often, they are given as oral medications. They may also be given as intravenous medications or as suppositories per rectum. None of these routes are of concern to the massage therapist because no increase in absorption rates with massage occurs. The drugs act specifically in the lungs on smooth muscle and in the brain's respiratory control centers. The effects of massage strokes are not changed by these mechanisms of action.

Side Effects

Common side effects of these drugs are dizziness, restlessness, and anxiety. These may decrease the response to massage strokes aimed at relaxation. The systemic reflex strokes, such as effleurage and rocking, may take longer to work. To meet a goal of relaxation for the client, slow and rhythmic effleurage and rocking to start may lead to a more effective massage. More stimulating strokes, such as tapotement or friction, may exacerbate the drug's side effects (see Sidebar: *Adverse Reactions to Methylxanthines*).

Other Asthma Drugs

Common Drug Names

albuterol: Apo-Salvent, Proventil, Ventolin

cromolyn sodium: Crolom, Gastrocrom, Intal, Nasalcrom, Rynacrom

ipratropium bromide: Apo-Ipravent, Atrovent (with albuterol: Combivent)

isoproterenol: Isuprel, Medihaler-Iso, Norisodrine

pirbuterol: Maxair

Other asthma drugs that relieve bronchospasm are the short acting beta-adrenergic agonists and anticholinergics discussed in Chapter 3. The most common are ipratropium bromide, albuterol, and isoproterenol. Other drugs commonly used are pirbuterol and cromolyn sodium.

Pharmacokinetics

The other asthma drugs are given either orally, or in many cases, as inhaled medications. Their absorption and distribution rates vary depending on the drugs.

Pharmacodynamics

Ipratropium bromide, albuterol, and isoproteranal relax bronchial smooth muscles by stimulating the sympathetic nervous system. They are used either alone or in combination with other asthma drugs or steroid therapy.

Pirbuterol acts also on the $beta_2$-adrenergic receptors to stimulate the nervous system and cause the bronchial smooth muscle to relax. It can prevent bronchospasm when used regularly and is given as an inhaled medication.

Cromolyn sodium stops the release of histamine by stabilizing the mast cell membrane. This slows the allergic reaction time and thus reduces bronchospasm. It is used to prevent bronchospasm in asthmatics but is not used in acute asthma attacks. It, too, is given as an inhaled medication.

Pharmacotherapeutics

These drugs are also used in the treatment of asthma, chronic bronchitis, and emphysema. Other uses include symptomatic relief of shortness of breath in patients with lung cancer.

MASSAGE IMPLICATIONS AND ASSESSMENT

The route of administration of these drugs is not of concern to the massage therapist. The beta-adrenergic agonists' action is to stimulate the sympathetic nervous system. Although they are very specific in their actions on the bronchial smooth

Adverse Reactions to Other Asthma Drugs

Side Effects
- Nervousness
- Tremors
- Dry mouth
- Cough
- Dizziness

Adverse Effects
- Palpitations
- Chest pain
- Tachycardia
- Diarrhea
- Wheezing
- Difficulty urinating
- Urinary retention
- Joint pain and swelling
- Rash

muscle and are not fully absorbed systemically as inhalants, there can be systemic effects. The effectiveness of systemic reflex strokes may be reduced by these drugs. Using slow, rhythmic effleurage and rocking to start a massage and for longer periods during the massage helps to counter this effect. Cromolyn sodium's action on mast cell membranes has no implications for changing the efficacy of massage strokes.

Side Effects

Common side effects of these other asthma drugs include nervousness, tremors, and dizziness. The above changes in the application of massage strokes assist in easing these side effects. Care should be taken when getting the client off the table to ensure that there is no dizziness and that he or she is safe (see Sidebar: *Adverse Reactions to Other Asthma Drugs*).

Expectorants

Expectorants thin mucus so it is cleared more easily out of airways. They also soothe mucous membranes in the respiratory tract.

Guaifenesin

Common Drug Names

guaifenesin: Anti-Tuss, Balminil, Breonesin (discontinued in the U.S.), Guiatuss, Humibid LA, Robitussin

The most commonly used expectorant is guaifenesin.

Pharmacokinetics

Guaifenesin is absorbed through the gastrointestinal (GI) tract, metabolized by the liver, and excreted primarily by the kidneys.

Pharmacodynamics

By increasing production of respiratory tract fluids, expectorants reduce the thickness, adhesiveness, and surface tension of mucus, making it easier to clear from the airways. Expectorants also provide a soothing effect on mucous membranes of the respiratory tract.

Pharmacotherapeutics

Guaifenesin is used for the relief of coughs from colds, minor bronchial irritation, bronchitis, influenza, sinusitis, bronchial asthma, emphysema, and other respiratory disorders. Guaifenesin may also be used to relieve a dry, hacking cough and is safe if taken as directed. It may be used alone or with antitussives, analgesics, or antihistamines.

MASSAGE IMPLICATIONS AND ASSESSMENT

Oral administration of guaifenesin is not a concern for absorption rate increases. The action of the drug is directly on the respiratory tract and does not change the efficacy of any of the massage strokes.

Side Effects

Guaifenesin may have a side effect of drowsiness. This means the usual relaxation of a massage may be increased. Using stimulating strokes at the end of the session counters this effect easily (see Sidebar: *Adverse Reactions to Guaifenesin*).

Adverse Reactions to Guaifenesin

Side Effects
- Drowsiness

Adverse Effects
- Nausea
- Vomiting
- Diarrhea
- Abdominal pain

Antitussives

Antitussive drugs suppress or inhibit coughing.

Types of Antitussives

Common Drug Names

benzonatate: Tessalon

codeine: methylmorphine, Paveral

dextromethorphan hydrobromide: Balminil DM, Benylin, Koffex, Pertussin

hydrocodone

Antitussives are typically used to treat dry, nonproductive coughs.

Pharmacokinetics

Antitussives are absorbed well through the GI tract, metabolized in the liver, and excreted in the urine.

Pharmacodynamics

Antitussives act in slightly different ways. Benzonatate acts by anesthetizing stretch receptors throughout the bronchi, alveoli, and pleura. Codeine, dextromethorphan, and hydrocodone suppress the cough reflex by direct action on the cough center in the medulla of the brain.

Pharmacotherapeutics

The uses of these drugs are slightly variable, but each treats a serious, nonproductive cough that interferes with a patient's ability to rest or carry out activities of daily living. Benzonatate relieves cough caused by pneumonia, bronchitis, the common cold, and chronic pulmonary diseases such as emphysema. It also can be used during bronchial diagnostic tests (such as bronchoscopy) when the patient must avoid coughing. Dextromethorphan is the most widely used cough suppressant in the United States and may provide better antitussive activity than codeine. Its popularity may stem from the fact that it produces few adverse reactions.

The narcotic antitussives (typically codeine and hydrocodone) are for treating intractable cough, usually associated with lung cancer. However, they are also used on occasion for coughs associated with colds or flu with acute bronchitis.

Adverse Reactions to Antitussives

Side Effects
- Dizziness
- Sedation
- Headache
- Nasal congestion
- Constipation
- Hypotension

Adverse Effects
- Rash
- Chills
- Chest numbness
- Arrhythmias
- Stupor
- Seizures
- Respiratory arrest

MASSAGE IMPLICATIONS AND ASSESSMENT

The route of administration is not of concern here, because antitussives are given orally. The action of these drugs is on the lung receptors or the cough center in the medulla. These actions do not change the effects of the massage strokes.

Side Effects

Dizziness, sedation, and constipation are the side effects that are of concern to the massage practitioner. The relaxing effect of the massage systemically will be increased by the drug side effects even if the client is not feeling them at the time of the massage. Once again, stimulating strokes (such as rapid effleurage and tapotement) should be used at the end of the session to help the client reorient and awaken. Care should be taken when the client is changing position and getting off the table. Constipation can be helped by abdominal massage (see Sidebar: *Adverse Reactions to Antitussives*).

Mucolytics

Mucolytics act directly on mucus, breaking down sticky, thick secretions so they are more easily eliminated.

Acetylcysteine

Common Drug Names

acetylcysteine: Airbron, Mucomyst, Mucosil, Parvolex

Acetylcysteine is the only thiol compound mucolytic used clinically in the United States for patients with abnormal or thick mucus.

Pharmacokinetics

Inhaled acetylcysteine is absorbed from the pulmonary epithelium. When taken orally, the drug is absorbed from the GI tract. Acetylcysteine is metabolized in the liver, and its excretion is unknown.

Pharmacodynamics

Acetylcysteine decreases the thickness of respiratory tract secretions by altering the molecular composition of mucus.

Pharmacotherapeutics

Mucolytics are used with other therapies to treat patients with abnormal or thick mucous secretions and may benefit patients with bronchitis, emphysema, pulmonary complications related to cystic fibrosis, and atelectasis caused by mucous obstruction as may occur in pneumonia, bronchiectasis, or chronic bronchitis. Mucolytics may also be used to prepare patients for bronchography and other bronchial studies.

Acetylcysteine is the antidote for acetaminophen overdose. However, it does not fully protect against liver damage caused by acetaminophen toxicity.

MASSAGE IMPLICATIONS AND ASSESSMENT

Mucolytics are either inhaled or taken orally. Increased absorption rates from massage are not a concern. The action is directly on the respiratory system and does not affect massage strokes.

Side Effects

Side effects of mucolytics include drowsiness and runny nose. Massage can be ended with some stimulating strokes to counter the increased sedation that can occur. Keeping tissues handy for the client is also helpful (see Sidebar: *Adverse Reactions to Acetylcysteine*).

Adverse Reactions to Acetylcysteine

Acetylcysteine has a "rotten egg" odor during administration that may cause nausea.

Side Effects
- Drowsiness
- Runny nose
- Nausea

Adverse Effects
- Bronchospasm
- Stomatitis
- Vomiting

Decongestants

Decongestants are classified as systemic or topical, depending on how they are administered.

Types of Decongestants

Common Drug Names

ephedrine: Kondon's Nasal (discontinued in the U.S.), Pretz-D

epinephrine: Bronchial Mist, Epifrin, Epinal, Primatene, Vaponefrin

naphazoline: AK-Con, Albalon, Allersol, Naphcon, Privine, VasoClear, Vasocon

oxymetazoline: Afrin, Dristan, Duramist, Visine

phenylephrine: Dionephrine, Neo-Synephrine, Prefrin, Rhinall

pseudoephedrine: Cenafed, Drixoral, Efidac, Maxenal, Myfedrine, Pseudofrin, Pseudo-
  gest, Robidrine, Sudafed

tetrahydrozoline: Collyrium Fresh, Eyesine, Murine, Tetrasine, Tyzine

xylometazoline: Decongest

As sympathomimetic drugs, systemic decongestants stimulate the sympathetic nervous system to reduce swelling of the respiratory tract's vascular network. Systemic decongestants include ephedrine, phenylephrine, and pseudoephedrine

Topical decongestants are also powerful vasoconstrictors. When applied directly to
swollen mucous membranes of the nose, they provide immediate relief from nasal congestion and include ephedrine, epinephrine, and phenylephrine (sympathomimetic
amines) as well as naphazoline, oxymetazoline, tetrahydrozoline, and xylometazoline (im-
idazoline derivatives of sympathomimetic amines).

Pharmacokinetics

The pharmacokinetic properties of decongestants vary. When taken orally, the systemic
decongestants are absorbed readily from the GI tract and widely distributed throughout
the body into various tissues and fluids, including the cerebrospinal fluid, placenta, and
breast milk. Systemic decongestants are slowly and incompletely metabolized by the liver
and excreted largely unchanged in the urine within 24 hours of oral administration. Topical decongestants act directly on the alpha-receptors of the vascular smooth muscle in the
nose, causing the arterioles to constrict. As a result of this direct vasoconstriction, absorption of the drug becomes negligible.

Pharmacodynamics

The properties of systemic and topical decongestants vary slightly. The systemic decongestants cause vasoconstriction by directly stimulating alpha-adrenergic receptors on the
blood vessels in the nasal mucosa. They also cause contraction of urinary and GI sphinc-
ters, dilation of the pupils of the eyes, and decreased secretion of insulin. These drugs may
also act indirectly, resulting in the release of norepinephrine from storage sites in the
body. This, in turn, results in peripheral vasoconstriction.

Like systemic decongestants, topical decongestants stimulate alpha-adrenergic receptors in the smooth muscle of the blood vessels in the nose, resulting in vasoconstriction. The combination of reduced blood flow to the nasal mucous membranes and decreased capillary permeability reduces swelling. This action improves respiration by
helping to drain sinuses, clear nasal passages, and open eustachian tubes.

Pharmacotherapeutics

Systemic and topical decongestants are used to relieve the symptoms of swollen nasal
membranes resulting from hay fever, allergic rhinitis, vasomotor rhinitis, acute coryza
(profuse discharge from the nose), sinusitis, and the common cold. Systemic decongestants are frequently given with other drugs, such as antihistamines, antimus-
carinics, antipyretic-analgesics, caffeine, and antitussives. Topical decongestants provide two major advantages over systemics: minimal adverse reactions and rapid
symptom relief.

MASSAGE IMPLICATIONS AND ASSESSMENT

Because these drugs are administered topically directly onto the mucous membrane or orally, no route of administration concerns exist for massage. The action of the oral systemic drugs is to stimulate the sympathetic nervous system and possibly to increase norepinephrine secretion. Both of these actions affect the systemic massage strokes. The ability of the strokes to bring the client to parasympathetic system relaxation is decreased. The increased use of slow and rhythmic effleurage and rocking, and a longer time of use of these strokes, may counteract these effects and help the client to relax. Topical decongestants cause vasoconstriction and are not systemically absorbed. Therefore, none of the above concerns exist.

Side Effects

Side effects occur most often with systemic oral decongestants. Nervousness, restlessness, and insomnia all occur as a result of the sympathetic stimulation and must be addressed by the massage therapist as described above (see Sidebar: *Adverse Reactions to Decongestants*).

Adverse Reactions to Decongestants

Side Effects
- Nervousness
- Restlessness
- Insomnia
- Dry mucosa

Adverse Effects
- Palpitations
- Urinary retention
- Hypertension
- Allergic reactions
- Topical decongestants

The most common adverse reaction associated with prolonged use (more than 5 days) of topical decongestants is rebound nasal congestion. Other reactions include:

- Burning and stinging of the nasal mucosa
- Sneezing
- Mucosal dryness or ulceration

Quick Quiz

1. Your client comes in for a massage and tells you he has had a bad cold and bronchitis. He is currently taking the decongestant Primatene and Guaifenesin with codeine for a cough. What are the massage implications?

2. Your massage client has asthma and is using Combivent Inhaler for acute attacks and Maxair twice a day for prevention. Will your client have a stimulated sympathetic systemic effect from these medications?

Gastrointestinal Drugs

Drugs and the GI System

The gastrointestinal (GI) tract is basically a hollow, muscular tube that begins at the mouth and ends at the anus. It encompasses the pharynx, esophagus, stomach, and the small and large intestines. Its primary functions are to digest and absorb foods and fluids and to excrete metabolic waste. Classes of drugs used to improve GI function include peptic ulcer drugs; adsorbent, antiflatulent, and digestive drugs; antidiarrheal and laxative drugs; and antiemetic and emetic drugs.

Peptic Ulcer Drugs

A peptic ulcer is a circumscribed lesion in the mucosal membrane, developing in the lower esophagus, stomach, or small intestine. There are three major causes of peptic ulcers: bacterial infection with *Helicobacter pylori* (*H. pylori*), use of nonsteroidal anti-inflammatory drugs (NSAIDs), and hypersecretory states such as Zollinger-Ellison syndrome (a condition in which excessive secretion of gastric acid causes peptic ulcers). Peptic ulcer drugs are used either to eradicate *H. pylori* or to restore the balance between acid and pepsin secretions and the GI mucosal defense. These drugs include systemic antibiotics, antacids, histamine-2 (H_2)-receptor antagonists, proton pump inhibitors, and other peptic ulcer drugs such as misoprostol and sucralfate.

Systemic Antibiotics

Common Drug Names

amoxicillin: Amoxicet, Amoxil, Apo-Amoxi, Gen-Amoxicillin, Moxilin, Novomoxin, Trimox, Wymox *clarithromycin:* Biaxin

metronidazole: Apo-Metronidazole, Flagyl, Noritate, Novo-Nidazol

tetracycline: Apo-Tetra, Brodspec, EmTet, Novo-Tetra, Sumycin, Wesmycin

H. pylori is a Gram-negative bacteria that is believed to be a major causative factor in the formation of peptic ulcers and gastritis (inflammation of the lining of the stomach). Eradication of the bacteria promotes ulcer healing and decreases their recurrence. Successful treatment involves the use of two or more antibiotics in combination with other drugs. Systemic antibiotics used to treat *H. pylori* include the drugs listed above.

Pharmacokinetics (how drugs circulate)

Systemic antibiotics are variably absorbed from the GI tract. Food, especially dairy products, decreases the absorption of tetracycline. All these antibiotics are distributed widely and are excreted primarily in the urine.

Pharmacodynamics (how drugs act)

Antibiotics act by destroying the *H. pylori* bacteria infection. They are usually combined with an H_2-receptor antagonist or a proton pump inhibitor (see below) to decrease stomach acid and to promote healing further.

Pharmacotherapeutics (how drugs are used)

Various combinations of antimicrobial drugs with either an H_2-receptor antagonist or a proton pump inhibitor have been clinically studied. Treatment plans that use at least two antimicrobial drugs and an antacid for 2 weeks are successful in curing up to 90% of patients with peptic ulcers.

Adverse Reactions to Antibiotics

Side Effects
- Nausea
- Diarrhea
- Altered taste

Adverse Effects
- Rash
- Anaphylactic shock

MASSAGE IMPLICATIONS AND ASSESSMENT

Massage will not affect the absorption of antibiotics given by mouth. The action of the drug is directly on the organism and does not affect how the body responds to massage. No change is needed in the application of massage strokes.

Side Effects

The main side effects of antibiotics are GI upset and diarrhea. This usually stops after a day or two of the medication and when the drug is taken with food. No change in application of massage strokes is needed (see Sidebar: *Adverse Reactions to Antibiotics*).

Antacids

Common Drug Names

aluminum hydroxide: AlternaGel, Alu-Cap, Amphojel, Basaljel (discontinued in the U.S.)

calcium carbonate: Alkamints, Amitone, Apo-Cal, Calci-Chew, Caltrate, Chooz, Florical, Mallamint, Rolaids Calcium Rich, Tums

magaldrate (aluminum-magnesium complex): Diovol, Gelusil, Maalox, Univol

magnesium hydroxide: magnesia magma, milk of magnesia

Pharmacokinetics

Antacids work locally in the stomach by neutralizing gastric acid. They do not need to be absorbed to treat peptic ulcers. Antacids are distributed throughout the GI tract and are eliminated primarily in the feces.

Pharmacodynamics

The acid-neutralizing action of antacids reduces the total amount of acid in the GI tract, allowing peptic ulcers time to heal. Because pepsin (an enzyme formed in the stomach that breaks down proteins) acts more effectively when the stomach is highly acidic, pepsin action is also reduced as acidity drops. Contrary to popular belief, antacids do not work by coating peptic ulcers or the lining of the GI tract.

Pharmacotherapeutics

Antacids, used alone or with other drugs, are primarily prescribed to relieve pain and to promote healing in peptic ulcer disease. Antacids also relieve symptoms of acid indigestion, heartburn, dyspepsia (burning or indigestion), or gastroesophageal reflux disease (GERD), a condition in which the contents of the stomach and duodenum flow back into the esophagus.

Antacids may also be used to prevent stress ulcers and GI bleeding in critically ill patients during times of severe physical stress. They may be used to control hyperphosphatemia (elevated blood phosphate levels) in kidney failure. Because calcium binds with phosphate in the GI tract, calcium carbonate antacids prevent phosphate absorption.

MASSAGE IMPLICATIONS AND ASSESSMENT

Massage does not affect the absorption of antacids. The action of the drug is directly on the acid in the stomach. These drugs do not affect how the body reacts to massage strokes.

Adverse Reactions to Antacids

All adverse reactions to antacids are dose-related.

Side Effects
- Diarrhea
- Constipation

Adverse Effects
- Electrolyte imbalances
- Kidney stones

Side Effects

Depending on the type of antacid and the frequency of use, constipation is a side effect of some of these drugs. The massage therapist can help to alleviate this problem by working on the abdomen to help stimulate movement along the intestinal tract and by encouraging increased fluid intake (see Sidebar: *Adverse Reactions to Antacids*).

H_2-Receptor Antagonists

Common Drug Names

cimetidine: Apo-Cimetidine, Nu-Cimet, Tagamet

famotidine: Alti-Famotidine, Apo-Famotidine, Novo-Famotidine, Pepcid, Rhoxal-famotidine, Ulcidine

nizatidine: Apo-Nizatidine, Axid, Novo-Nizatidine

ranitidine: Alti-Ranitidine, Apo-Ranitidine, Novo-Ranitidine, Nu-Ranit, Zanta, Zantac

H_2-receptor antagonists are commonly prescribed antiulcer drugs in the United States. They are also available in OTC forms in lower doses.

Pharmacokinetics

Cimetidine, nizatidine, and ranitidine are absorbed rapidly and completely from the GI tract. Famotidine is not completely absorbed. Food and antacids may reduce the absorption of H_2-receptor antagonists. H_2-receptor antagonists are distributed widely throughout the body, metabolized by the liver, and excreted primarily in the urine.

Pharmacodynamics

H_2-receptor antagonists block histamine from stimulating the acid-secreting parietal cells of the stomach. Acid secretion in the stomach depends on the binding of gastrin, acetylcholine, and histamine to receptors on the parietal cells. If the binding of any one of these substances is blocked, acid secretion is reduced. The H_2-receptor antagonists, by binding with H_2 receptors, block the action of histamine in the stomach and reduce acid secretion.

Pharmacotherapeutics

H_2-receptor antagonists are used therapeutically to promote healing of duodenal and gastric ulcers as well as provide long-term treatment of pathologic GI hypersecretory conditions such as Zollinger-Ellison syndrome. These agents are also used to reduce gastric acid production and to prevent stress ulcers in severely ill patients and in those with reflux esophagitis or upper GI bleeding

MASSAGE IMPLICATIONS AND ASSESSMENT

As with the previously mentioned GI drugs, H$_2$ receptor antagonists act directly on the stomach and do not affect how the body reacts to the various massage strokes.

Side Effects

One common side effect of using H$_2$-receptor antagonists is constipation. Again, the massage therapist can help the client to deal with this by performing abdominal massage aimed at stimulating the intestinal tract. Other side effects must be reported to a physician (see Sidebar: *Adverse Reactions to H$_2$-Receptor Antagonists*).

Adverse Reactions to H$_2$-Receptor Antagonists

Side Effects
- Headache
- Dizziness
- Nausea
- Constipation

Adverse Effects
- Rash
- Itching
- Muscle pain
- Impotence
- Loss of sexual desire
- Diarrhea

Proton Pump Inhibitors

Common Drug Names

esomeprazole: Nexium

lansoprazole: Prevacid

omeprazole: Losec, Prilosec

pantoprazole: Panto IV, Pantoloc, Protonix

rabeprazole: Aciphex

Proton pump inhibitors disrupt chemical binding in stomach cells to reduce acid production, lessening irritation and allowing peptic ulcers to heal.

Pharmacokinetics

Proton pump inhibitors are given orally in enteric-coated formulas to bypass the stomach, because they are highly acid labile (easily destroyed). When in the small intestine, they dissolve and their absorption is rapid. These medications are extensively metabolized by the liver to inactive compounds and then eliminated in urine.

Pharmacodynamics

Proton pump inhibitors block the last step in the secretion of gastric acid by combining with hydrogen, potassium, and adenosine triphosphate in the parietal cells of the stomach. This effectively blocks the secretion of acid and reduces the total acid present in the stomach.

Pharmacotherapeutics

Proton pump inhibitors are indicated for short-term treatment of active gastric ulcers, active ulcers in the small intestines, and erosive esophagitis (when the lining of the esophagus is worn away). These agents are also used for treating symptomatic GERD that is not responsive to other therapies. Proton pump inhibitors are used in combination with antibiotics to treat active peptic ulcers associated with *H. pylori* infection. Finally, these drugs are used in the long-term treatment of hypersecretory states such as Zollinger-Ellison syndrome (excessive acid secretion).

MASSAGE IMPLICATIONS AND ASSESSMENT

Proton pump inhibitors act directly on the stomach cells to decrease acid production. This action does not affect the response of the body to the various massage strokes. No alteration or changes in application are needed.

Side Effects

Constipation and flatulence are side effects of this category of drugs. The massage therapist may be able to aid the client by performing abdominal massage to help increase movement of stool through the intestines. The client should be encouraged to drink extra water (see Sidebar: *Adverse Reactions to Proton Pump Inhibitors*).

Other Peptic Ulcer Drugs

Common Drug Names

misoprostol: Cytotec

sucralfate: Apo-Sucralfate, Carafate, Novo-Sucralfate, Sulcrate

Research continues on the usefulness of other drugs in treating peptic ulcer disease. Misoprostol and sucralfate are currently in use.

Pharmacokinetics

Each of these drugs has slightly different pharmacokinetic properties. After an oral dose, misoprostol is absorbed extensively and rapidly. It ss metabolized to misoprostol acid, which is clinically active (meaning it is able to produce a pharmacologic effect). Misoprostol acid is excreted primarily in the urine. Sucralfate is minimally absorbed from the GI tract and is excreted in the feces.

Pharmacodynamics

The actions of these drugs vary. Misoprostol protects against peptic ulcers caused by NSAIDs by reducing the secretion of gastric acid and by boosting the production of gastric mucus, a natural defense against peptic ulcers. Sucralfate works locally in the stomach, rapidly reacting with hydrochloric acid to form a thick, pastelike substance that adheres to the gastric mucosa and, especially, to ulcers. By binding to the ulcer site, sucralfate actually protects the ulcer from the damaging effects of acid and pepsin (a stomach enzyme that breaks down proteins) to promote healing.

Pharmacotherapeutics

Each of these drugs has its own therapeutic use. Misoprostol prevents gastric ulcers caused by NSAIDs in patients at high risk for complications resulting from gastric ulcers. Sucralfate is used for short-term treatment (up to 8 weeks) of duodenal or gastric ulcers as well as for prevention of recurrent ulcers or stress ulcers.

MASSAGE IMPLICATIONS AND ASSESSMENT

Neither of the above drugs' actions will affect the response of the body to massage.

Side Effects

Most commonly, constipation and flatulence are side effects of these drugs. Massage of the abdomen to encourage movement through the intestines and advisement to drink more fluids are indicated (see Sidebar: *Adverse Reactions to Other Peptic Ulcer Drugs*).

Adverse Reactions to Other Peptic Ulcer Drugs

Side Effects
- Gas
- Constipation
- Metallic taste

Adverse Effects
- Nausea/vomiting
- Diarrhea
- Abdominal pain

Adsorbent, Antiflatulent, and Digestive Drugs

Adsorbent, antiflatulent, and digestive drugs are used to fight undesirable toxins, acids, and gases in the GI tract, aiding healthy GI function.

Adsorbent Drugs

Common Drug Names

activated charcoal: Actidose, Actidose-Aqua, activated carbon, Charcadole, Liqui-Char

Natural and synthetic adsorbents are prescribed as antidotes for the ingestion of toxins, substances that can lead to poisoning or overdose. The most commonly used clinical adsorbent is activated charcoal, a black powder residue obtained from the distillation of various organic materials.

Pharmacokinetics

Activated charcoal must be administered soon after toxic ingestion because it can only bind with drugs or poisons that have not yet been absorbed from the GI tract. After initial absorption, some poisons move back into the intestines, where they are reabsorbed. Activated charcoal may be administered repeatedly to break this cycle. Activated charcoal, which is not absorbed or metabolized by the body, is excreted unchanged in the feces.

Pharmacodynamics

Because adsorbents attract and bind toxins in the intestine, they inhibit toxins from being absorbed from the GI tract. However, this binding does not change any toxic effects caused by earlier absorption of the poison.

Pharmacotherapeutics

Activated charcoal is a general-purpose antidote used for many types of acute oral poisoning. It is not indicated in acute poisoning from cyanide, ethanol, methanol, iron, sodium chloride alkalies, inorganic acids, or organic solvents.

MASSAGE IMPLICATIONS AND ASSESSMENT

Because these drugs are used in poison ingestion, massage is contraindicated until treatment is complete and the physician releases the client for massage. Changes in the massage protocols depend on whether the client has any permanent damage resulting from the poisoning.

Antiflatulent Drugs

Common Drug Names

simethicone: Flatulex, Gas-X, Mylanta Gas, Mylicon, Ovol, Phazyme

Antiflatulents disperse gas pockets in the GI tract. They are available alone or in combination with antacids. A major antiflatulent drug currently in use is simethicone.

Pharmacokinetics

Antiflatulents are not absorbed from the GI tract. They are distributed only in the intestinal lumen and are eliminated intact in the feces.

Pharmacodynamics

Antiflatulents provide defoaming action in the GI tract. By producing a film in the intestines, simethicone disperses mucus-enclosed gas pockets and helps prevent their formation.

Pharmacotherapeutics

Antiflatulents are prescribed to treat conditions in which excess gas is a problem, such as functional gastric bloating, postoperative gaseous bloating, diverticular disease, spastic or irritable colon, and air swallowing.

MASSAGE IMPLICATIONS AND ASSESSMENT

Because this drug works in the GI tract, it does not affect the application of massage strokes and how the body receives them.

Side Effects

The main side effect of simethicone is belching and rectal gas release. Massage of the abdomen may help with releasing this gas and increase the comfort of the client. If the client consents and is not sensitive to scents, aromatherapy may be used.

Digestive Drugs

Common Drug Names

dehydrocholic acid: Cholan-HMB

lactase: Dairyaid, Dairy Ease, Lactaid, Lactrase

pancreatin: Creon Capsules, Digepepsin (discontinued in the U.S.), Dizymes, Donnazyme (discontinued in the U.S.), Entozyme, Pancrezyme

pancrelipase: Cotazym Capsules, Creon, Ilozyme, Ku-Zyme HP, Pancrease, Pancrelipase Capsules

Protilase, Ultrase, Viokase, Zymase (discontinued in the U.S.)

Digestive drugs (digestants) aid digestion in patients who are missing enzymes or other substances needed to digest food. Digestants that function in the GI tract, liver, and pancreas include dehydrocholic acid as well as pancreatin and pancrelipase (pancreatic enzymes).

Pharmacokinetics

Digestants are not absorbed. They act locally in the GI tract and are excreted in feces.

Pharmacodynamics

The action of digestants resembles the action of the body substances they replace. Dehydrocholic acid, a bile acid, increases the output of bile in the liver. The pancreatic enzymes pancreatin and pancrelipase replace normal pancreatic enzymes. Digestants contain trypsin to digest proteins, amylase to digest carbohydrates, and lipase to digest fats.

Pharmacotherapeutics

Because their action resembles the action of the body substances they replace, each digestant has its own indication. Dehydrocholic acid, a bile acid, provides temporary relief from constipation and promotes the flow of bile. Pancreatic enzymes are given to patients with insufficient levels of pancreatic enzymes, such as those with pancreatitis and cystic fibrosis. They may also be used to treat steatorrhea (disorder of fat metabolism characterized by fatty, foul-smelling stools).

MASSAGE IMPLICATIONS AND ASSESSMENT

These drugs act specifically in the digestive system to aid in digestion. There is no effect on how the body receives and reacts to massage strokes. No changes in application of massage are needed.

Side Effects

The most common side effects of digestive drugs are cramping, nausea, and diarrhea. A relaxing massage may help to calm these effects, especially a massage using the systemic reflex strokes that can help the body to relax. Other adverse effects, such as epigastric pain, may indicate gallstones and must be referred to a physician for evaluation and massage withheld (see Sidebar: *Adverse Reactions to Digestive Drugs*).

Adverse Reactions to Digestive Drugs

Side Effects
- Cramping
- Diarrhea
- Nausea

Adverse Effects
- Biliary colic
- Gallstones

Antidiarrheal and Laxative Drugs

Diarrhea and constipation represent the two major symptoms related to disturbances of the large intestine. Antidiarrheals act systemically or locally and include opioid-related drugs and other antidiarrheal drugs.

Laxatives stimulate defecation and include hyperosmolar drugs, dietary fiber and related bulk-forming substances, emollients, stimulants, and lubricants.

Opioid-Related Antidiarrheal Drugs

Common Drug Names

difenoxin: Motofen

diphenoxylate with atropine: Diphenatol, Lomocot, Lomotil, Lonox

loperamide: Apo-Loperamide, Diamode, DiarrEze, Imodium, Imogen, Imotil, Imperim, Kaodene, Kao-Paverin, K-Pec, Lopercap

---

Opioid-related drugs decrease peristalsis (involuntary, progressive, wavelike intestinal movement that pushes fecal matter along) in the intestines.

Pharmacokinetics

Difenoxin with atropine and diphenoxylate with atropine are readily absorbed from the GI tract. However, loperamide is not absorbed well after oral administration. All three medications are distributed in the serum, metabolized in the liver, and excreted primarily in the feces. Diphenoxylate is metabolized to difenoxin, its biologically active major metabolite.

Pharmacodynamics

Difenoxin, diphenoxylate, and loperamide slow GI motility by depressing the circular and longitudinal muscle action (peristalsis) in the large and small intestines. These drugs also decrease expulsive contractions throughout the colon.

Pharmacotherapeutics

Difenoxin, diphenoxylate, and loperamide are used to treat acute, nonspecific diarrhea. Loperamide also is used to treat chronic diarrhea.

MASSAGE IMPLICATIONS AND ASSESSMENT

Absorption of these drugs is not affected by massage. The action of the opioid-related antidiarrheals is mostly local, on the smooth muscle of the intestinal tract. However, the close relationship of these drugs to opiates can lead to central nervous system (CNS) depression. The systemic reflex strokes (such as effleurage, rocking, and friction) that normally bring increased endorphins and relaxation are enhanced; the local reflex strokes may be slowed in their effects on the muscles. Using increased speed with reflexive strokes and/or using stimulating strokes at the end of the massage helps prevent the client from being too relaxed, dizzy, or ungrounded from the massage. Mechanical strokes are most effective on the local muscles.

Side Effects

The most common side effects of the opioid-related antidiarrheal drugs—fatigue, dizziness, and drowsiness—are caused by CNS depression. The above changes in massage protocols assist in minimizing problems related to these side effects and massage. Abdominal pain and distention could be serious complications and should be referred to a physician for evaluation immediately and massage withheld. Constipation should be referred for physician evaluation as well. Dosage adjustments may need to be made to prevent more serious reactions (see Sidebar: *Adverse Reactions to Opioid-Related Antidiarrheal Drugs*).

> **Adverse Reactions to Opioid-Related Antidiarrheal Drugs**
>
> **Side Effects**
> - Nausea/vomiting
> - Drowsiness
> - Fatigue
> - Dizziness
>
> **Adverse Effects**
> - Abdominal distention
> - CNS depression
> - Tachycardia
> - Paralytic ileus

Other Antidiarrheal Drugs

Common Drug Names

attapulgite: Diasorb, Kaopectate, K-Pek

bismuth subgallate: Devrom

bismuth subsalicylate: Bismatrol, Diotame, Pepto-Bismol

kaolin and pectin: Kaodene, Kaolinpec, Kao-Spen, Kapectolin, Kaolin with Pectin, K-C, K-P

These antidiarrheal drugs are locally acting, OTC antidiarrheals. They work by adsorbing irritants and soothing the intestinal mucosa. Kaolin and pectin mixtures are used much less frequently because they seem to be less effective.

Pharmacokinetics

These other antidiarrheal drugs are not absorbed; therefore, they are not distributed throughout the body. They are excreted in the feces.

Pharmacodynamics

These drugs act as adsorbents, binding with bacteria, toxins, and other irritants on the intestinal mucosa. They decrease the pH in the intestinal lumen and provide a soothing effect on the irritated mucosa.

Pharmacotherapeutics

These antidiarrheal drugs are used to relieve mild to moderate acute diarrhea. They also may be used to temporarily relieve chronic diarrhea until the cause can be determined and definitive treatment begun.

Adverse Reactions to Other Antidiarrheal Drugs

Side Effects
- Dark stools
- Constipation

Adverse Effects
- Bowel obstruction (rare)

MASSAGE IMPLICATIONS AND ASSESSMENT

These drugs act directly on the GI tract and do not affect the body's reaction to massage.

Side Effects

The most common side effect is constipation, usually only occurring with use for chronic diarrhea. Because these drugs are most often used for acute episodes, it is rare to encounter it in a massage client. Referral for physician evaluation is appropriate, however, because dosage adjustments may need to be made (see Sidebar: *Adverse Reactions to Other Antidiarrheal Drugs*).

Hyperosmolar Laxatives

Common Drug Names

glycerin: Fleet Babylax, Glycerin Suppositories, glycerol, Osmoglyn, Sani-Supp

lactulose: Acilac, Cholac, Constilac, Constulose, Enulose, Generlac, Kristalose, Laxilose

polyethylene glycol (PEG): Colyte, GoLYTELY, Klean-Prep, Lyteprep, MiraLax, NuLytely, PegLyte

saline compounds (magnesium salts): Citro-Mag, Magonate, milk of magnesia

sodium biphosphate: Fleet enema, Phospho-soda, Visicol

Hyperosmolar laxatives work by drawing water into the intestine, thereby promoting bowel distention and peristalsis.

Pharmacokinetics

The pharmacokinetic properties of the hyperosmolar laxatives vary. Glycerin is placed directly into the colon by enema or suppository and is not absorbed systemically. Lactulose enters the GI tract orally and is minimally absorbed. As a result, the drug is distributed only in the intestine. It is metabolized by bacteria in the colon and excreted in the feces. After saline compounds are introduced into the GI tract orally or as an enema, some of their ions are absorbed. Absorbed ions are excreted in the urine, the unabsorbed drug in the feces. PEG is a nonabsorbable solution that acts as an osmotic drug but does not alter electrolyte balance.

Pharmacodynamics

Hyperosmolar laxatives produce a bowel movement by drawing water into the intestine. Fluid accumulation distends the bowel and promotes peristalsis and a bowel movement.

Pharmacotherapeutics

The uses of hyperosmolar laxatives vary. Glycerin is helpful in bowel retraining. Lactulose is used to treat constipation and help reduce ammonia production and absorption from the intestines in liver disease. Saline compounds are used when prompt and complete bowel evacuation is required.

MASSAGE IMPLICATIONS AND ASSESSMENT

Glycerin and lactulose are more gentle and act in the intestines. No effect occurs that changes the action of the massage strokes on the body. The saline compounds are stronger and quicker in their actions and are often used to prepare the client for tests and procedures such as colonoscopy. The client is likely to be more comfortable at home. It is best to give the massage before the client takes the laxative.

Side Effects

The most common side effects of using these laxatives are fatigue, weakness, and lethargy. They are related to the fluid shifts into the intestine and occur most often with the saline compounds after evacuation of the bowels. Massage is not indicated when side effects are present because of bowel preparation.

When giving massage to someone using lactulose for chronic or acute constipation, gentle abdominal massage can be used. Glycerin is usually given per rectum. Massage of the abdomen may help with stimulating evacuation. Obviously, this would be appropriate for working at home with a family member or in a hospital setting, but not in a massage office (see Sidebar: *Adverse Reactions to Hyperosmolar Laxatives*).

Adverse Reactions to Hyperosmolar Laxatives

Side Effects
- Fatigue
- Weakness
- Lethargy

Adverse Effects
- Abdominal distention
- Cramps
- Nausea/vomiting
- Diarrhea
- Hypokalemia
- Dehydration
- Increase blood glucose (with lactulose)
- Electrolyte imbalances
- Arrhythmias

Dietary Fiber and Related Bulk-Forming Laxatives

Common Drug Names

methylcellulose: Citrucel

polycarbophil: Equalactin, Fiberall, FiberCon, Fiber-Lax, FiberNorm, Mitolax

psyllium hydrophilic mucilloid: Hydrocil, Konsyl-D, Metamucil, Mondone, Novo-Mucilax Reguloid, Serutan, Syllact

A high-fiber diet is the most natural way to prevent or treat constipation. Dietary fiber is the part of plants not digested in the small intestine. Bulk-forming laxatives, which resemble dietary fiber, contain natural and semisynthetic polysaccharides and cellulose.

Pharmacokinetics

Dietary fiber and bulk-forming laxatives are not absorbed systemically. Dietary fiber and bulk-forming laxatives are excreted in the feces.

Pharmacodynamics

Dietary fiber and bulk-forming laxatives increase stool mass and the amount of water drawn into the large intestine, promoting peristalsis.

Pharmacotherapeutics

Bulk-forming laxatives are used to treat simple cases of constipation, especially constipation resulting from a low-fiber or low-fluid diet, and to aid patients recovering from acute myocardial infarction (MI) or cerebral aneurysms who need to avoid Valsalva's maneuver (forced expiration against a closed airway) and maintain soft feces. These drugs are also used to manage patients with irritable bowel syndrome and diverticulosis.

Adverse Reactions to Fiber and Bulk-Forming Laxatives

Side Effects
- Gas
- Diarrhea

Adverse Effects
- Intestinal obstruction
- Fecal impaction
- Esophageal obstruction

MASSAGE IMPLICATIONS AND ASSESSMENT

These drugs do not change how the body reacts to massage strokes. Many people use these daily to maintain regularity. Gentle abdominal massage and reminders to drink water will help the client with this goal.

Side Effects

Gas is the most common side effect with the fiber laxatives. Gentle abdominal massage can help to alleviate this effect. Abdominal pain or worsening constipation must be referred for immediate evaluation by a physician and massage withheld (see Sidebar: *Adverse Reactions to Fiber and Bulk-Forming Laxatives*).

Emollient Laxatives

Common Drug Names

dioctyl sulfosuccinate: Docusate calcium, docusate sodium, Colace, Colax-C, DOS Softgel, D-S-S, Ryalex, Surfak

docusate with casanthrol: Doxidan, Peri-Colace

Emollients—also known as stool softeners—include the calcium, potassium, and sodium salts of docusate.

Pharmacokinetics

Administered orally, emollients are absorbed and excreted through bile in the feces.

Pharmacodynamics

Emollients soften the stool and make bowel movements easier by emulsifying the fat and water components of feces in the small and large intestines. This detergent action allows water and fats to penetrate the stool, making it softer and easier to eliminate. Emollients also stimulate electrolyte and fluid secretion from intestinal mucosal cells.

Pharmacotherapeutics

Emollients are the drugs of choice for softening stools in patients who should avoid straining during a bowel movement, including those with recent MI or surgery, disease of the anus or rectum, increased intracranial pressure (ICP), and hernias.

MASSAGE IMPLICATIONS AND ASSESSMENT

The action of emollient drugs does not affect the response of the body to massage. Clients taking these drugs may benefit from gentle abdominal massage.

Side Effects

Side effects are infrequent with these drugs and are generally mild (see Sidebar: *Adverse Reactions to Emollient Laxatives*).

Adverse Reactions to Emollient Laxatives

Side Effects
- Bitter taste
- Diarrhea
- Throat irritation
- Cramps

Stimulant Laxatives

Common Drug Names

bisacodyl: Alophen, Apo-Bisacodyl, Bisac-Evac, Dulcolax, Feen-A-Mint, Femilax

cascara sagrada: cascara

castor oil: Emulsoil, Neoloid, Purge

phenolphthalein: Espotabs, Evac-U-Gen, Ex-Lax

senna: Black Draught, Senexon, Senna-Gen, Senokot, X-Prep

Stimulant laxatives are also known as irritant cathartics.

Pharmacokinetics

Stimulant laxatives are minimally absorbed and are metabolized in the liver. The metabolites are excreted in the urine and feces.

Pharmacodynamics

Stimulant laxatives stimulate peristalsis and produce a bowel movement by irritating the intestinal mucosa or stimulating nerve endings of the intestinal smooth muscle. Castor oil and phenolphthalein also increase peristalsis in the small intestine.

Pharmacotherapeutics

Stimulant laxatives are the preferred drugs for emptying the bowel before general surgery, sigmoidoscopic or proctoscopic procedures, and radiologic procedures such as barium studies of the GI tract. Stimulant laxatives are also used to treat constipation caused by prolonged bed rest, neurologic dysfunction of the colon, and constipating drugs such as narcotics.

Adverse Reactions to Stimulant Laxatives

Side Effects
- Weakness
- Nausea
- Cramps
- Inflamed rectum

Adverse Effects
- Dehydration

MASSAGE IMPLICATIONS AND ASSESSMENT

These drugs do not interfere with the response to massage strokes. Depending on dosage and on route (per rectum is the quickest), response to the drugs may occur quickly.

Side Effects

Commonly, these drugs cause cramping with evacuation of the bowel and may cause weakness. Gentle massage of the abdomen may help if the setting is appropriate (see Sidebar: *Adverse Reactions to Stimulant Laxatives*).

Lubricant Laxatives

Common Drug Names

mineral oil: Fleet Mineral Oil Enema, Kondremul, Lanosyl, Liqui-Doss, Milkinol, Petrogalar Plain

Mineral oil is the main lubricant laxative in current clinical use.

Pharmacokinetics

Absorbed mineral oil is distributed to the abdominal lymph nodes, intestinal mucosa, liver, and spleen. Mineral oil is metabolized by the liver and excreted in the feces.

Pharmacodynamics

Mineral oil lubricates the stool and the intestinal mucosa and prevents water reabsorption from the lumen of the bowel. The increased fluid content of the feces increases peristalsis. Rectal administration by enema also produces distention.

Pharmacotherapeutics

Mineral oil is used to treat constipation and maintain soft stools when straining is contraindicated, such as after recent MI (to avoid Valsalva's maneuver), eye surgery (to prevent increased pressure in the eye), or cerebral aneurysm repair (to avoid increased ICP). Administered orally or by enema, this lubricant laxative is also used to treat patients with fecal impaction.

MASSAGE IMPLICATIONS AND ASSESSMENT

Massage strokes are not affected by the action of this drug.

Side Effects

The main side effect is cramping and diarrhea, especially with rectal administration. Gentle abdominal massage may be helpful if the setting is appropriate (see Sidebar: *Adverse Reactions to Mineral Oil*).

> **Adverse Reactions to Mineral Oil**
>
> **Side Effects**
> - Nausea
> - Vomiting
> - Diarrhea
> - Abdominal cramping

Antiemetic and Emetic Drugs

Antiemetics and emetics represent two groups of drugs with opposing actions. Emetic drugs, which are derived from plants, produce vomiting. Antiemetic drugs decrease nausea, reducing the urge to vomit.

Antiemetic Drugs

Common Drug Names: Antihistamines

diphenhydramine: Allerdryl, Benadryl

dimenhydrinate: Dramamine, Gravol, Hydrate, TripTone

cyclizine hydrochloride: Marezine (discontinued in the U.S.)

hydroxyzine pamoate: Vistaril

meclizine hydrochloride: Antivert, Bonamine, Bonine, Dramamine II, Meni-D

trimethobenzamide: Benzacot, Tigan

> ### *Common Drug Names:* Phenothiazines
>
> *chlorpromazine hydrochloride:* Chlorpromanyl, Largactil, Thorazine
> *perphenazine:* Apo-Perphenazine, Trilafon
> *prochlorperazine maleate:* Compazine, Compro, Nu-Prochlor, Stemetil
>
> ### *Common Drug Names:* Serotonin Receptor Agonists
>
> *granisetron:* Kytril
> *ondansetron:* Zofran

Pharmacokinetics

The pharmacokinetic properties of antiemetics vary slightly. Oral antihistamine antiemetics are absorbed well from the GI tract and are metabolized primarily by the liver. Their inactive metabolites are excreted in the urine. Phenothiazine antiemetics and serotonin receptor antagonists are absorbed well, extensively metabolized by the liver, and excreted in the urine and feces.

Pharmacodynamics

The action of antiemetics may vary. The mechanism of action that produces the antiemetic effect of antihistamines is unclear.

Phenothiazines produce their antiemetic effect by blocking the dopaminergic receptors in the chemoreceptor trigger zone in the brain (the area of the brain that stimulates vomiting). The serotonin receptor antagonists block serotonin stimulation centrally in the chemoreceptor trigger zone and peripherally in the vagal nerve terminals, both of which stimulate vomiting.

Pharmacotherapeutics

The uses of antiemetics vary. With the exception of trimethobenzamide, the antihistamines are specifically used for nausea and vomiting caused by inner ear stimulation. As a consequence, these drugs prevent or treat motion sickness. They usually are most effective when given before activities that produce motion sickness and are much less effective when nausea or vomiting has already begun.

Phenothiazine antiemetics and serotonin receptor antagonists control severe nausea and vomiting from various causes. They are used when vomiting becomes severe and potentially hazardous, such as postsurgical or viral nausea and vomiting. Both types of drugs are also prescribed to control the nausea and vomiting resulting from cancer chemotherapy and radiation therapy.

MASSAGE IMPLICATIONS AND ASSESSMENT

The actions of these drugs vary, but all have effects on the CNS. The relaxing effects of massage can be significantly enhanced, taking place more quickly and with deeper changes in consciousness. Stimulating strokes at the end of the massage (such as tapotement and rapid effleurage) and care in getting the client off the table are essential. If the drugs have been given by injection or by patch (transdermal), massage is contraindicated in that local area. For the most part, side effects are caused by CNS effects (see Sidebar: *Adverse Reactions to Antiemetic Drugs*).

Other Antiemetic Drugs

Common Drug Names

benzquinamide

diphenidol

dronabinol: Marinol

metoclopramide: Apo-Metoclop, Clopra, Maxeran, Maxolon (discontinued in the U.S.), Octamide, Pramin, Reclomide, Reglan

scopolamine: Isopto Hyoscine, Scopace, Transderm Scōp, Transderm-V

Benzquinamide

Benzquinamide hydrochloride is used to prevent or treat nausea and vomiting caused by anesthesia and surgery. This drug may be preferred in some circumstances because it does not produce CNS or respiratory depression. Plus, benzquinamide does not produce the extrapyramidal effects (abnormal involuntary movements) or hypotension that may occur with the phenothiazines.

Scopolamine

Scopolamine prevents motion sickness, but its use is limited because of its sedative and anticholinergic effects. One scopolamine transdermal preparation, Transderm Scōp, is highly effective without producing the usual adverse effects.

Metoclopramide

Metoclopramide hydrochloride has been used for many years in Europe to prevent motion sickness. It is being used in the United States to prevent chemotherapy-induced nausea and vomiting.

Diphenidol

Diphenidol effectively prevents vertigo (whirling sensation), in addition to preventing or treating generalized nausea and vomiting. However, its use is limited because of the auditory and visual hallucinations, confusion, and disorientation that may occur.

Adverse Reactions to Antiemetic Drugs

Antihistamines

Side Effects
- Drowsiness
- Dry mouth

Adverse Effects
- Paradoxical CNS stimulation

Phenothiazines

Side Effects
- Headache
- Insomnia
- Restlessness
- Constipation
- Dry mouth
- Dizziness
- Hypotension

Adverse Effects
- Confusion
- Agitation
- Euphoria
- Urinary retention
- Impotence
- Visual and auditory disturbances

Serotonin Receptor Agonists

Side Effects
- Anxiety
- Depression
- Headache
- Weakness
- Insomnia

Adverse Effects
- Confusion
- Euphoria
- Agitation
- Hypotension
- Tachycardia

Dronabinol

Dronabinol, a purified derivative of the cannabis, is a schedule II drug (meaning it has a potential for abuse). It is used to treat nausea and vomiting resulting from cancer chemotherapy in patients whose conditions do not respond adequately to conventional antiemetics. It is also been used to stimulate appetite in patients with acquired immune deficiency syndrome (AIDS). However, dronabinol can accumulate in the body, and tolerance or physical and psychological dependence can develop.

MASSAGE IMPLICATIONS AND ASSESSMENT

These drugs have varying actions but all affect the CNS. As with the previously mentioned antiemetic drugs, the therapist must be aware that increased and quick response to the relaxation effects of massage can occur. Also, these drugs can be used with serious illnesses. Therefore, physician consultation should be obtained.

Emetics

Emetics are used to induce vomiting in a person who has ingested toxic substances. Ipecac syrup is an OTC emetic. Its effectiveness varies, and it has potential for abuse in those with eating disorders. The use of ipecac syrup has become controversial because it delays the use of charcoal or can reduce the effectiveness of oral antidotes used in the emergency department for specific poisons. The U.S. Federal Drug Administration is reviewing its OTC status and may make it available by prescription only.

Pharmacokinetics

Little information exists concerning the absorption, distribution, and excretion of ipecac syrup. Vomiting occurs within 10 to 30 minutes of administration of ipecac syrup. The success of treatment is directly linked to fluid intake with ipecac administration.

Pharmacodynamics

Ipecac syrup induces vomiting by stimulating the vomiting center located in the brain's medulla.

Pharmacotherapeutics

Ipecac syrup is considered the therapy of choice for emptying the stomach because of its effectiveness and low incidence of adverse effects.

MASSAGE IMPLICATIONS AND ASSESSMENT

Because ipecac is given in the event of poisoning, massage is contraindicated until the physician has released the client and any possible long-term damages have been determined.

Quick Quiz

1. Your client tells you she has been very constipated. Her doctor has given her Lactulose twice a day until she has a bowel movement. She took her first dose that morning. What are the implications for massage?

2. Your client has irritable bowel syndrome and has been taking Lomotil for chronic diarrhea. Today he tells you he has not had a bowel movement in more than a week and is complaining of severe abdominal pain. What should you do?

Anti-Infective Drugs

10

Selecting an Antimicrobial Drug

Selecting an appropriate antimicrobial drug to treat a specific infection involves several important steps. First, the microorganism must be isolated and identified. This generally is achieved through growing a culture. Second, the susceptibility of the microorganism to various drugs must be determined. Because culture and sensitivity testing takes 48 hours, treatment usually starts at the assessment stage and then is reevaluated when test results are obtained. Third, the location of the infection must be considered. For therapy to be effective, an adequate concentration of the antimicrobial agent must be delivered to the infection site. Fourth, the cost of the drug must be considered, as well as its potential adverse effects and the possibility of patient allergies.

Preventing Pathogen Resistance

The usefulness of antimicrobial drugs is limited by pathogens that may develop resistance to a drug's action. Resistance is the ability of a microorganism to live and grow in the presence of an antimicrobial drug that is usually bacteriostatic (inhibits the growth or multiplication of bacteria) or bactericidal (kills bacteria). Resistance usually results from genetic mutation of the microorganism, often caused by overusing antibiotics or stopping antibiotic therapy too soon. This allows the bacteria that was not completely destroyed to develop resistance to the antibiotic.

Antibacterial Drugs

The number and variety of antibacterial drugs in use today are quite astonishing. New and more potent forms are being discovered all the time. Because all antibacterial drugs have basically the same implications for massage, all the various classes will be explored and the massage implications addressed together at the end of this section.

Antibacterial drugs are used mainly to treat systemic (involving the whole body rather than a localized area) bacterial infections. The antibacterial classes include:

- aminoglycosides
- penicillins
- cephalosporins
- tetracyclines
- clindamycin and lincomycin
- macrolides
- vancomycin
- carbapenems
- monobactams
- fluoroquinolones
- sulfonamides
- nitrofurantoin

Aminoglycosides

Common Drug Names

amikacin: Amikin

gentamicin: Alcomicin, Garamycin

kanamycin: Kantrex

neomycin: Myciguent, Neo-Fradin

netilmicin

streptomycin

tobramycin

Aminoglycosides provide effective bactericidal activity against aerobic Gram-negative bacilli, some aerobic Gram-positive bacteria, mycobacteria, and some protozoa.

Pharmacokinetics (how drugs circulate)

Because aminoglycosides are absorbed poorly from the gastrointestinal (GI) tract, they are usually given parenterally. After intravenous or intramuscular administration, aminoglycoside absorption is rapid and complete. Aminoglycosides are distributed widely in extracellular fluid. They are excreted primarily by the kidneys.

Pharmacodynamics (how drugs act)

Aminoglycosides act as bactericidal drugs (this means they kill bacteria) against susceptible organisms. Bacterial resistance to an aminoglycoside may be related to failure of the drug to cross the cell membrane or destruction of the drug by bacterial enzymes. Some Gram-positive cocci (enterococci) resist aminoglycoside transport across the cell membrane. When penicillin is used with aminoglycoside therapy, the cell wall is altered, allowing the aminoglycoside to penetrate the bacterial cell.

Pharmacotherapeutics (how drugs are used)

Aminoglycosides are most useful in treating serious nosocomial (hospital-acquired) infections, urinary tract infections (UTIs), infections of the central nervous system (CNS) and the eye (treated with local instillation), and general infections caused by a wide variety of bacteria (see Sidebar: *Adverse Reactions to Aminoglycosides*).

Penicillins

Penicillins remain one of the most important and useful antibacterials, despite the availability of numerous others. The penicillins can be divided into four groups: natural penicillins, aminopenicillins, penicillinase-resistant penicillins, and extended-spectrum penicillins.

Common Drug Names: Natural Penicillins

penicillin G benzathine: Bicillin L-A, Permapen

penicillin G potassium: Megacillin, Pfizerpen

penicillin G procaine: Wycillin, Ayercillin, Crysticillin

penicillin G sodium: Crystapen

penicillin V: Apo-Pen VK, Suspen, V-Cillin, Truxcillin, Veetids, Nadopen-V, Novo-Pen- VK

Common Drug Names: Aminopenicillins

amoxicillin-clavulanate potassium: Augmentin, Clavulin, Gen-Amoxicillin, Trimox, Wymox

ampicillin: Apo-Ampi, Marcillin, Novo-Ampicillin, Principen

Common Drug Names: Penicillinase-Resistant Penicillins

cloxacillin: Alclox, Apo-Cloxi, Cloxapen, Novo-Cloxin

dicloxacillin: Dycill (discontinued in the U.S.), Dynapen, Pathocil (discontinued in the U.S.)

nafcillin: Nafcil (discontinued in the U.S.), Nallpen (discontinued in the U.S.), Unipen

oxacillin: Bactocill (discontinued in the U.S.), Prostaphlin (discontinued in the U.S.)

Common Drug Names: Extended-Spectrum Penicillins

carbenicillin: Geocillin

mezlocillin: Mezlin

piperacillin: Pipracil, Pipril

piperacillin and tazobactam: Tazocin, Zosyn

ticarcillin: Ticar, Ticillin

Adverse Reactions to Aminoglycosides

Serious adverse reactions limit the use of aminoglycosides and include:

- Neuromuscular reactions, ranging from peripheral nerve toxicity to neuro-muscular blockade
- Ototoxicity
- Kidney toxicity

Adverse reactions to oral aminoglycosides include:

- Nausea
- Vomiting
- Diarrhea

**Adverse Reactions
to Penicillins**

Hypersensitivity
reactions are the major
adverse reactions to
penicillins and include:

- Anaphylactic
  reactions
- Serum sickness (a
  hypersensitivity
  reaction occurring 1
  to 2 weeks after
  injection of a foreign
  serum)
- Drug fever
- Various skin rashes

Adverse GI reactions
are associated with oral
penicillins and include:

- Tongue inflammation
- Nausea or vomiting
- Diarrhea

The aminopenicillins
and extended-spectrum
penicillins can produce
pseudomembranous
colitis (diarrhea caused
by a change in the
flora of the colon or an
overgrowth of a toxin-
producing strain of
Clostridium difficile).
Oxacillin therapy may
cause liver toxicity.

Pharmacokinetics

After oral administration, penicillins are absorbed mainly in the small intestine. Absorption of oral penicillin varies and depends on such factors as particular penicillin used, pH of the patient's stomach and intestine, and presence of food in the GI tract. Penicillins are distributed widely to most areas of the body, including the lungs, liver, kidneys, muscle, bone, and placenta. High concentrations also appear in the urine, making penicillins useful in treating UTIs. Penicillins are metabolized to a limited extent in the liver to inactive metabolites and are excreted 60% unchanged by the kidneys. Nafcillin also is excreted in bile.

Pharmacodynamics

Penicillins usually are bactericidal (they kill bacteria) by destroying the cell wall of the organism.

Pharmacotherapeutics

No other class of antibacterial drugs provides as wide a spectrum of antimicrobial activity as the penicillins. Penicillin is given by intramuscular injection when oral administration is inconvenient or a patient's compliance is questionable. Because long-acting preparations of penicillin G (penicillin G benzathine and penicillin G procaine) are relatively insoluble, they must be administered by the intramuscular route (see Sidebar: *Adverse Reactions to Penicillins*).

Cephalosporins

Many antibacterial drugs introduced for clinical use in recent years have been cephalosporins. Cephalosporins are grouped into generations according to their effectiveness against different organisms, their characteristics, and their development.

Common Drug Names: First Generation

cefadroxil: Apo-Cefadroxil, Duricef, Novo-Cefadroxil

cefazolin: Ancef, Kefzol

cephalexin: Apo-Cephalex, Biocef, Keflex, Novo-Lexin

cephradine: Velosef

Common Drug Names: Second Generation

cefaclor: Apo-Cefaclor, Ceclor

cefamandole: Mandol

cefmetazole: Zefazone (discontinued in the U.S.)

cefprozil: Cefzil

ceftibuten

cefuroxime axetil

cefuroxime sodium

Common Drug Names: Third Generation

cefdinir: Omnicef

cefixime: Suprax

cefoperazone: Cefobid

cefpodoxime: Vantin

ceftazidime: Ceptaz, Fortaz, Tazicef, Tazidime

ceftizoxime: Cefizox

ceftriaxone: Rocephin

Common Drug Names: Fourth Generation

cefepime: Maxipime

cephalosporin

Loracarbef is a synthetic beta-lactam antibiotic that belongs to a new class of drugs known as the carbacephem antibiotics. Because it is similar to second-generation cephalosporins, it is included with the cephalosporins.

Because penicillins and cephalosporins are chemically similar (they both have what is called a beta-lactam molecular structure), some cross-sensitivity occurs. This means that someone who has had a reaction to penicillin is also at risk for a reaction to cephalosporins in approximately 5% of cases.

Pharmacokinetics

Many cephalosporins are administered parenterally because they are not absorbed from the GI tract. Some cephalosporins are absorbed from the GI tract and can be administered orally, but food usually delays the absorption of these drugs. After absorption, cephalosporins are distributed widely. Many cephalosporins, including loracarbef, are not

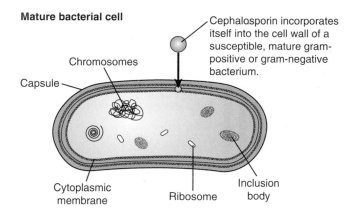

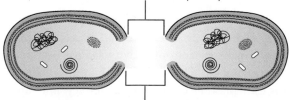

Figure 10-1 Action of Cephalosporins in Attacking Bacteria. The antibacterial action of cephalosporins depends on their ability to penetrate the bacterial wall and bind with proteins on the cytoplasmic membrane.

metabolized at all. All cephalosporins are excreted primarily unchanged by the kidneys with the exception of cefoperazone and ceftriaxone, which are excreted in the feces via bile.

Pharmacodynamics

Cephalosporins inhibit cell wall synthesis by binding to the bacterial enzymes known as penicillin-binding proteins (PBPs), located on the cell membrane. After the drug damages the cell wall by binding with the PBPs, the body's natural defense mechanisms destroy the bacteria (Fig. 10-1).

Pharmacotherapeutics

The four generations of cephalosporins have particular therapeutic uses. First-generation cephalosporins are used to treat pneumonia, cellulitis (skin infection), and osteomyelitis (bone infection). Second-generation cephalosporins act against a variety of bacteria. Third-generation cephalosporins also act against a wide variety of bacteria. Fourth-generation cephalosporins are active against a wide range of Gram-positive and Gram-negative bacteria (see Sidebar: *Adverse Reactions to Cephalosporins*).

Tetracyclines

Common Drug Names

demeclocycline: Declomycin

doxycycline: Adoxa, Apo-Doxy, Doxycin, Monodox, Vibramycin

minocycline: Alti-Minocycline, Apo-Minocycline, Dynacin, Minocin

tetracycline: Apo-Tetra, Brodspec, EmTet, Sumycin, Wesmycin

Tetracyclines are broad-spectrum antibiotics. They are classified as short-acting compounds (such as chlortetracycline hydrochloride), intermediate-acting compounds (such as demeclocycline hydrochloride), and long-acting compounds (such as doxycycline hyclate and minocycline hydrochloride).

Pharmacokinetics

Tetracyclines are absorbed from the small intestines when taken orally. Tetracyclines are distributed widely into body tissues and fluids, concentrated in bile, and excreted primarily by the kidneys

Pharmacodynamics

All tetracyclines are primarily bacteriostatic, meaning they inhibit the growth or multiplication of bacteria.

Pharmacotherapeutics

Tetracyclines provide a broad spectrum of activity against bacteria and other microorganisms. The long-acting compounds doxycycline and minocycline provide more action against various organisms than other tetracyclines. Tetracyclines are used to treat Rocky Mountain spotted fever, Q fever, and Lyme disease. They are the drugs of choice for treating some UTIs. Tetracyclines in low dosages, administered either orally or topically, effectively treat acne because they can decrease the fatty acid content of sebum (see Sidebar: *Adverse Reactions to Tetracyclines*).

Adverse Reactions to Cephalosporins

Adverse reactions to cephalosporins include:

- Confusion
- Seizures
- Bleeding
- Nausea
- Vomiting
- Diarrhea

Hypersensitivity reactions are the most common systemic adverse reactions to cephalosporins and include:

- Hives
- Itching
- Rash that looks like the measles
- Serum sickness (reaction after injection of a foreign serum characterized by edema, fever, hives, and inflammation of the blood vessels and joints)
- Anaphylaxis (in rare cases)

Adverse Reactions to Tetracyclines

Tetracyclines produce many of the same adverse reactions as other antibacterials, such as:

- Superinfection (overgrowth of resistant organisms)
- Nausea
- Vomiting
- Abdominal distress and distention
- Diarrhea

Other adverse reactions include:

- Photosensitivity reactions (red rash on areas exposed to sunlight)
- Liver toxicity
- Kidney toxicity

Clindamycin

Common Drug Names

clindamycin: Alti-Clindamycin, Cleocin, Clindagel, Clindets, Dalacin

Because of its high potential for serious adverse effects, clindamycin is another antibacterial drug that is prescribed only when there is no therapeutic alternative.

Pharmacokinetics

When taken orally, clindamycin is absorbed well and distributed widely in the body. It is metabolized by the liver and excreted by the kidney and biliary pathways.

Pharmacodynamics

Clindamycin is primarily bacteriostatic (slows growth and replications) against most organisms.

Pharmacotherapeutics

Because of its potential for serious toxicity and pseudomembranous colitis (characterized by severe diarrhea, abdominal pain, fever, and mucus and blood in the stools), clindamycin is limited to a few clinical situations in which safer alternative antibacterials are not available. It is used primarily to treat abdominal and pulmonary infections. It may also be used as an alternative to penicillin in treating staphylococcal infections in a patient with penicillin allergy (see Sidebar: *Adverse Reactions to Clindamycin*).

Adverse Reactions to Clindamycin

Pseudomembranous colitis may occur with clindamycin use. This syndrome can be fatal and requires prompt discontinuation of the drug. Although this is the most serious reaction to clindamycin and limits its use, other reactions may also occur, such as:

- Diarrhea
- Stomatitis (mouth inflammation)
- Nausea
- Vomiting
- Hypersensitivity reactions

Macrolides

Common Drug Names

erythromycin: Akne-Mycin, Erygel, Apo-Erythro Base, Diomycin

erythromycin estolate: Ilosone, Novo-Rhythro

erythromycin ethylsuccinate: Apo-Erythro-ES, E.E.S., EryPed

erythromycin gluceptate: Ilotycin Gluceptate

erythromycin lactobionate: Erythrocin

erythromycin stearate: Apo-Erythro-S, MY-E

Macrolides are used to treat a number of common infections. They include the above-mentioned erythromycin derivatives. Other macrolides include azithromycin and clarithromycin.

Pharmacokinetics

Because erythromycin is acid-sensitive, it must be buffered or have enteric coating to prevent destruction by gastric acid. Erythromycin is absorbed in the small intestine. It is distributed to most tissues and body fluids. Erythromycin is metabolized by the liver and excreted in bile in high concentrations; small amounts are excreted in the urine.

Pharmacodynamics

Macrolides inhibit bacterial growth and replication, much like clindamycin.

Pharmacotherapeutics

Erythromycin has a range of therapeutic uses. Erythromycin is the drug of choice for treating Legionnaires disease. In patients who are allergic to penicillin, erythromycin is effective to treat gonorrhea and syphilis. Erythromycin may also be used to treat minor staphylococcal infections of the skin. Other macrolides are used to treat a wide variety of infections (see Sidebar: *Adverse Reactions to Macrolides*).

Vancomycin

Common Drug Names

vancomycin: Vancocin, Vancoled

Vancomycin hydrochloride is used increasingly to treat methicillin-resistant *Staphylococcus aureus*, which has become a major concern in the United States and other parts of the world. Because of the emergence of vancomycin-resistant enterococci, vancomycin must be used judiciously.

Pharmacokinetics

Because vancomycin is absorbed poorly from the GI tract, it must be given intravenously to treat systemic infections. Vancomycin diffuses well into pleural (around the lungs), pericardial (around the heart), synovial (joint), and ascitic (in the abdominal cavity) fluids.

The metabolism of vancomycin is unknown. Approximately 85% of the dose is excreted unchanged in urine within 24 hours. A small amount may be eliminated through the liver and biliary tract.

Pharmacodynamics

Vancomycin inhibits bacterial cell wall synthesis. When the bacterial cell wall is damaged, the body's natural defenses can attack the organism.

Pharmacotherapeutics

Vancomycin is active against a wide variety of organisms. Intravenous vancomycin is the therapy of choice for patients with serious resistant staphylococcal infections who are hypersensitive to penicillins. Vancomycin, when used with an aminoglycoside, is also the treatment of choice for infections of the heart in patients who are allergic to penicillin (see Sidebar: *Adverse Reactions to Vancomycin*).

Carbapenems

Common Drug Names

imipenem-cilastatin: Primaxin

meropenem: Merrem

Adverse Reactions to Macrolides

Although erythromycin produces few adverse effects, it may produce:
- Epigastric distress
- Nausea
- Vomiting
- Diarrhea (especially with large doses)
- Rashes
- Fever
- Eosinophilia (an increase in the number of eosinophils, a type of white blood cell)
- Anaphylaxis

Adverse Reactions to Vancomycin

Adverse reactions to vancomycin, although rare, include:
- Hypersensitivity and anaphylactic reactions
- Drug fever
- Eosinophilia (an increased number of eosinophils, a type of white blood cell)
- Neutropenia (reduced number of neutrophils, another type of white blood cell)

Severe hypotension may occur with rapid intravenous administration of vancomycin and may be accompanied by a red rash with flat and raised lesions on the face, neck, chest, and arms.

Carbapenems are a class of beta-lactam antibacterials. The antibacterial spectrum of activity for these drugs is broader than that of any other antibacterial studied to date.

Pharmacokinetics

The pharmacokinetic properties of carbapenems slightly vary. Imipenem must be given with cilastatin because imipenem alone is rapidly metabolized in the tubules of the kidneys, rendering it ineffective. After parenteral administration, imipenem-cilastatin is distributed widely. It is metabolized by several mechanisms and excreted primarily in the urine.

Meropenem is distributed widely after parenteral administration. Metabolism is insignificant; 70% of the drug is excreted unchanged in the urine.

Pharmacodynamics

Imipenem and meropenem usually are bactericidal (they kill the bacteria).

Pharmacotherapeutics

Imipenem is effective against many skin infections and intestinal infections. It also may be used as therapy for serious nosocomial (hospital-acquired) infections or infections in immunocompromised hosts.

Meropenem is indicated in the treatment of intra-abdominal infections and for the management of bacterial meningitis caused by susceptible organisms (see Sidebar: *Adverse Reactions to Carbapenems*).

Monobactam

Common Drug Names

aztreonam: Azactam

Aztreonam is the first member in the class of monobactam antibiotics. It is a synthetic monobactam with a narrow spectrum of activity that includes many Gram-negative aerobic bacteria.

Pharmacokinetics

After parenteral administration, aztreonam is rapidly and completely absorbed and distributed widely. It is metabolized partially and is excreted primarily in the urine as unchanged drug.

Pharmacodynamics

Aztreonam's bactericidal activity results from inhibition of bacterial cell wall synthesis. It preferentially binds to the PBP-3 of susceptible Gram-negative bacteria. As a result, division of the cell wall is inhibited and lysis occurs.

Pharmacotherapeutics

Aztreonam is indicated in a range of therapeutic situations. It is effective against a wide variety of organisms. It is also used to treat complicated and uncomplicated UTIs, septicemia

---

Adverse Reactions to Carbapenems

Common adverse reactions to imipenem-cilastatin and meropenem include:

- Nausea
- Vomiting
- Diarrhea

Hypersensitivity reactions such as rashes may occur, particularly in patients with known hypersensitivity to penicillins.

Adverse Reactions to Monobactams

- Diarrhea
- Hypersensitivity and skin reactions
- Hypotension
- Nausea and vomiting
- Transient electrocardiogram changes (including ventricular arrhythmias)
- Transient increases in serum liver enzyme levels

(infection in the blood), as well as lower respiratory tract, skin and skin-structure, intra-abdominal, and gynecologic infections (see Sidebar: *Adverse Reactions to Monobactams*).

Fluoroquinolones

Common Drug Names

alatrofloxacin: Trovafloxacin, Trovan
ciprofloxacin: Ciloxan, Cipro
enoxacin: Penetrex
gatifloxacin: Tequin
levofloxacin: Levaquin
lomefloxacin: Maxaquin
moxifloxacin: ABC Pack, Avelox
norfloxacin: Apo-Norflox, Noroxin, Riva-Norfloxacin
ofloxacin: Floxin, Ocuflox
sparfloxacin: Zagam
trovafloxacin: Trovan

Fluoroquinolones are structurally similar synthetic antibiotics. They are primarily administered to treat UTIs as well as upper respiratory infections, pneumonia, and gonorrhea.

Pharmacokinetics

Fluoroquinolones are absorbed well after oral administration. Fluoroquinolones are minimally metabolized in the liver and are excreted primarily in the urine. Sparfloxacin is excreted equally in the urine and feces; trovafloxacin is primarily eliminated in feces.

Pharmacodynamics

Fluoroquinolones work by interrupting deoxyribonucleic acid (DNA) synthesis during bacterial replication. As a result, the bacteria are prevented from replicating.

Pharmacotherapeutics

Fluoroquinolones can be used to treat a wide variety of infections. Some drugs in this class also have specific indications. Ciprofloxacin is used to treat lower respiratory tract infections, infectious diarrhea, and skin, bone, or joint infections. Trovafloxacin mesylate and its intravenous form, alatrofloxacin mesylate, are used to treat community- and hospital-acquired pneumonia, sinusitis, gonorrhea, and complicated diabetic foot ulcers. Sparfloxacin is used to treat bronchitis and community-acquired pneumonia. Lomefloxacin also is used to treat lower respiratory tract infections and to prevent UTIs in patients who are undergoing procedures through the urethra (the tube from the bladder to the outside of the body). Ofloxacin is used to treat selected sexually transmitted diseases, lower respiratory infections, skin and skin-structure infections, and prostatitis (inflammation of the prostate gland). Levofloxacin is also indicated for treatment of lower respiratory infections (see Sidebar: *Adverse Reactions to Fluoroquinolones*).

Adverse Reactions to Fluoroquinolones

Well tolerated by most patients, fluoroquinolones produce few adverse reactions but may produce:

- Nausea
- Vomiting
- Diarrhea
- Abdominal pain

Sulfonamides

Common Drug Names

co-trimoxazole (sulfamethoxazole and trimethoprim): Bactrim, Septra DS, SMX-TMP, Sulfatrim

sulfadiazine: Alti-Sulfasalazine, Azulfidine, Salazopyrin, S.A.S.

sulfamethoxazole: Apo-Sulfamethoxazole, Gantanol (discontinued in the U.S.)

sulfisoxazole: Gantrisin, Sulfizole, Truxazole

Sulfonamides were the first effective systemic antibacterial drugs.

Pharmacokinetics

Most sulfonamides are absorbed well and distributed widely in the body. They are metabolized in the liver to inactive metabolites and are excreted by the kidneys.

Pharmacodynamics

Sulfonamides are bacteriostatic drugs that prevent the growth of microorganisms.

Pharmacotherapeutics

Sulfonamides are frequently used to treat acute UTIs. Sulfonamides also are used to treat infections caused by a wide variety of bacteria (see Sidebar: *Adverse Reactions to Sulfonamides*).

Nitrofurantoin

Common Drug Names

nitrofurantoin: Apo-Nitrofurantoin, Furadantin, Macrobid, Macrodantin

Nitrofurantoin is used primarily to treat acute and chronic UTIs.

Pharmacokinetics

After oral administration, nitrofurantoin is absorbed rapidly and well from the GI tract. Nitrofurantoin is partially metabolized by the liver, and 30% to 50% is excreted unchanged in the urine.

Pharmacodynamics

Usually bacteriostatic (slowing growth), nitrofurantoin may become bactericidal (killing the bacteria), depending on its urinary concentration and the susceptibility of the infecting organisms.

Pharmacotherapeutics

Because the absorbed drug concentrates in the urine, nitrofurantoin is used to treat UTIs. It has a higher antibacterial activity in acid urine. Nitrofurantoin is not effective against systemic bacterial infections (see Sidebar: *Adverse Reactions to Nitrofurantoin*).

Adverse Reactions to Sulfonamides

Excessively high doses of less water-soluble sulfonamides can produce crystals in the urine and deposits of sulfonamide crystals in the renal tubules. This complication is not a problem with the newer water-soluble sulfonamides. Hypersensitivity reactions may occur and appear to increase as the dosage increases.

A reaction that resembles serum sickness may occur, producing fever, joint pain, hives, bronchospasm, and leukopenia (reduced white blood cell count). Sulfonamides also can produce photosensitivity.

Adverse Reactions to Nitrofurantoin

Adverse reactions to nitrofurantoin include:
- GI irritation
- Anorexia
- Nausea
- Vomiting
- Diarrhea
- Dark yellow or brown urine
- Abdominal pain
- Chills
- Fever
- Joint pain
- Anaphylaxis
- Hypersensitivity reactions involving the skin, lungs, blood, and liver

MASSAGE IMPLICATIONS AND ASSESSMENT

Any antibacterial drug given by the parenteral route presents a local contraindication for massage. The actions of the antibacterial drugs do not affect the way the body receives and responds to massage. There is no contraindication to massage just because a client is taking an antibacterial drug. However, the type, location, and severity of infection; the toxicity of the antibacterial drug; and the client's general condition must be taken into account. It is the client's condition that contraindicates massage in some cases. The side effects of antibacterials are most commonly nausea, vomiting, and diarrhea. The more severe adverse effects are always cause for concern. Massage is contraindicated, and these effects should be reported to a physician immediately. In a case of severe infection, a physician's consent for massage must be obtained.

A good rule to use when deciding whether to massage a client with any infection is as follows. If the client is in control of the infection, then perform massage; if the infection is in control of the client (severe symptoms that are affecting functioning), then do not perform massage.

Antiviral Drugs

Antiviral drugs are used to prevent or treat viral infections. Major antiviral drugs used to treat systemic infections include:

- acyclovir
- amantadine hydrochloride
- didanosine
- famciclovir
- foscarnet
- ganciclovir
- nelfinavir
- zalcitabine
- zidovudine

Antiherpesvirus Drugs

Common Drug Names

acyclovir: Apo-Acyclovir, Avirax, Zovirax
famciclovir: Famvir
ganciclovir: Cytovene, Vitrasert
valacyclovir: Valtrex

Acyclovir sodium, an antiherpesvirus drug, is an effective antiviral drug that causes minimal toxicity to cells. A derivative of acyclovir, ganciclovir has potent antiviral activity against herpes simplex virus (HSV) and cytomegalovirus (CMV).

Famciclovir is a prodrug (a precursor of a drug) that undergoes rapid change to the active antiviral compound penciclovir. It enters viral cells (HSV types 1 and 2 and varicella zoster), where it inhibits viral replication.

Pharmacokinetics

Each of these antiherpesvirus drugs travels its own route through the body. When given orally, absorption of acyclovir is slow and only 15% to 30% complete. It is distributed throughout the body and metabolized primarily inside the infected cells; the majority of the drug is excreted in the urine. Ganciclovir is administered intravenously because it is absorbed poorly from the GI tract. More than 90% of ganciclovir is not metabolized and is excreted unchanged by the kidneys. Famciclovir is extensively metabolized in the liver and excreted in urine.

Pharmacodynamics

To be effective, acyclovir and ganciclovir must be metabolized to their active forms in cells infected by the herpesvirus. Acyclovir enters virus-infected cells, where it is changed through a series of steps to acyclovir triphosphate. Acyclovir disrupts viral replication. On entry into CMV-infected cells, ganciclovir is converted to ganciclovir triphosphate, which also disrupts viral replication and growth.

Pharmacotherapeutics

Acyclovir is used to treat infection caused by herpes viruses. Oral acyclovir is used primarily to treat initial and recurrent genital herpes infections. Intravenous acyclovir is used to treat severe initial herpes in patients with normal immune systems, initial and recurrent skin and mucus membrane herpes infections in immunocompromised patients, herpes zoster infections (shingles), disseminated varicella-zoster virus in immunocompromised patients, and varicella infections (chickenpox) in immunocompromised patients.

Ganciclovir is used to treat CMV retinitis in immunocompromised patients, including those with acquired immune deficiency syndrome (AIDS) and other infections such as encephalitis.

Famciclovir is used to treat acute herpes zoster and recurrent genital herpes.

MASSAGE IMPLICATIONS AND ASSESSMENT

Because the antiviral drugs are most often given by mouth, there is no concern regarding absorption and massage. The actions of these drugs are directly on the virus-infected cells and do not affect massage strokes. The client's condition (severity of symptoms) may contraindicate massage, as will the presence of open skin lesions.

Adverse Reactions to Antiherpesvirus Drugs

Treatment with each of these antiherpesvirus drugs may lead to particular adverse reactions.

Acyclovir
Reversible kidney impairment may occur with rapid intravenous injection or infusion of acyclovir. Common reactions to oral acyclovir include headache, nausea, vomiting, and diarrhea. Hypersensitivity reactions may also occur with both IV and oral acyclovir.

Ganciclovir
The most common adverse reactions to ganciclovir are granulocytopenia and thrombocytopenia.

Famciclovir
Common adverse reactions to famciclovir include headache and nausea.

Adverse Reactions to Foscarnet

Adverse reactions to foscarnet may include:

- Fatigue, depression, fever, confusion, headache, numbness and tingling, dizziness, and seizures
- Nausea and vomiting, diarrhea, and abdominal pain
- Granulocytopenia and leukopenia
- Involuntary muscle contractions, neuropathy
- Difficulty breathing
- Rash
- Altered kidney function

Side Effects

Headache is a common side effect of these drugs and may be helped by gentle, relaxing massage of the face and scalp. Other adverse effects must be referred to a physician and massage withheld (see Sidebar: *Adverse Reactions to Antiherpesvirus Drugs*).

Foscarnet

Common Drug Names

foscarnet: Foscavir

The antiviral drug foscarnet is used to treat CMV retinitis in patients with AIDS. It is also used to treat acyclovir-resistant HSV infections in immunocompromised patients.

Pharmacokinetics

The majority of foscarnet is excreted unchanged in the urine in patients with normal renal function.

Pharmacodynamics

Foscarnet prevents viral replication and growth.

Pharmacotherapeutics

The primary therapeutic use of foscarnet is treatment of retinitis (eye infections) in patients with AIDS.

MASSAGE IMPLICATIONS AND ASSESSMENT

The action of foscarnet will not affect the action of massage strokes. The client's condition may require changes in massage protocol.

Side Effects

Common side effects of foscarnet are fatigue, dizziness, and neuropathies. Neuropathies contraindicate deep tissue massage. Fatigue and dizziness can be relieved by using more stimulating strokes and more rapid systemic reflex strokes such as effleurage (see Sidebar: *Adverse Reactions to Foscarnet*).

Amantadine, Rimantadine, and Influenza (Flu) Drugs

Common Drug Names

amantadine: Antadine, Endantadine, Symadine (discontinued in the U.S.), Symmetrel
oseltamivir: Tamiflu
rimantadine: Flumadine
zanamivir: Relenza

Amantadine and its derivative rimantadine hydrochloride are used to prevent or treat influenza A infections as well as other viral infections. Newer drugs that can treat both influenza A and B are zanamivir and oseltamivir.

Pharmacokinetics

After oral administration, amantadine and rimantadine are absorbed well in the GI tract and distributed widely throughout the body. Amantadine is eliminated primarily in the urine; rimantadine is extensively metabolized and then excreted in urine. Zanamivir is inhaled directly into the lungs, and oseltamivir is given orally.

Pharmacodynamics

Although the exact mechanism of action of amantadine is unknown, the drug appears to inhibit an early stage of viral replication. Rimantadine inhibits viral replication.

Pharmacotherapeutics

Amantadine and rimantadine are used to prevent and treat respiratory tract infections caused by strains of the influenza A virus. They can reduce the severity and duration of fever and other symptoms in patients already infected with influenza A. They also protect patients undergoing immunization during the 2 weeks needed for immunity to develop or patients who cannot receive the influenza vaccine because of hypersensitivity. Amantadine is also used to treat Parkinsonism and drug-induced extrapyramidal reactions (abnormal involuntary movements). Both amantadine and rimantadine can be used to treat hepatitis B and C.

The newer drugs zanamivir and oseltamivir, when taken within 2 days of onset of flu symptoms, lessen severity of symptoms and the length of the illness by 1 to 3 days.

MASSAGE IMPLICATIONS AND ASSESSMENT

Neither amantadine nor rimantadine affect massage stroke actions on the body. The client's condition is more of a deciding factor regarding changes to massage protocols.

Side Effects

The common side effects of concern to the massage therapist are fatigue, depression, nervousness, and insomnia. The first two are approached by the therapist with a somewhat more stimulating massage, especially using systemic reflex strokes. The second two are approached by using slow, less stimulating systemic reflex strokes. A good evaluation of the client's symptoms is required here (see Sidebar: *Adverse Reactions to Amantadine, Rimantadine, and Influenza Drugs*).

Ribavirin

Common Drug Names

ribavirin: Rebetol, Tribavirin, Virazole

ribaviron and interferon: Rebetron

Ribavirin currently is available only to treat respiratory syncytial virus (RSV) infections in children.

Special Note: The combination drug Rebetron (ribavirin and interferon) is used to treat hepatitis C. It is administered by aerosol inhalation only.

Pharmacokinetics

Ribavirin is administered by nasal or oral inhalation and is absorbed well. It has a limited, specific distribution, with the highest concentration level found in the respiratory tract and in red blood cells (RBCs). Ribavirin is metabolized in the liver and by RBCs. It is excreted primarily by the kidneys, with some excreted in the feces.

Pharmacodynamics

The mechanism of action of ribavirin is not known completely, but the drug's metabolites inhibit viral DNA and RNA synthesis, subsequently halting viral replication.

Pharmacotherapeutics

Ribavirin therapy is used to treat severe lower respiratory tract infections in infants and young children.

MASSAGE IMPLICATIONS AND ASSESSMENT

The action of this drug does not interfere with massage stroke responses in the body. The client's condition may, however, require changes in massage protocols.

Side Effects

Hypotension is a side effect of ribavirin. The massage therapist needs to be aware of this and stimulate the client at the end of the massage with tapotement and/or rapid effleurage. Using care when getting the client off the table is important (see Sidebar: *Adverse Reactions to Ribavirin*).

Nucleoside Reverse Transcriptase Inhibitors

Common Drug Names

abacavir: Ziagen

didanosine: Videx

zalcitabine: Dideoxycytidine, Hivid

zidovudine: Apo-Zidovudine, AZT, Retrovir

Didanosine, abacavir, and zalcitabine are nucleoside reverse transcriptase inhibitors (NRTIs) used in the treatment of advanced human immunodeficiency virus (HIV) infections. Zidovudine, another NRTI, was the first drug to receive Food and Drug Administration approval for treating AIDS or AIDS-related complex.

Pharmacokinetics

Each of the NRTIs has its own pharmacokinetic properties. Zidovudine is absorbed well from the GI tract, distributed widely throughout the body, metabolized by the liver, and excreted by the kidneys. The exact route of metabolism is not fully understood. Approximately half of an absorbed dose is excreted in the urine. Oral zalcitabine is absorbed well from the GI tract when administered on an empty stomach. Absorption is reduced when the drug is given with food. Abacavir is rapidly and extensively absorbed after oral administration. Abacavir is metabolized by the enzymes and primarily excreted in the urine with the remainder excreted in feces. Didanosine is poorly absorbed in the stomach. Absorption is increased in its buffered forms. It is excreted in urine.

Pharmacodynamics

NRTIs must undergo conversion to their active metabolites to produce their action. Zidovudine is converted by cellular enzymes to an active form, zidovudine triphosphate, which prevents HIV (the virus that causes AIDS) from replicating (Fig. 10-2). Didanosine and zalcitabine undergo cellular enzyme conversion to their active antiviral metabolites to block the replication of HIV. Abacavir is converted to an active metabolite that inhibits viral replication.

Pharmacotherapeutics

NRTIs are used in the treatment of HIV and AIDS. Intravenous zidovudine is used to help patients who are hospitalized and unable to take oral medication. It is also used to prevent transmission of HIV from mother to fetus and to treat AIDS-related dementia. Oral zidovudine is used as part of a multidrug regimen for treating HIV infection. Didanosine is an alternative initial treatment of HIV infection. Zalcitabine and abacavir are used in combination with other antiretroviral agents to treat HIV infection.

MASSAGE IMPLICATIONS AND ASSESSMENT

The actions of these drugs do not affect how the body receives and responds to the various massage strokes. Nevertheless, the client's condition may necessitate changes in massage protocol.

Side Effects

Side effects of concern to the massage therapist are headache, dizziness, muscle pain, fatigue, and peripheral neuropathies. Deep tissue massage is not used in the presence of neuropathy. Changes in the massage application depend on the symptoms the client is experiencing that day. If fatigue and dizziness are present, a shorter session may be needed and/or a slightly more stimulating massage with systemic reflex strokes may help to balance out the effects of medication (see Sidebar: *Adverse Reactions to Nucleoside Reverse Transcriptase Inhibitors*).

Adverse Reactions to Nucleoside Reverse Transcriptase Inhibitors

Each of the nucleoside reverse transcriptase inhibitors (NRTIs) can cause adverse reactions.

Zidovudine

- Blood-related reactions
- Headache and dizziness
- Muscle pain, fever, and rash
- Nausea, vomiting, abdominal pain, diarrhea

Didanosine

- Diarrhea, nausea, vomiting, abdominal pain, constipation, stomatitis, unusual taste or loss of taste, dry mouth, pancreatitis
- Headache, peripheral neuropathy, dizziness
- Muscle weakness, rash, itching, muscle pain, hair loss

Zalcitabine

- Peripheral neuropathy, mouth ulcers, nausea, rash, headache, muscle pain, fatigue

Abacavir

- Potentially fatal hypersensitivity reactions

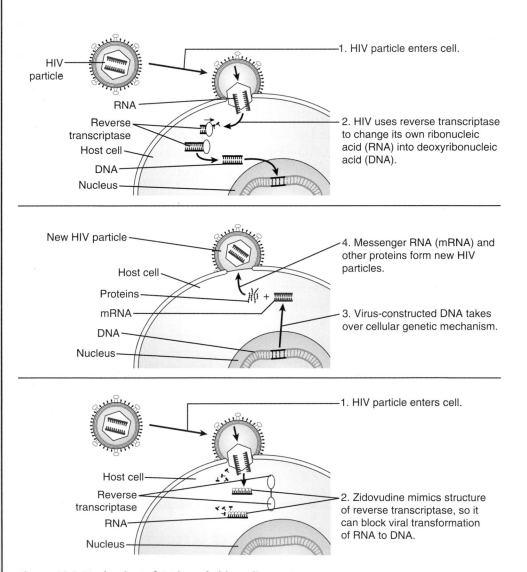

Figure 10-2 Mechanism of Action of Zidovudine. Zidovudine can inhibit replication of human immunodeficiency virus (HIV). The first two illustrations show how HIV invades cells and then replicates itself. The bottom illustration shows how zidovudine blocks viral transformation.

Protease Inhibitors

Common Drug Names

indinavir: Crixivan

nelfinavir: Viracept

ritonavir: Norvir

saquinavir: Fortovase, Invirase

Protease inhibitors are drugs that act against an enzyme, HIV protease, to prevent the enzyme from dividing a larger viral precursor protein into the active smaller enzymes the virus needs to mature fully. The result is an immature, noninfectious cell.

Pharmacokinetics

Protease inhibitors may have different pharmacokinetic properties. Saquinavir and saquinavir mesylate are poorly absorbed from the GI tract. They are widely distributed, metabolized by the liver, and excreted mainly by the kidneys. Ritonavir is well absorbed, metabolized by the liver, and broken down into at least five metabolites. It is mainly excreted in the feces, with some elimination through the kidneys. Indinavir is rapidly absorbed. The drug is excreted mainly through feces. Nelfinavir's bioavailability (the degree to which it becomes available to target tissue after administration) is not determined. Food increases its absorption. It is metabolized in the liver and excreted primarily in the feces.

Pharmacodynamics

All these drugs inhibit the growth and replication of HIV.

Pharmacotherapeutics

Protease inhibitors are indicated for use in combination with other drugs for treatment of HIV infection.

MASSAGE IMPLICATIONS AND ASSESSMENT

The action of these drugs is on the virus itself and does not affect how the body receives and responds to massage.

Side Effects

Some of the side effects of the protease inhibitors that are of concern to the massage therapist are fatigue, headache, acid reflux, dizziness, and insomnia. Each presents a different problem that could be encountered during a massage session. Fatigue and dizziness are balanced with a slightly more stimulating massage using systemic reflex strokes and stimulating massage. Headache can be helped with face and scalp massage. Reflux may require different positioning, and insomnia can be addressed using systemic reflex strokes applied very slowly and rhythmically (rocking and effleurage). The massage therapist has the opportunity to be very ingenious in approaching the massage and meeting the needs of the client (see Sidebar: *Adverse Reactions to Protease Inhibitors*).

Antitubercular Drugs

Common Drug Names

ethambutol: Etibi, Myambutol

isoniazid: Isotamine, Nydrazid

pyrazinamide: Tebrazid

rifampin: Rifadin, Rimactane, Rofact

Antitubercular drugs are used to treat tuberculosis (TB), which is caused by *Mycobacterium tuberculosis*. Not always curative, these drugs can halt the progression of a mycobacterial infection. Unlike most antibiotics, antitubercular drugs may need to be administered over many months. This creates problems, such as patient noncompliance, development of bacterial resistance, and drug toxicity.

Traditionally, isoniazid, rifampin, and ethambutol were the mainstays of multidrug TB therapy and successfully prevented the emergence of drug resistance. Because of the current incidence of drug-resistant TB strains, however, a four-drug regimen is now recommended for initial treatment. A newer drug, rifapentine, is a longer acting drug that is sometimes being used in place of rifampin.

Antitubercular drugs should be modified if local testing shows resistance to one or more of them. If local outbreaks of TB resistant to isoniazid and rifampin are occurring in institutions (e.g., health care or correctional facilities), then five-drug or six-drug regimens are recommended as initial therapy.

Pharmacokinetics

Most antitubercular drugs are administered orally. When administered orally, these drugs are absorbed well from the GI tract and distributed widely throughout the body. They are metabolized primarily in the liver and excreted by the kidneys.

Pharmacodynamics

Antitubercular drugs are specific for mycobacteria. At usual doses, ethambutol and isoniazid are tuberculostatic, meaning they inhibit the growth of *M. tuberculosis*. In contrast, rifampin is tuberculocidal and destroys the mycobacteria. Because bacterial resistance to isoniazid and rifampin can develop rapidly, they should always be used with other antitubercular drugs.

The exact mechanism of ethambutol remains unclear, but it may stop multiplication and cause cell death. Ethambutol acts only against replicating bacteria. Although isoniazid's exact mechanism of action is not known, it is believed that the drug disrupts the cell wall, thus stopping replication. Only replicating, not resting, bacteria appear to be inhibited.

Rifampin inhibits RNA synthesis in susceptible organisms. The drug is effective primarily in replicating bacteria but may have some effect on resting bacteria as well. The exact mechanism of action of pyrazinamide is not known, but the antimycobacterial activity appears to be linked to the drug's conversion to the active metabolite pyrazinoic acid. Pyrazinoic acid, in turn, creates an acidic environment.

Pharmacotherapeutics

Isoniazid usually is used with ethambutol, rifampin, or streptomycin. This is because combination therapy for TB and other mycobacterial infections can prevent or delay the development of resistance. Ethambutol is used with isoniazid and rifampin to treat patients with uncomplicated pulmonary TB.

Although isoniazid is the most important drug for treating TB, bacterial resistance develops rapidly if it is used alone. However, resistance does not pose a problem when isoniazid is used alone to *prevent* TB in individuals who have been exposed to the disease, and no evidence exists of cross-resistance between isoniazid and other antitubercular drugs. Isoniazid is typically given orally, but may be given intravenously if necessary.

Rifampin is a first-line drug for treating pulmonary TB with other antitubercular drugs. Pyrazinamide is currently recommended as a first-line TB drug in combination with ethambutol, rifampin, and isoniazid. Pyrazinamide is a highly specific drug that is active only against *M. tuberculosis*. Resistance to pyrazinamide may develop rapidly when pyrazinamide is used alone.

MASSAGE IMPLICATIONS AND ASSESSMENT

The action of the antitubercular drugs does not affect the application of massage strokes.

Side Effects

There are several side effects of these drugs that need to be addressed by the massage therapist. These are headache, dizziness, cramps, and flatulence as well as peripheral neuropathies. Deep tissue massage is contraindicated with peripheral neuropathies. Abdominal massage can help cramping and gas. If dizziness is present, care needs to be taken when the client is changing positions and getting off the massage table (see Sidebar: *Adverse Reactions to Antitubercular Drugs*).

Antimycotic Drugs

Common Drug Names

amphotericin B

flucytosine

fluconazole

Adverse Reactions to Antitubercular Drugs

Ethambutol
- Itching
- Joint pain
- GI distress
- Malaise
- Leukopenia
- Headache
- Dizziness
- Numbness
- Tingling of the extremities
- Confusion

  Although rare, hypersensitivity reactions to ethambutol may produce rash and fever. Anaphylaxis may also occur.

Isoniazid
Peripheral neuropathy is the most common adverse reaction.

Rifampin
The most common adverse reactions include:
- Epigastric pain
- Nausea
- Vomiting
- Abdominal cramps
- Flatulence
- Anorexia
- Diarrhea

Pyrazinamide
Liver toxicity is the major limiting adverse reaction. GI disturbances include nausea, vomiting, and anorexia.

functioning, which has the opposite effect and interferes with physiologic functions) that acts as an antimycotic (suppressing the growth of fungi). It is used primarily with another antimycotic drug, such as amphotericin B, to treat systemic fungal infections.

Pharmacokinetics

After oral administration, flucytosine is absorbed well from the GI tract and distributed widely. It undergoes little metabolism and is excreted primarily by the kidneys.

Pharmacodynamics

Flucytosine penetrates fungal cells, where it is converted to its active metabolite fluorouracil. Fluorouracil causes cell death.

Pharmacotherapeutics

Although amphotericin B is effective in treating candidal and cryptococcal meningitis alone, flucytosine is given with it to reduce the dosage and the risk of toxicity. This combination therapy is the treatment of choice for cryptococcal meningitis. Flucytosine can be used alone to treat lower urinary tract *Candida* infections because it reaches a high urinary concentration.

Adverse Reactions to Flucytosine

Flucytosine may produce unpredictable adverse reactions, including:
- Confusion
- Headache
- Drowsiness
- Vertigo
- Hallucinations
- Difficulty breathing
- Respiratory arrest
- Rash
- Nausea
- Vomiting
- Abdominal distention
- Diarrhea
- Anorexia

MASSAGE IMPLICATIONS AND ASSESSMENT

The action of flucytosine does not affect the application of massage.

Side Effects

Headache, drowsiness, and vertigo are common side effects of flucytosine. The massage therapist can help the client by taking care when he or she is changing positions and getting off the table, as well as by stimulating the client at the end of the massage (see Sidebar: *Adverse Reactions to Flucytosine*).

Itraconazole

Common Drug Names

itraconazole: Sporanox

Itraconazole belongs to a class of drugs known as the synthetic triazoles. It inhibits the synthesis of ergosterol, a vital component of fungal cell membranes.

Pharmacokinetics

Oral bioavailability is maximal when itraconazole is taken with food. It is extensively metabolized in the liver into a large number of metabolites. It is excreted in the feces.

Pharmacodynamics

Itraconazole interferes with fungal wall synthesis, making the fungus susceptible to the body's immune system.

Pharmacotherapeutics

Itraconazole is used to treat a wide variety of fungal infections.

MASSAGE IMPLICATIONS AND ASSESSMENT

Itraconazole does not interfere with the response of the body to massage.

Side Effects

Dizziness can be a side effect of this drug. Care should be taken with changes of position for the massage client taking this drug (see Sidebar: *Adverse Reactions to Itraconazole*).

Adverse Reactions to Itraconazole

- Dizziness
- Headache
- Hypertension
- Impaired liver function

Ketoconazole

Common Drug Names

ketoconazole: Apo-Ketoconazole, Nizoral

Ketoconazole is an effective oral antimycotic drug with a broad spectrum of activity.

Pharmacokinetics

When given orally, ketoconazole is absorbed variably and distributed widely. It undergoes extensive liver metabolism and is excreted through the bile and feces.

Pharmacodynamics

Within the fungal cells, ketoconazole damages the cell membrane. This inhibits cell growth. Ketoconazole usually produces fungistatic effects but also can produce fungicidal effects under certain conditions.

Pharmacotherapeutics

Ketoconazole is used to treat topical and systemic infections caused by susceptible fungi, which include dermatophytes and most other fungi.

MASSAGE IMPLICATIONS AND ASSESSMENT

Ketoconazole doe not interfere with the body's response to massage.

Side Effects

Ketoconazole has no side effects of concern to the massage therapist. Any adverse reactions must be reported to the physician and massage withheld (see Sidebar: *Adverse Reactions to Ketoconazole*).

Nystatin

Common Drug Names

nystatin: Bio-Statin, Candistatin, Mycostatin, Nilstat, Nyaderm, Nystat-Rx

Nystatin is used only topically or orally to treat local fungal infections because it is extremely toxic when administered parenterally.

Pharmacokinetics

Oral nystatin undergoes little or no absorption, distribution, or metabolism. It is excreted unchanged in the feces. Topical nystatin is not absorbed through the skin or mucous membranes.

Pharmacodynamics

Nystatin can act as a fungicidal or fungistatic drug, depending on the organism present.

Pharmacotherapeutics

Nystatin is used primarily to treat fungal skin infections. The drug is effective for candidal infections. Topical nystatin is used to treat skin or mucous membrane candidal infections, such as oral thrush, diaper rash, vaginal and vulvar candidiasis, and candidiasis between skin folds. Oral nystatin is used to treat GI infections.

MASSAGE IMPLICATIONS AND ASSESSMENT

Topical nystatin is a local contraindication for massage because of absorption and localized infection. The action of the drug, however, does not affect the application of massage strokes.

Side Effects

There are no side effects of concern to the massage practitioner regarding nystatin. Any adverse effects must be reported to the physician and massage withheld (see Sidebar: *Adverse Reactions to Nystatin*).

Antimalarial and Antiprotozoal Drugs

Malaria is a protozoal infection of the genus *Plasmodium* that produces severe chills, fever, and profuse sweating. Malaria is transmitted by the bite of the infected female Anopheles mosquito.

Antimalarial Drugs

Common Drug Names

chloroquine: Aralen, Chlorquin

hydroxychloroquine: Plaquenil

mefloquine: Lariam

primaquine: Prymaccone

pyrimethamine: Daraprim

quinidine: Biquin Durules, Cardioquin (discontinued in the U.S.), Cin-Quin, Kinidin Durules, Quinaglute, Quinalan (discontinued in the U.S.), Quinate (discontinued in the U.S.)

(Note: Sulfonamides, sulfones, and tetracyclines also may be used in combination with these drugs.)

Pharmacokinetics

After oral administration, antimalarial drugs are absorbed well and distributed widely throughout the body. The extent of metabolism among these drugs varies, and excretion occurs primarily in the urine.

Pharmacodynamics

The actions of these antimalarial drugs vary. Chloroquine and hydroxychloroquine are believed to destroy parasites. Other antimalarial drugs have similar actions. Quinine's antimalarial action may result from its incorporation into the DNA of the parasite, rendering it ineffective. Its action also may result from depression of oxygen uptake and carbohydrate metabolism in the parasite. In addition, quinine acts as a skeletal muscle relaxant, a local anesthetic, an antipyretic, and an analgesic, thus relieving malarial symptoms. The exact mechanism of mefloquine's antimalarial effects remains unknown. Because it is a structural analog of quinine, it may have similar pharmacodynamic effects.

Pharmacotherapeutics

The effectiveness of each antimalarial drug toward different strains of malaria varies. Chloroquine remains the oral drug of choice to prevent and treat all malaria strains, except chloroquine-resistant or multidrug-resistant strains. Hydroxychloroquine is an alternative when chloroquine is not available. For treatment of malaria caused by chloroquine-resistant or multidrug-resistant strains, quinine is the drug of choice and is given with slower-acting antimalarial drugs. Primaquine is the drug of choice in combination with chloroquine to treat several strains of malaria. Mefloquine is used to treat malaria caused by resistant strains. It is also administered to prevent malaria infections. Quinidine is the parenteral drug of choice for the treatment of malaria in patients who cannot tolerate oral therapy.

MASSAGE IMPLICATIONS AND ASSESSMENT

The actions of these drugs are directly on the parasite that infects the blood. They do not affect the response of the body to the various massage strokes.

Side Effects

Cramps, muscle pain, and fatigue are side effects of antimalarial drugs. The massage therapist can assist the client in dealing with these side effects by using gentle mechanical local strokes and systemic reflex strokes (see Sidebar: *Adverse Reactions to Antimalarial Drugs*).

Other Antiprotozoal Drugs

Common Drug Names

atovaquone: Malarone, Mepron

furazolidone: Furoxone

Iodoquinol: Diodoquin, Diquinol, Yodoxin

metronidazole: Apo-Metronidazole, Flagyl, Metro-Gel, Nidagel, Noritate

pentamidine: NebuPent, Pentacarinat, Pertam

trimetrexate: Neutrexin

Although many other drugs are used to treat protozoal infections, few are readily obtainable. The most frequently used is metronidazole. Amphotericin B, paromomycin, and co-trimoxazole are also sometimes used as antiprotozoals.

Pharmacokinetics

These antiprotozoal drugs may have differing pharmacokinetic properties. After oral administration, the absorption of atovaquone varies. The bioavailability increases approximately threefold when it is administered with meals. Atovaquone is not metabolized and is excreted primarily in the feces. Iodoquinol is poorly absorbed; however, it exerts its effects locally in the lower GI tract. Its metabolism is unknown, and it is excreted primarily in the feces. The absorption of pentamidine is limited after aerosol administration; however, it is absorbed well after intramuscular administration. Its metabolism is unknown, and it is excreted unchanged in the urine. After oral administration, furazolidone is absorbed poorly and is inactivated in the intestine. Approximately 5% of an oral dose of furazolidone is excreted in the urine as unchanged drug and metabolites. The majority of a metronidazole dose is absorbed after oral administration. It is distributed widely, is metabolized partially in the liver, and is excreted in the urine and, to a lesser degree, in the feces.

Pharmacodynamics

Antiprotozoal drugs produce their effects through various actions. Atovaquone is thought to inhibit protozoal growth and replication. Furazolidone kills bacteria and protozoa. Iodoquinol is a contact amebicide that acts directly to kill protozoa in the GI tract. Metronidazole destroys bacteria, amoebas, and *Trichomonas*. Pentamidine and trimetrexate cause cell death. Trimetrexate must be administered concurrently with folinic acid to protect the patient's normal cells.

Pharmacotherapeutics

Antiprotozoal drugs are used for a wide range of disorders caused by single-celled parasitic animals invading many parts of the body.

MASSAGE IMPLICATIONS AND ASSESSMENT

The action of the antiprotozoal drugs does not affect the application of massage strokes. Local contraindications for massage exist for parenteral injections or topical applications of the drugs.

Side Effects

Constipation is a side effect of antiprotozoal drugs. The massage practitioner can address this with abdominal massage (see Sidebar: *Adverse Reactions to Antiprotozoal Drugs*).

Adverse Reactions to Antiprotozoal Drugs

Antiprotozoal drugs may result in a variety of adverse reactions.

Atovaquone
- Rash
- Nausea and vomiting
- Diarrhea
- Headache
- Fever
- Cough

Furazolidone
- Nausea and vomiting

Iodoquinol
- Anorexia
- Vomiting
- Diarrhea
- Abdominal cramps
- Constipation
- Itching around the anus

Pentamidine
- Kidney toxicity
- Pain or hardness at the injection site
- Elevated liver function test results
- Leukopenia (reduced white blood cell count)
- Nausea
- Anorexia
- Bronchospasm and cough

Quick Quiz

1. Your client tells you she is taking Bactrim for a UTI for the past 3 days. She states she has some frequency still but no other symptoms and has experienced no side effects from the drug. What should you do?

2. A new client comes to see you. In the health history he indicates that he has TB and has been taking the standard four-drug treatment of isoniazid, rifampin, pyrazinamide, and ethambutol for the past 2 months. He has returned to work but gets fatigued easily and has a little shortness of breath on exertion. Should you give massage?

3. A client has a fungal skin infection being treated with topical nystatin. The rash is under the breasts, on the abdomen, and in the groin area. Can you give massage?

Anti-Inflammatory Drugs, Anti-Allergy Drugs, and Immunosuppressants

11

Drugs and the Immune System

Immune and inflammatory responses protect the body from invading foreign substances. These responses can be modified by certain classes of drugs. Antihistamines block the effects of histamine on target tissues. Corticosteroids suppress immune responses and reduce inflammation. Noncorticosteroid immunosuppressants prevent rejection of transplanted organs and treat autoimmune diseases. Uricosurics prevent or control the frequency of gouty arthritis attacks.

Antihistamines

Antihistamines primarily act to block histamine effects that occur in an immediate (type I) hypersensitivity reaction, commonly called an allergic reaction. They are available alone or in combination products by prescription or over the counter.

Histamine-1-Receptor Antagonists

Common Drug Names: Ethanolamines

clemastine fumarate: Tavist, Dayhist

dimenhydrinate: Apo-Dimenhydrinate, Calm-X, Dramamine, Gravol, Hydrate, Triptone

diphenhydramine hydrochloride: Acot-Tussin, Alercap, Allerdryl, Benadryl, Dephenadryl, Hydramine

Common Drug Names: Ethylenediamines

pyrilamine maleate

tripelennamine citrate: PBZ

tripelennamine hydrochloride: PBZ-SR, Pelamine, Pyribenzamine

Common Drug Names: Alkylamines

brompheniramine maleate: Colhist Solution, Dimetane, Dimetapp, Lodrane

chlorpheniramine maleate: Aller-Chlor, Chlor-Trimeton, Chlor-Tropolon, (with Tylenol: Coricidin)

dexchlorpheniramine maleate: Polaramine

triprolidine (usually in combination with pseudoephedrine): Actanol, Actifed, Allerfed, Aphedrid, Triacin

Common Drug Names: Phenothiazines

methdilazine hydrochloride

promethazine hydrochloride: Anergan, Phenergan

trimeprazine tartrate: Panectyl (available only in Canada)

Common Drug Names: Piperidines

azatadine maleate: Optimine (with pseudoephedrine), Rynatan, Trinalin

cetirizine: Zyrtec, Zyrtec-D

cyclizine hydrochloride: Marezine (discontinued in the U.S.)

cyproheptadine hydrochloride: Periactin

desloratadine: Clarinex

fexofenadine hydrochloride: Allegra, Allegra-D

loratadine: Alavert, Claritin, Claritin-D, Claritin RediTab

meclizine hydrochloride: Antivert, Bonamine, Bonine, Dramamine II, Meni-D

Common Drug Names: Miscellaneous

azelastine: Astelin (a nasal spray antihistamine)

hydroxyzine hydrochloride: Atarax, Hyzine-50, Restall

hydroxyzine pamoate: Vistacot, Vistaril

The term antihistamine refers to drugs that act as histamine-1 (H_1)-receptor antagonists; that is, they compete with histamine for binding to H_1-receptor sites throughout the body. However, they do not displace histamine already bound to the receptor.

Pharmacokinetics (how drugs circulate)

H_1-receptor antagonists are absorbed well after oral or parenteral administration. Some can also be given rectally. Antihistamines are distributed widely throughout the body and central nervous system (CNS), with the exception of loratadine. Fexofenadine, loratadine, desloratadine, and cetirizine (nonsedating antihistamines) minimally penetrate the blood–brain barrier. Therefore, little of the drug is distributed in the CNS, producing fewer effects there than other antihistamines. Antihistamines are metabolized by liver enzymes and excreted in the urine, with small amounts secreted in breast milk. Fexofenadine, mainly excreted in feces, is an exception.

Pharmacodynamics (how drugs act)

H_1-receptor antagonists compete with histamine for H_1 receptors on effector cells (the cells that cause allergic symptoms), blocking histamine from producing its effects (Fig. 11-1). H_1-receptor antagonists produce their effects by:

- Blocking the action of histamine on the small blood vessels
- Decreasing dilation of arterioles and engorgement of tissues

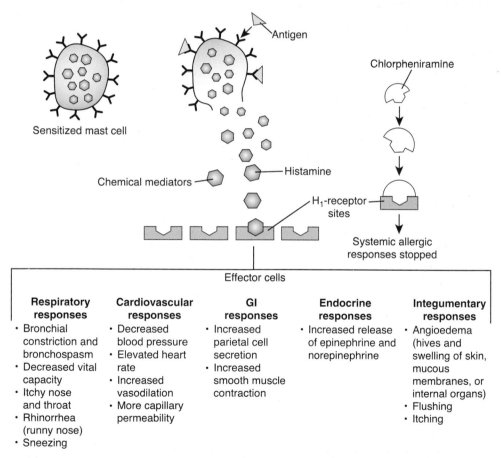

Respiratory responses	Cardiovascular responses	GI responses	Endocrine responses	Integumentary responses
• Bronchial constriction and bronchospasm • Decreased vital capacity • Itchy nose and throat • Rhinorrhea (runny nose) • Sneezing	• Decreased blood pressure • Elevated heart rate • Increased vasodilation • More capillary permeability	• Increased parietal cell secretion • Increased smooth muscle contraction	• Increased release of epinephrine and norepinephrine	• Angioedema (hives and swelling of skin, mucous membranes, or internal organs) • Flushing • Itching

Figure 11-1 Stopping an Allergic Response With Chlorpheniramine. Although chlorpheniramine cannot reverse symptoms of an allergic response, it can stop the progression of the response. When sensitized to an antigen (substance causing an allergic reaction), a mast cell reacts to repeated antigen exposure by releasing chemical mediators. One of these mediators, histamine, binds to histamine-1 (H_1) receptors found on the effector cells (the cells responsible for allergic symptoms). This initiates the allergic response that affects respiratory, cardiovascular, gastrointestinal, endocrine, and integumentary (skin) systems. Chlorpheniramine competes with histamine for H_1-receptor sites on the effector cells. By attaching to these sites first, the drug prevents more histamine from binding to the effector cells and causing further allergic symptoms.

- Reducing the leaking of plasma proteins and fluids out of the capillaries (capillary permeability), thereby lessening edema
- Inhibiting most smooth muscle responses to histamine (in particular, blocking the constriction of bronchial, gastrointestinal [GI], and vascular smooth muscle)
- Relieving symptoms by acting on the terminal nerve endings in the skin that flare and itch when stimulated by histamine
- Suppressing lacrimal and salivary secretion

Several antihistamines have a high affinity for H_1 receptors in the brain and are used for their CNS sedative effects. These drugs include diphenhydramine, dimenhydrinate, promethazine, and various piperidine derivatives.

Pharmacotherapeutics (how drugs are used)

Antihistamines are used to treat the symptoms of type I hypersensitivity reactions, such as allergic rhinitis (runny nose and itchy eyes caused by a local sensitivity reaction), vasomotor rhinitis (rhinitis not caused by allergy or infection), allergic conjunctivitis (inflammation of the membranes of the eye), urticaria (hives), and angioedema (submucosal swelling in the hands, face, and feet).

Antihistamines have other therapeutic uses. Many are used primarily as antiemetics (to control nausea and vomiting). They can also be used as adjunctive therapy to treat an anaphylactic reaction after serious symptoms are controlled. Diphenhydramine can help treat Parkinson's disease and drug-induced extrapyramidal reactions (abnormal involuntary movements). Because of its antiserotonin qualities, cyproheptadine may be used to treat Cushing's disease, serotonin-associated diarrhea, vascular cluster headaches, and anorexia nervosa.

MASSAGE IMPLICATIONS AND ASSESSMENT

H_1-receptor antagonists have multiple actions in the body. If they are given parenterally (by injection), the site of injection should not be massaged for 2 to 4 hours after the injection. Oral administration absorption rates are not affected by massage. These drugs block histamine, decrease blood vessel dilation and permeability, decrease smooth muscle response and nerve sensitivity in the skin, and stop the release of certain endocrine and exocrine substances. In the case of dermatologic symptoms such as hives or rash, massage is contraindicated in the areas affected. Massage strokes mechanically increase the dilation of blood vessels and flow of blood to the tissues; therefore, they could work against the drug actions and exacerbate the symptoms. If the drugs are being used to prevent reactions, to treat respiratory conditions, or to treat other systemic problems, the massage implications are more related to the side effects of the drugs rather than the actions.

Side Effects

Side effects of the H_1-receptor antagonists that are of most concern to the massage therapist are related to CNS depression. Dizziness, lethargy, hypotension, and constipation occur. The massage practitioner needs to take care in getting the client to change positions and should utilize more stimulating systemic strokes, such as rapid effleurage and tapotement, during the massage. In a few cases, hypertension can be an effect of these drugs. Monitoring blood pressure is important. Elevated blood pressure should be reported to a physician and, if severe, no massage should be done (see Sidebar: *Adverse Reactions to H_1-Receptor Antagonists*).

Adverse Reactions to H_1-Receptor Antagonists

Side Effects
- Dizziness
- Lassitude
- Disturbed coordination
- Muscle weakness
- Epigastric distress
- Loss of appetite
- Nausea and vomiting
- Constipation
- Diarrhea
- Dryness of the mouth, nose, and throat
- Hypotension
- Hypertension
- Rapid heart rate

Adverse Effects
- Arrhythmias
- Allergic reactions

Corticosteroids

Corticosteroids suppress immune responses and reduce inflammation. They are available as natural or synthetic steroids. Natural corticosteroids are hormones produced by the adrenal cortex; most corticosteroid drugs are synthetic forms of these hormones. Natural and synthetic corticosteroids are classified according to their biologic activities. Glucocorticoids, such as cortisone acetate and dexamethasone, affect carbohydrate and protein metabolism. Mineralocorticoids, such as aldosterone and fludrocortisone acetate, regulate electrolyte and water balance.

Glucocorticoids

Common Drug Names

beclomethasone: Alti-Beclomethasone, Beconase, Propaderm, QVAR, Vancenase, Vanceril

betamethasone: Alphatrex, Betaderm, Betamethacot, Beta-Val, Betnovate, Prevex, Valisone

cortisone: Compound E, Cortone

dexamethasone: Alti-Dexamethasone, Decadron, Dexacort, Dexasone, Dexone, Hexadrol

hydrocortisone: A-HydroCort, Anusol Suppositories, Cortef, Hydrocortone, Solu-Cortef

methylprednisolone: A-methaPred, Depo-Medrol, Depopred, Medrol, Solu-Medrol

prednisolone: Delta-Cortef, deltacortisone, Orapred, Inflamase Forte, Key-Pred-SP, Pred Forte, Prednicot, Prednisol, Prelone

prednisone: Deltasone, Prednicot, Apo-Prednisone, Sterapred, Winpred *triamcinolone:* Aristocort Forte, Aristospan, Azmacort, Kenalog, Nasacort, Tac-3, Triam Forte, Trinasal

Most glucocorticoids are synthetic analogs of hormones secreted by the adrenal cortex. They exert anti-inflammatory, metabolic, and immunosuppressant effects.

Pharmacokinetics

Glucocorticoids are absorbed well when administered orally. After intramuscular administration, they are absorbed completely. Glucocorticoids are metabolized in the liver and excreted by the kidneys.

Pharmacodynamics

Glucocorticoids suppress hypersensitivity and immune responses through a process that is not entirely understood. Glucocorticoids suppress the redness, edema, heat, and tenderness associated with the inflammatory response (Fig. 11-2).

Pharmacotherapeutics

In addition to their use as replacement therapy for patients with adrenocortical insufficiency, glucocorticoids are prescribed for immunosuppression and reduction of inflammation as well as for their effects on the blood and lymphatic systems.

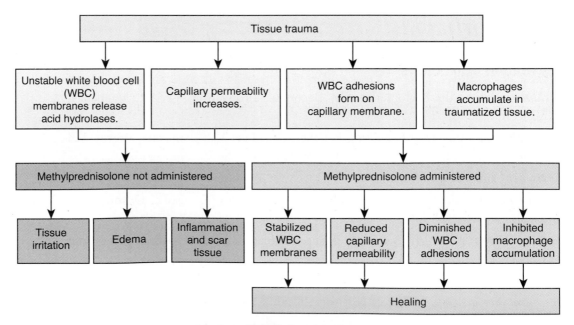

Figure 11-2 Mechanism of Action of Methylprednisolone. Tissue trauma normally leads to tissue irritation, edema, inflammation, and production of scar tissue. Methylprednisolone counteracts the initial effects of tissue trauma, promoting healing.

MASSAGE IMPLICATIONS AND ASSESSMENT

Absorption of oral glucocorticoids is not affected by massage. Injection sites, however, are avoided for several hours. The actions of these drugs are not completely understood. They have multiple effects on metabolism, cellular activity, fluid balance, and tissue density. If the drug is given for a short time because of an acute inflammatory reaction or allergic reaction, major effects of the tissues of the body are not of concern. The client's condition must be evaluated to see if massage is contraindicated (skin eruptions) or if gentle, supportive massage will be helpful. When glucocorticoids are used long term for chronic diseases, multiple and major changes in tissue take place. Excess adipose tissue is deposited, connective tissue is weakened, muscle wasting can occur, and decreased bone density may be seen. Deep tissue massage is contraindicated.

Because local mechanical strokes may not be as effective and may even be damaging, the client will often best be served by using systemic reflex strokes such as rhythmic, gentle effleurage and rocking. This helps to balance the body. Each individual will react differently, depending on the length of treatment with glucocorticoids and the dosage. Mechanical strokes such as pétrissage, compression, and friction are evaluated based on each client's response. These strokes are approached with caution until the response of the client is clear. A physician's release must always be obtained for a client receiving long-term glucocorticoid treatment.

Side Effects

There are many side effects of glucocorticoids. Those of concern for the massage practitioner include hypertension, fluid retention, osteoporosis, cushingoid symptoms (moon face, buffalo hump), easy bruising, and impaired tissue regeneration. If hypertension and fluid retention are severe, they may be contraindications for massage. Check with the physician before continuing with massage. If the side effects are milder, gentle, rhythmic effleurage may help to alleviate them.

Deep tissue work is contraindicated. Myofascial techniques and traction are contraindicated if bruising, tissue weakness, or osteoporosis are severe (see Sidebar: *Adverse Reactions to Glucocorticoids*).

Adverse Reactions to Glucocorticoids

- Insomnia
- Increased sodium and water retention
- Increased potassium excretion
- Suppressed immune and inflammatory responses

Adverse Effects
- Osteoporosis
- Intestinal perforation
- Peptic ulcers
- Impaired wound healing
- Diabetes mellitus
- Hyperlipidemia
- Adrenal atrophy
- Hypothalamic-pituitary axis suppression
- Cushingoid signs and symptoms (buffalo hump, moon face, and elevated blood glucose levels)

Mineralocorticoids

Common Drug Names

aldosterone

fludrocortisone acetate: Florinef

Mineralocorticoids affect electrolyte and water balance. Fludrocortisone acetate is a synthetic analog of hormones secreted by the adrenal cortex. Aldosterone is a natural mineralocorticoid. The use of aldosterone has been curtailed by high cost and limited availability.

Pharmacokinetics

Fludrocortisone acetate is absorbed well and distributed to all parts of the body. This drug is metabolized in the liver to inactive metabolites and is excreted by the kidneys.

Pharmacodynamics

Fludrocortisone acetate affects fluid and electrolyte balance by acting on the kidney to increase sodium reabsorption as well as potassium and hydrogen secretion.

Pharmacotherapeutics

Fludrocortisone acetate is used as replacement therapy for patients with adrenocortical insufficiency (reduced secretion of glucocorticoids, mineralocorticoids, and androgens). Fludrocortisone acetate may also be used to treat salt-losing congenital adrenogenital syndrome (characterized by a lack of cortisol and deficient aldosterone production) after the patient's electrolyte balance has been restored.

Adverse Reactions to Mineralocorticoids

Side Effects
- Sodium and water retention
- Bruising
- Diaphoresis

Adverse Effects
- Hypertension
- Cardiac hypertrophy
- Edema
- Heart failure
- Hypokalemia
- Urticaria
- Allergic rash

MASSAGE IMPLICATIONS AND ASSESSMENT

Absorption of oral mineralocorticoids is not affected by massage. The action of the drug is in the kidneys, increasing sodium and water retention. These drugs do not affect the various massage strokes.

Side Effects

The main side effects of mineralocorticoids are edema and hypertension. Easy bruising is also a frequent side effect. As with the glucocorticoids, if edema and hypertension are severe, massage is contraindicated and a physician should be notified. If they are mild, gentle, rhythmic effleurage may help to relieve the symptoms. Deep tissue work is contraindicated. A physician's release must be obtained for any client taking these drugs (see Sidebar: *Adverse Reactions to Mineralocorticoids*)

Other Immunosuppressants

Common Drug Names

azathioprine: Alti-Azathioprine, Imuran

cyclosporine: Gengraf, Neoral, Sandimmune

lymphocyte immune globulin (ATG equine): Atgam

muromonab-CD3: Orthoclone, monoclonal antibody, OKT3

tacrolimus: Prograf, Protopic

The above drugs are used for their immunosuppressant effects in patients undergoing allograft transplantation (between two people who are not identical twins). They are also used experimentally to treat autoimmune diseases (diseases resulting from an inappropriate immune response directed against the self).

Cyclophosphamide, although classified as an alkylating drug, also is used as an immunosuppressant. Cyclophosphamide is used primarily to treat cancer.

Pharmacokinetics

Different immunosuppressants take different paths through the body. When administered orally, azathioprine is absorbed readily from the GI tract, whereas absorption of cyclosporine is varied and incomplete. ATG and muromonab-CD3 are administered only by intravenous injection.

The distribution of azathioprine is not understood fully. Cyclosporine and muromonab-CD3 are distributed widely throughout the body. The distribution of ATG is not clear.

Azathioprine and cyclosporine are metabolized in the liver. Muromonab-CD3 is consumed by T cells circulating in the blood. The metabolism of ATG is unknown. Azathioprine and ATG are excreted in the urine; cyclosporine is excreted principally in the bile. How muromonab-CD3 is excreted is unknown.

Pharmacodynamics

How certain immunosuppressants achieve their desired effects has yet to be determined precisely. The exact mechanism of action of azathioprine, cyclosporine, and ATG is unknown but may be explained by the following:

- Azathioprine antagonizes metabolism of the amino acid purine and, therefore, may inhibit ribonucleic acid and deoxyribonucleic acid structure and synthesis. It also may inhibit coenzyme formation and function.
- Cyclosporine is believed to inhibit helper T cells and suppressor T cells.
- ATG may eliminate antigen-reactive T cells in the blood, alter T-cell function, or both.

In patients receiving kidney allografts, azathioprine suppresses cell-mediated hypersensitivity reactions and produces various alterations in antibody production. Muromonab-CD3, a monoclonal antibody, blocks the function of T cells.

Pharmacotherapeutics

Immunosuppressants are used mainly to prevent rejection in patients who undergo organ transplantation.

MASSAGE IMPLICATIONS AND ASSESSMENT

The action of the immunosuppressants is not clearly understood. What is known does not seem to have any implications for the action of the various massage strokes in the body. It is important to realize that these clients have faced life-threatening illnesses and are very susceptible to infection. Great care should be

Adverse Reactions to Other Immunosuppressants

Azathioprine
- Bone marrow suppression
- Nausea and vomiting
- Liver toxicity

Cyclosporine
- Kidney toxicity
- Hyperkalemia
- Infection
- Liver toxicity
- Nausea and vomiting

Lymphocyte Immune Globulin
- Fever and chills
- Reduced white blood cell or platelet count
- Infection
- Nausea and vomiting

Muromonab-CD3
- Fever and chills
- Nausea and vomiting
- Tremor
- Pulmonary edema
- Infection

used in the application of massage of any kind until the individual response can be determined. Physician release must always be obtained.

Side Effects

The immunosuppressants have many serious adverse reactions. Often these are related to susceptibility to infections and hematologic changes. Great care should be taken not to expose the client to any infection. The appearance of any adverse reaction must be reported immediately to the physician, and massage should not be done until the client is evaluated (see Sidebar: *Adverse Reactions to Other Immunosuppressants*).

Uricosurics and Other Antigout Drugs

Uricosurics, along with other antigout drugs, exert their effects through their anti-inflammatory actions.

Uricosurics

Common Drug Names

probenecid: Benuryl

sulfinpyrazone: Anturane, Apo-Sulfinpyrazone, Nu-Sulfinpyrazone

Uricosurics act by increasing uric acid excretion in the urine. The primary goal in using uricosurics is to prevent or control the frequency of gouty arthritis attacks.

Pharmacokinetics

Uricosurics are absorbed from the GI tract. Distribution of the two drugs is widespread. Metabolism of the drugs occurs in the liver, and excretion is primarily by the kidneys. Only small amounts of these drugs are excreted in the feces.

Pharmacodynamics

Probenecid and sulfinpyrazone reduce the reabsorption of uric acid in the kidneys. This results in excretion of uric acid in the urine, reducing serum urate levels.

Pharmacotherapeutics

Probenecid and sulfinpyrazone are indicated for treatment for chronic gouty arthritis and tophaceous gout (the deposition of tophi or urate crystals under the skin and into joints). Probenecid is also used to promote uric acid excretion in patients experiencing hyperuricemia. Probenecid and sulfinpyrazone should not be given during an acute gouty attack. If taken at that time, these drugs prolong inflammation. Because these drugs may increase the chance of an acute gouty attack when therapy begins and whenever the serum urate level changes rapidly, colchicine is administered during the first 3 to 6 months of probenecid or sulfinpyrazone therapy.

MASSAGE IMPLICATIONS AND ASSESSMENT

Absorption of the uricosurics is not affected by massage. Because the action of these drugs is directly on the kidneys, there is no change in the effect of massage strokes. Local contraindications may exist if there are still uric acid crystals in the joint or under the skin. In this case, no deep tissue or friction are used and only light effleurage applied to the area.

Side Effects

Side effects that may occur with the uricosurics are dizziness and hypotension. Stimulating strokes at the end of the massage help prevent problems related to these side effects. On occasion, alopecia (hair loss) occurs. Scalp massage is avoided in these cases. Other adverse reactions are referred to the physician (see Sidebar: *Adverse Reactions to Uricosurics*).

Adverse Reactions to Uricosurics

Probenecid
- Headache
- Anorexia
- Nausea and vomiting
- Hypersensitivity reactions

Sulfinpyrazone
- Nausea
- Indigestion
- GI pain
- GI blood loss

Other Antigout Drugs

Common Drug Names

allopurinol: Aloprim, Apo-Allopurinol, Zyloprim

colchicine: Colchicine MR, Colgout

Allopurinol is used to reduce production of uric acid, thus preventing gouty attacks. Colchicine is used to treat acute gouty attacks.

Pharmacokinetics

Allopurinol and colchicine take somewhat different paths through the body. When given orally, allopurinol is absorbed from the GI tract. Allopurinol and its metabolite oxypurinol are distributed throughout the body. It is metabolized by the liver and excreted in the urine.

Colchicine is also absorbed from the GI tract. Colchicine is partially metabolized in the liver. The drug and its metabolites then reenter the intestinal tract through biliary secretions. After reabsorption from the intestines, colchicine is distributed to various tissues. The drug is excreted primarily in the feces and to a lesser degree in the urine.

Pharmacodynamics

Allopurinol and its metabolite oxypurinol inhibit xanthine oxidase, the enzyme responsible for the production of uric acid. By reducing uric acid formation, allopurinol eliminates the hazards of hyperuricuria.

Colchicine appears to reduce the inflammatory response to monosodium urate crystals deposited in joint tissues. Colchicine may produce its effects by inhibiting migration of white blood cells (WBCs) to the inflamed joint. This reduces phagocytosis and lactic acid production by WBCs, decreasing urate crystal deposits and reducing inflammation.

Pharmacotherapeutics

Allopurinol is used to treat primary gout; thus, it is hoped also to prevent acute gouty attacks. It is prescribed with uricosurics when smaller dosages of each drug are needed. It is also used to treat gout or hyperuricemia that may occur with blood abnormalities and during treatment of tumors or leukemia, to treat primary or secondary uric acid nephropathy (with or without the accompanying symptoms of gout), and to treat and prevent recurrent uric acid stone formation. Additionally, it is used to treat patients whose conditions respond poorly to maximum dosages of uricosurics or who have allergic reactions or intolerance to uricosuric drugs.

Colchicine is used to relieve the inflammation of acute gouty arthritis attacks. If given promptly, it is especially effective in relieving pain. Also, giving colchicine during the first several months of allopurinol, probenecid, or sulfinpyrazone therapy may prevent the acute gouty attacks that sometimes accompany the use of these drugs.

MASSAGE IMPLICATIONS AND ASSESSMENT

The absorption of these drugs is not affected by massage. The actions of these drugs also do not affect how the body reacts to the various massage strokes. The client's condition may require a local contraindication to massage, because inflammation may be severe and painful. If massage is given, deep tissue and friction to the local area are contraindicated until all uric acid crystals and inflammation are resolved.

Side Effects

The only side effect of concern to massage therapists is alopecia. If this is present, scalp massage is avoided. All other adverse reactions must be reported to the physician immediately and massage withheld (see Sidebar: *Adverse Reactions to Other Antigout Drugs*).

Adverse Reactions to Other Antigout Drugs

Side Effects
- Nausea/vomiting
- Diarrhea
- Abdominal pain
- Rash

Adverse Effects
- Bone marrow suppression

Quick Quiz

1. Your client tells you that she has been taking Benadryl for the past 5 days for a severe allergic reaction. She states she had a rash all over her arms and chest, but it is "almost all gone now" and only slightly itchy. She only had a small amount of rash on her legs. Should you do massage and if so, what strokes should you use?

2. You are working at a salon and a new client comes in for a massage. He tells you that he had a liver transplant two and a half months ago. His incision is well healed and he is feeling pretty good. He is taking prednisone, Sandimmune, and Atgam. He would like a relaxation massage. What should you do?

Psychiatric Drugs

Drugs and Psychiatric Disorders

This chapter presents drugs that are used to treat various sleep and psychogenic disorders, such as anxiety, depression, and psychotic disorders.

Sedative and Hypnotic Drugs

Sedatives reduce activity or excitement. Some degree of drowsiness commonly accompanies sedative use. When given in large doses, sedatives are considered hypnotics and induce a state resembling natural sleep. The three main classes of synthetic drugs used as sedatives and hypnotics are benzodiazepines, barbiturates, and nonbenzodiazepine-nonbarbiturate drugs. Other sedatives include alcohol and over-the-counter sleep aids.

Benzodiazepines

Common Drug Names: Sedatives/Hypnotics

estazolam: ProSom

flurazepam: Apo-Flurazepam, Dalmane

lorazepam: Apo-Lorazepam, Ativan, Novo-Lorazepam, Nu-Loraz, Riva-Lorazepam

quazepam: Doral

temazepam: Apo-Temazepam, Gen-Temazepam, Novo-Temazepam, Restoril

triazolam: Gen-Triazolam, Halcion

Common Drug Names: Antianxiety

alprazolam: Alprazolam Intensol, Alti-Alprazolam, Apo-Alpraz, Novo-Alprazol, Nu-Alprax, Xana TS, Xanax

chlordiazepoxide: Apo-Chlordiazepoxide, Librium, methaminodiazepoxide

clorazepate dipotassium: Apo-Clorazepate, Novo-Clopate, Tranxene

diazepam: Valium, Apo-Diazepam, Diastat, Diazemuls, Diazepam Intensol

halazepam: Paxipam

lorazepam: Apo-Lorazepam, Ativan, Novo-Lorazepam, Nu-Loraz, Riva-Lorazepam

oxazepam: Apo-Oxazepam, Serax

Benzodiazepines produce many therapeutic effects, including daytime sedation, sedation before anesthesia, sleep inducement, relief of anxiety and tension, skeletal muscle relaxation, and anticonvulsant activity. Benzodiazepines are used in various clinical situations and exert either a primary or a secondary sedative or hypnotic effect. Benzodiazepines used primarily for their sedative or hypnotic effects include:

- estazolam
- flurazepam hydrochloride
- lorazepam
- quazepam
- temazepam
- triazolam

Benzodiazepines used primarily for the treatment of anxiety include:

- alprazolam
- chlordiazepoxide hydrochloride
- clorazepate dipotassium
- diazepam
- halazepam
- lorazepam
- oxazepam
- prazepam

Pharmacokinetics (how drugs circulate)

Benzodiazepines are absorbed well from the gastrointestinal (GI) tract and are distributed widely in the body. Some may also be given parenterally. All benzodiazepines are metabolized in the liver and excreted primarily in the urine.

Pharmacodynamics (how drugs act)

Researchers believe that benzodiazepines work by stimulating gamma-aminobutyric acid (GABA) receptors in the brain associated with wakefulness and attention (Fig. 12-1). At low dosages, benzodiazepines decrease anxiety by acting on the limbic system and other areas of the brain that help regulate emotional activity. The drugs can usually calm or sedate the patient without causing drowsiness. At higher dosages, benzodiazepines induce sleep, probably because they depress the brain. Benzodiazepines increase total sleep time and produce a deep, refreshing sleep.

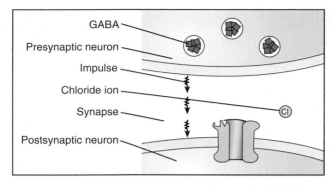

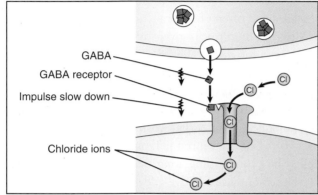

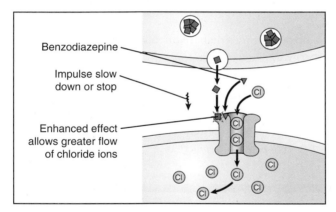

Figure 12-1. Mechanism of Action of the Benzodiazepines.
The speed of impulses from a presynaptic neuron across a
synapse is influenced by the amount of chloride ions in the
postsynaptic neuron. The passage of chloride ions into the
postsynaptic neuron depends on the inhibitory
neurotransmitter called gamma-aminobutyric acid (GABA).
When GABA is released from the presynaptic neuron, it
travels across the synapse and binds to GABA receptors on
the postsynaptic neuron. This binding allows the chloride
ions to flow into the postsynaptic neuron and causes the
nerve impulses to slow. The result is decreased impulses
stimulating the nerves. Benzodiazepines bind to receptors
on or near the GABA receptor, enhancing the effect of
GABA and allowing more chloride ions to flow into the
postsynaptic neuron. This depresses the nerve impulses,
causing them to slow or stop.

Pharmacotherapeutics (how drugs are used)

Clinical indications for benzodiazepines include relaxing the patient during the day of or before surgery, treating insomnia, for inducing intravenous anesthesia, treating alcohol withdrawal symptoms, treating anxiety and seizure disorders, and producing skeletal muscle relaxation.

Adverse Reactions to Benzodiazepines

Side Effects
- Fatigue
- Muscle weakness
- Dry mouth
- Nausea and vomiting
- Dizziness
- Daytime sedation
- Hangover effect (residual drowsiness and impaired reaction time on awakening)
- Rebound insomnia

Adverse Effects
- Amnesia
- Ataxia
- Drug abuse
- Drug tolerance
- Drug dependence

MASSAGE IMPLICATIONS AND ASSESSMENT

Benzodiazepines are most often given orally, and massage does not affect the absorption of the drug. If the drug is given by injection, the site of the injection should not be massaged for at least 2 hours. The action of the benzodiazepines is that of slowing or depressing certain receptors in the brain. This includes the motor cortex. The massage strokes that work through local reflex and local mechanical action are more effective. These include pétrissage, compression, vibration, and myofascial techniques. Strokes that work through systemic reflex action give an additive effect to the drug's central nervous system (CNS) depression. These strokes are applied in a more stimulating manner, such as rapid effleurage and tapotement, to counteract these additive effects.

Side Effects

Side effects of benzodiazepines that are of concern to the massage practitioner are fatigue, dizziness, drowsiness, and hypotension. These should be addressed as discussed above. Stimulation during and at the end of the massage with systemic reflex strokes should alleviate any problems. The effects of these drugs may last from 12 to 24 hours. Therefore, even if the client is taking the drug as a nighttime sleep aid, effects may still be seen and potentiated by massage during the day (see Sidebar: *Adverse Reactions to Benzodiazepines*).

Barbiturates

Common Drug Names

amobarbital: Amytal

butabarbital: Butisol

mephobarbital: Mebaral

pentobarbital: Nembutal

phenobarbital: Luminal

secobarbital: Seconal

The major pharmacologic action of barbiturates is to reduce overall CNS alertness. Barbiturates are used primarily as sedatives and hypnotics.

Low doses of barbiturates depress the sensory and motor cortex in the brain, causing drowsiness. High doses may cause respiratory depression and death because of their ability to depress all levels of the CNS.

Pharmacokinetics

Barbiturates are absorbed well from the GI tract, distributed rapidly, metabolized by the liver, and excreted in the urine.

Pharmacodynamics

As sedative-hypnotics, barbiturates depress the sensory cortex of the brain, decrease motor activity, and produce drowsiness, sedation, and hypnosis.

Pharmacotherapeutics

Barbiturates have many clinical indications, including daytime sedation (for short periods only, typically less than 2 weeks), hypnotic effects for patients with insomnia, preoperative sedation and anesthesia, relief of anxiety, and anticonvulsant effects. With prolonged use of barbiturates, the patient can develop drug tolerance as well as psychological and physical dependence. In comparison, benzodiazepines are relatively effective and safe and for these reasons have replaced barbiturates as the sedatives and hypnotics of choice.

Adverse Reactions to Barbiturates

Side Effects
- Drowsiness
- Lethargy
- Headache
- Mild bradycardia
- Hypotension
- Vertigo
- Nausea and vomiting
- Diarrhea
- Epigastric pain

Adverse Effects
- Depression
- Hypoventilation
- Spasm of the larynx and bronchi
- Respiratory depression
- Allergic reactions

MASSAGE IMPLICATIONS AND ASSESSMENT

The barbiturate drugs have a very strong CNS depressant effect. As with the benzodiazepines, systemic reflex strokes and relaxation effects of massage are increased. When applied for stimulation, the systemic reflex strokes take longer to achieve the desired effects. Rapid effleurage and tapotement are used during and at the end of the massage. The muscles respond to the local reflex and mechanical strokes.

Side Effects

Drowsiness, lethargy, dizziness, and hypotension are side effects of barbiturate drugs. These can be alleviated by using the massage strokes as described above. Other adverse effects must be reported to a physician and massage withheld until the client can be assessed (see Sidebar: *Adverse Reactions to Barbiturates*).

Nonbenzodiazepines-Nonbarbiturates

Common Drug Names

chloral hydrate: Aquachloral, PMS-Chloral Hydrate, Somnote

ethchlorvynol: Placidyl

zaleplon: Sonata

zolpidem: Ambien

Nonbenzodiazepine-nonbarbiturate drugs act as hypnotics for short-term treatment of simple insomnia. These drugs offer no special advantages over other sedatives. With the exception of zolpidem, which may be effective for up to 35 days, nonbenzodiazepines-nonbarbiturates lose their effectiveness by the end of the second week of treatment.

Pharmacokinetics

Nonbenzodiazepines-nonbarbiturates are absorbed rapidly from the GI tract, metabolized in the liver, and excreted in the urine.

Pharmacodynamics

The mechanism of action for nonbenzodiazepines-nonbarbiturates is not fully known, but they produce depressant effects similar to barbiturates.

Pharmacotherapeutics

Nonbenzodiazepines-nonbarbiturates are typically used for short-term treatment of simple insomnia, sedation before surgery, and sedation before electroencephalogram (EEG) studies.

Adverse Reactions to Nonbenzodiazepines-Nonbarbiturates

Side Effects
- Nausea and vomiting
- Gastric irritation
- Hangover effects
- Lethargy
- Hypotension
- Drowsiness
- Dizziness

Adverse Effects
- Respiratory depression
- Respiratory arrest

MASSAGE IMPLICATIONS AND ASSESSMENT

Although the action of these drugs is not fully understood, they have CNS depressant activity similar to benzodiazepines and barbiturates. The massage therapist uses stimulating systemic reflex strokes (tapotement and rapid effleurage) to counteract the additive effects of both the massage and the drugs.

Side Effects

Side effects of the nonbenzodiazepine-nonbarbiturate sedative drugs are drowsiness, hypotension, dizziness, and lethargy. They can be alleviated as discussed above (see Sidebar: *Adverse Reactions to Nonbenzodiazepines-Nonbarbiturates*).

Antidepressant and Antimanic Drugs

Antidepressant and antimanic drugs are used to treat affective disorders, that is, disturbances in mood characterized by depression or elation. Unipolar disorders, characterized by periods of clinical depression, are treated with monoamine oxidase (MAO) inhibitors, tricyclic antidepressants, or other antidepressants.

Lithium is used to treat bipolar disorders, which are characterized by alternating periods of manic behavior and clinical depression.

Monoamine Oxidase Inhibitors

MAO inhibitors are divided into two classifications based on chemical structure: hydrazines, which include phenelzine sulfate, and nonhydrazines, which includes a single drug, tranylcypromine sulfate.

Common Drug Names: Hydrazines

isocarboxazid: Marplan

moclobemide (available only in Canada): Alti-Moclobemide, Manerix

phenelzine: Nardil

Common Drug Names: Nonhydrazines

tranylcypromine: Parnate

Pharmacokinetics

MAO inhibitors are absorbed rapidly and completely from the GI tract and are metabolized in the liver. They are excreted mainly by the GI tract and to a lesser degree by the kidneys.

Pharmacodynamics

The exact mechanism of action of MAO inhibitors is unclear. These drugs appear to work by inhibiting monoamine oxidase, the enzyme that normally metabolizes the neurotransmitters norepinephrine and serotonin. By doing so, these drugs make more norepinephrine and serotonin available and relieve the symptoms of depression.

Pharmacotherapeutics

MAO inhibitors are the treatment of choice for atypical depression, which produces signs opposite of those of typical depression. In cases of atypical depression, the patient gains weight, lacks suicidal tendencies, and has increased sexual drive. MAO inhibitors may be used to treat typical depression resistant to other therapies or when other therapies are contraindicated. Other uses include treatment of phobic anxieties, neurodermatitis (an itchy skin disorder seen in anxious, nervous people), hypochondriasis (abnormal concern about health), and refractory narcolepsy (sudden sleep attacks).

Certain foods can interact with MAO inhibitors and produce severe reactions. Severe hypertensive crises are the most common and can be life-threatening. The most serious reactions involve tyramine-rich foods (such as red wines, aged cheeses, and fava beans) and sympathomimetic drugs. Foods with moderate tyramine contents (e.g., yogurt and ripe bananas) may be eaten occasionally but with care. Because of the serious side effects and multiple drug and food interactions, MAO inhibitors are rarely used unless other therapies have failed.

MASSAGE IMPLICATIONS AND ASSESSMENT

MAO inhibitors are taken orally. Therefore, massage does not affect the rate at which the drug is absorbed. The action of the drugs is on an enzyme in the CNS. It does not interfere with the effectiveness of the massage strokes.

Side Effects

MAO inhibitors have many common side effects. If the client is experiencing restlessness and insomnia, systemic reflex strokes designed to relax and calm (e.g., slow, rhythmic effleurage, rocking or gentle touch) are used. If the client is experiencing drowsiness, dizziness, or hypotension, the use of more stimulating systemic reflex strokes (rapid effleurage, tapotement, or shaking) is more appropriate. If constipation is a side effect, abdominal massage may help to alleviate this problem. In some cases, skin and mucous membranes may bruise or there may be bleeding under the skin. If such cases are severe, massage may be contraindicated. If such cases are mild, deep tissue should not be used or used only with great caution (see Sidebar: _Adverse Reactions to MAO Inhibitors_).

Tricyclic Antidepressants

Common Drug Names

amitriptyline: Apo-Amitriptyline, Elavil, Emitrip (discontinued in the U.S.), Endep, Enovil (discontinued in the U.S.), Levate, Novotriptyn, Vanatrip

amoxapine: Asendin (discontinued in the U.S.)

clomipramine: Anafranil, Apo-Clomipramine, Gen-Clomipramine

desipramine: Alti-Desipramine, Norpramin, Novo-Desipramine

doxepin: Alti-Doxepin, Apo-Doxepin, Sinequan

imipramine: Apo-Imipramine, Tofranil

nortriptyline: Alti-Nortriptyline, Apo-Nortriptyline, Aventyl, Norventyl, Pamelor

protriptyline: Vivactil

trimipramine: Apo-Trimip, Novo-Tripramine, Rhotrimine, Surmontil

Tricyclic antidepressants are used to treat depression.

Pharmacokinetics

Tricyclic antidepressants are metabolized extensively in the liver and eventually excreted as inactive compounds (only small amounts of active drug are excreted) in the urine. The extreme fat solubility of these drugs accounts for their wide distribution throughout the body, slow excretion, and long half-lives.

Pharmacodynamics

Researchers believe that tricyclic antidepressants increase the amount of norepinephrine, serotonin, or both by preventing their reuptake in the presynaptic nerves. After a neurotransmitter has performed its job, several fates are possible, including rapidly reentering the neuron from which it was released (called reuptake). Preventing reuptake results in increased levels of these neurotransmitters in the synapses, relieving depression.

Pharmacotherapeutics

Tricyclic antidepressants are used to treat episodes of major depression. They are especially effective in treating depression of insidious onset accompanied by weight loss, anorexia, or insomnia. Physical signs and symptoms may respond after 1 to 2 weeks of therapy; psychologic symptoms, after 2 to 4 weeks.

Tricyclic antidepressants are much less effective in patients with hypochondriasis, atypical depression, or depression accompanied by delusions. However, they may be helpful in treating acute episodes of depression.

Tricyclic antidepressants also are being investigated for use in preventing migraine headaches and in treating phobias, urinary incontinence, attention deficit disorder, duodenal or peptic ulcer disease, and diabetic neuropathy.

MASSAGE IMPLICATIONS AND ASSESSMENT

Absorption of the tricyclic drugs is not affected by massage. Their action in the CNS synapses does not affect how the body reacts to any of the massage strokes.

Side Effects

Side effects of sedation and hypotension may occur with the use of tricyclic drugs, especially when the client is starting therapy. Care in changing positions and stimulation at the end of the massage can prevent any problems with these side effects worsening due to the relaxation effects of massage (see Sidebar: *Adverse Reactions to Tricyclic Antidepressants*).

Adverse Reactions to Tricyclic Antidepressants

Side Effects
- Orthostatic hypotension (a drop in blood pressure on standing)
- Sedation
- Rashes
- Photosensitivity reactions
- Fine resting tremor
- Decreased sexual desire
- Inhibited ejaculation

Adverse Effects
- Transient eosinophilia
- Reduced white blood cell count
- Granulocytopenia
- Palpitations
- Conduction delays
- Rapid heartbeat

Selective Serotonin Reuptake Inhibitors

Common Drug Names

citalopram: Celexa

escitalopram: Lexapro

fluoxetine: Alti-Fluoxetine, Apo-Fluoxetine, Prozac, Rhoxal-fluoxetine, Sarafem

fluvoxamine: Alti-Fluvoxamine, Apo-Fluvoxamine, Luvox

paroxetine: Paxil

sertraline: Apo-Sertraline, Zoloft

Developed to treat depression with fewer adverse effects, selective serotonin reuptake inhibitors (SSRIs) are chemically different from tricyclic antidepressants and MAO inhibitors.

Pharmacokinetics

SSRIs are absorbed almost completely after oral administration. SSRIs are primarily metabolized in the liver and are excreted in the urine.

Pharmacodynamics

SSRIs inhibit the nerve reuptake of the neurotransmitter serotonin. By increasing serotonin, symptoms of depression are decreased.

Pharmacotherapeutics

SSRIs are used to treat the same major depressive episodes as tricyclic antidepressants and have the same degree of effectiveness. Fluvoxamine, fluoxetine, sertraline, and paroxetine are also used to treat obsessive-compulsive disorder. Paroxetine is also indicated for social anxiety disorder. SSRIs may also be useful in treating panic disorders, eating disorders, personality disorders, impulse control disorders, and premenstrual syndrome.

Adverse Reactions to SSRIs

Side Effects
- Anxiety
- Insomnia
- Somnolence
- Palpitations
- Orthostatic hypotension
- Constipation

Adverse Effects
- Extreme agitation
- Suicidal thoughts
- Self-mutilation
- Suicide attempts

MASSAGE IMPLICATIONS AND ASSESSMENT

Massage does not affect the absorption rate of the SSRIs. Because the SSRIs act in the synapses of the brain to prevent the reuptake of serotonin, the drugs do not affect the reaction of the body to the various massage strokes.

Side Effects

The side effects of the SSRIs that are of concern to the massage therapist include orthostatic hypotension, sleepiness, anxiety, and insomnia. Massage is applied depending on what side effects (if any) the client is experiencing. Anxiety and insomnia are approached with slow, rhythmic effleurage and rocking, both systemic reflex strokes. Hypotension and sleepiness require more stimulating systemic reflex strokes, like tapotement (see Sidebar: *Adverse Reactions to SSRIs*).

Miscellaneous Antidepressants

Common Drug Names

bupropion: Wellbutrin, Zyban

maprotiline: Ludiomil

mirtazapine: Remeron

nefazodone: Serzone

trazodone: Alti-Trazodone, Apo-Trazodone, Desyrel, Trazorel

venlafaxine: Effexor

Bupropion is a dopamine reuptake blocking agent. Maprotiline and mirtazapine are tetracyclic antidepressants. Nefazodone is a phenylpiperazine agent. Trazodone is a triazopyridine agent. Venlafaxine is a serotonin-norepinephrine reuptake inhibitor.

Pharmacokinetics

The paths these antidepressants take through the body vary. Maprotiline and mirtazapine are absorbed from the GI tract, distributed widely in the body, metabolized by the liver, and excreted by the kidneys. Bupropion's absorption is unknown. It is probably metabolized in the liver and is primarily excreted in urine. Venlafaxine is rapidly absorbed after oral administration, partially bound to plasma proteins, metabolized in the liver, and excreted in urine. Trazodone is absorbed well from the GI tract, distributed widely in the body, and metabolized by the liver. Approximately 75% is excreted in urine, and the remainder is excreted in feces. Nefazodone is rapidly and completely absorbed and is excreted in the urine.

Pharmacodynamics

Much about how these drugs work has yet to be understood fully. Maprotiline and mirtazapine probably increase the amount of norepinephrine, serotonin, or both in the CNS by blocking their reuptake by presynaptic neurons (nerve terminals). Bupropion is believed to inhibit the reuptake of the neurotransmitter dopamine. Venlafaxine is thought to inhibit the nerve reuptake of serotonin and norepinephrine. Trazodone, although its effect is unknown, is thought to exert antidepressant effects by inhibiting the reuptake of norepinephrine and serotonin in the presynaptic neurons. Nefazodone's action is not precisely defined. It inhibits neuronal uptake of serotonin and norepinephrine. It also occupies serotonin and alpha$_1$-adrenergic receptor sites.

Pharmacotherapeutics

These miscellaneous drugs are all used to treat depression. Trazodone may also be effective in treating aggressive behavior and panic disorder.

MASSAGE IMPLICATIONS AND ASSESSMENT

As with the other antidepressants, no effect on the reaction of the body to the various massage strokes is of concern.

Side Effects

Orthostatic hypotension, constipation, dizziness, and drowsiness are all side effects of these various antidepressants. They all require the application of the stimulating systemic reflex strokes (rapid effleurage, tapotement, shaking) at the end of the massage or even during the entire massage if side effects are severe. Abdominal massage helps with any constipation problems (see Sidebar: *Adverse Reactions to Miscellaneous Antidepressants*).

Adverse Reactions to Miscellaneous Antidepressants

Maprotiline
- Seizures
- Orthostatic hypotension
- Tachycardia
- Electrocardiographic changes

Mirtazapine
- Tremors
- Confusion
- Nausea
- Constipation

Bupropion
- Headache
- Confusion
- Tremor
- Agitation
- Tachycardia
- Anorexia
- Nausea and vomiting

Venlafaxine and nefazodone
- Headache
- Somnolence
- Dizziness
- Nausea

Trazodone
- Drowsiness
- Dizziness

Lithium

Common Drug Names

lithium carbonate: Carbolith, Duralith, Eskalith, Lithane, Lithizine, Lithobid, Lithonate (discontinued in the U.S.), Lithotabs (discontinued in the U.S.)

lithium citrate: Cibalith-S

Lithium carbonate and lithium citrate are the drugs of choice to prevent or treat mania. The discovery of lithium was a milestone in treating mania and bipolar disorders.

Pharmacokinetics

When taken orally, lithium is absorbed rapidly and completely and is distributed to body tissues. An active drug, lithium is not metabolized and is excreted from the body unchanged.

Pharmacodynamics

In mania, the patient experiences excessive catecholamine stimulation. In bipolar disorder, the patient is affected by swings between the excessive catecholamine stimulation of mania and the diminished catecholamine stimulation of depression.

Lithium may regulate catecholamine release in the CNS by increasing norepinephrine and serotonin uptake, reducing the release of norepinephrine in the presynaptic neuron, or inhibiting norepinephrine's action in the postsynaptic neuron.

Pharmacotherapeutics

Lithium is used primarily to treat acute episodes of mania and to prevent relapses of bipolar disorders. Other uses of lithium being researched include preventing unipolar depression and migraine headaches as well as treating depression, alcohol neutropenia dependence, anorexia nervosa, and syndrome of inappropriate antidiuretic hormone (a condition in which the kidneys do not excrete enough fluid).

Lithium has a narrow therapeutic margin of safety. A blood level that is even slightly higher than the therapeutic level can be dangerous.

MASSAGE IMPLICATIONS AND ASSESSMENT

The absorption rate of lithium is not affected by massage. The actions of the drug are not fully understood but do not seem to directly affect how the body receives and reacts to the various massage strokes. However, because of the narrow margins of safety with this drug, it is best to discuss with and receive a release from the client's physician before doing any kind of massage.

Side Effects

The narrow therapeutic safety margin of lithium causes many problems for the client who is taking this drug. Side effects are frequent and multiple. Some of those that concern the massage practitioner during a session are hypotension, dizziness, drowsiness, weakness, changes in reflex reactions, and rash.

Rash is a local contraindication for massage and must be reported to the physician. Multiple CNS effects and exaggerated reflexes may make local reflex strokes less effective. Parts of the nervous system are sluggish and others may be overstimulated. The best approach is to use systemic reflex strokes in a slightly more rapid application if the client is depressed or drowsy, but more slowly and for relaxation if the client is more restless and anxious. Changes in the client's symptoms or other adverse effects must be reported to the physician immediately and massage withheld (see Sidebar: *Adverse Reactions to Lithium*).

Antianxiety Drugs

Antianxiety drugs, also called anxiolytics, include some of the most commonly prescribed drugs in the United States. They are used primarily to treat anxiety disorders. The three main types of antianxiety drugs are benzodiazepines (discussed in a previous section), barbiturates (also discussed in a previous section), and buspirone.

Buspirone

Common Drug Names

buspirone: Apo-Buspirone, BuSpar, Buspirex, Gen-Buspirone

Buspirone hydrochloride is the first anxiolytic in a class of drugs known as azaspirodecanedione derivatives. This drug's structure and mechanism of action differ from those of other antianxiety drugs. Buspirone has several advantages, including less sedation, no increase in CNS depressant effects when taken with alcohol or sedative-hypnotics, and lower abuse potential.

Pharmacokinetics

Buspirone is absorbed rapidly. The drug is eliminated in the urine and feces.

Pharmacodynamics

The mechanism of action of buspirone is not known. However, it is known that buspirone does not affect GABA receptors like the benzodiazepines. Buspirone seems to produce various effects in the midbrain and acts as a midbrain modulator, possibly because of its high affinity for serotonin receptors.

Pharmacotherapeutics

Buspirone is used to treat generalized anxiety states. Patients who have not received benzodiazepines seem to respond better to buspirone. Because of its slow onset of action, buspirone is ineffective when quick relief from anxiety is needed.

Adverse Reactions to Lithium

Side Effects
- Drowsiness
- Tremors
- Dizziness
- Incoordination
- Hypotension
- Metallic taste
- Dry mouth
- Blurred vision
- Tinnitus
- Indigestion
- Thinning hair
- Acne
- Reversible electrocardiographic changes
- Thirst
- Polyuria
- Elevated white blood cell count

Adverse Effects
- Confusion
- Lethargy
- Slurred speech
- Increased reflex reactions
- Seizures
- Psychomotor retardation
- Stupor
- Blackouts
- Coma
- Impaired speech
- Arrhythmias
- Renal toxicity
- Leukocytosis
- Hypothyroidism
- Hyponatremia
- Diminished or absent sensation

MASSAGE IMPLICATIONS AND ASSESSMENT

The actions of the drug buspirone are not known to affect the reaction of the body to massage strokes in any way. No change in application of massage is needed because of this drug's effects

Side Effects

The main side effects of this drug are dizziness and drowsiness, although some people experience restlessness and insomnia. The approach to dizziness and drowsiness is to stimulate with systemic reflex strokes. Restlessness and insomnia, however, are better approached by calming the nervous system with slow, relaxing systemic reflex strokes (see Sidebar: *Adverse Reactions to Buspirone*).

Antipsychotic Drugs

Antipsychotic drugs can control psychotic symptoms, such as delusions, hallucinations, and thought disorders, that can occur with schizophrenia, mania, and other psychoses. Drugs used to treat psychoses have several different names, including:

- antipsychotic, because they can eliminate signs and symptoms of psychoses
- major tranquilizer, because they can calm an agitated patient
- neuroleptic, because they have an adverse neurobiologic effect that causes abnormal body movements.

Regardless of what they are called, all antipsychotic drugs belong to one of two major groups: typical antipsychotics (which include phenothiazines and nonphenothiazines) and atypical antipsychotics (which include the newer agents, clozapine, olanzapine, and risperidone).

Typical Antipsychotics

Common Drug Names: Phenothiazines

chlorpromazine: Chlorpromanyl, Largactil, Thorazine

fluphenazine decanoate: Modecate, Prolixin Decanoate

fluphenazine enanthate: enanthate, Moditen, Prolixin Enanthate

fluphenazine hydrochloride: Anatensol, Apo-Fluphenazine, Permitil, Prolixin

mesoridazine besylate: Serentil

perphenazine: Trilafon, Apo-Perphenazine

thioridazine: Apo-Thioridazine, Mellaril

trifluoperazine: Apo-Trifluoperazine, Stelazine

Common Drug Names: *Nonphenothiazines*

haloperidol: Apo-Haloperidol, Haldol, Novo-Peridol, Peridol

loxapine succinate: Loxapac, Loxitane

molindone: Moban

pimozide: Orap

thiothixene: Navane

Typical antipsychotics, which include phenothiazines and nonphenothiazines, can be broken down into smaller classifications.

Many clinicians believe that the phenothiazines should be treated as three distinct drug classes because of the differences in the adverse reactions they cause. Aliphatics primarily cause sedation and anticholinergic effects. These are moderately potent drugs that include chlorpromazine hydrochloride and promazine hydrochloride. Piperazines primarily cause extrapyramidal reactions and include acetophenazine maleate, fluphenazine decanoate, fluphenazine enanthate, fluphenazine hydrochloride, perphenazine, and trifluoperazine hydrochloride. Piperidines primarily cause sedation and include mesoridazine besylate and thioridazine hydrochloride.

Based on their chemical structure, nonphenothiazine antipsychotics can be divided into several drug classes, including butyrophenones, such as haloperidol and haloperidol decanoate; dibenzoxazepines, such as loxapine succinate; dihydroindolines, such as molindone hydrochloride; diphenylbutylpiperidines, such as pimozide; and thioxanthenes, such as chlorprothixene, thiothixene, and thiothixene hydrochloride.

Pharmacokinetics

Although phenothiazines are absorbed erratically, they are distributed to many tissues and are highly concentrated in the brain. Like phenothiazines, nonphenothiazines are absorbed erratically. They are also distributed throughout the tissues and are highly concentrated in the brain.

All phenothiazines are metabolized in the liver and excreted in urine and bile. Because fatty tissues slowly release accumulated phenothiazine metabolites into the plasma, phenothiazines may produce effects up to 3 months after they are stopped. Nonphenothiazines are also metabolized in the liver and excreted in the urine and bile.

Pharmacodynamics

Although the mechanism of action of phenothiazines is not understood fully, researchers believe that these drugs work by blocking postsynaptic dopaminergic receptors in the brain. The mechanism of action of nonphenothiazines resembles that of phenothiazines.

Pharmacotherapeutics

Phenothiazines are used primarily to treat schizophrenia, to calm anxious or agitated patients, to improve a patient's thought processes, and to alleviate delusions and hallucinations. Additionally, there are other therapeutic uses for phenothiazines. They are administered to treat other psychiatric disorders, such as brief reactive psychosis, atypical psychosis, schizoaffective psychosis, autism, and major depression with psychosis. In combination with lithium, they are used in the treatment of bipolar disorder until the slower-acting lithium produces its therapeutic effect. They are also prescribed to quiet mentally challenged children and agitated geriatric patients, particularly those with dementia. Phenothiazines may increase the effects of analgesics. Finally, they are helpful in the management of pain, anxiety, and nausea in patients with cancer.

As a group, nonphenothiazines are used to treat psychotic disorders. Thiothixene is also used to control acute agitation. Haloperidol and pimozide may be used to treat Tourette's syndrome as well.

MASSAGE IMPLICATIONS AND ASSESSMENT

Any antipsychotic given by injection presents a contraindication for massage at the site of the injection. The length of this contraindication depends on the medication. Looking up the peak effect times for the intramuscular injection of the drug in question provides a good indication of how long the area should be avoided.

Because of the serious nature of the illness for which these drugs are prescribed and because of the multiple effects on the CNS, a physician release must be obtained before massage is performed. Because these drugs affect the neurotransmitter dopamine, many nerve–muscle pathways are affected. These effects are considered side effects or adverse reactions and are often dose-dependent. Changes in the application of massage are discussed below with the side effects.

Side Effects

Neurologic side effects are the most common with the use of typical antipsychotics. Muscle rigidity is frequent. Tardive dyskinesia and extrapyramidal symptoms may also occur. Local reflex strokes may be less effective. The best approach is to use local mechanical strokes (pétrissage, friction, and myofascial techniques) and the systemic reflex strokes to calm the nervous system. Severe symptoms or changes noted in the client should be reported immediately to the physician and massage withheld (see Sidebar: *Adverse Reactions to Typical Antipsychotics*).

Adverse Reactions to Typical Antipsychotics

- Extrapyramidal symptoms
- Tardive dyskinesia
- Neuroleptic malignant syndrome
- Muscle rigidity
- Extreme EPS
- Severely elevated body temperature
- Hypertension
- Rapid heart rate
- Respiratory failure
- Cardiovascular collapse

Atypical Antipsychotics

Common Drug Names

aripiprazole: Abilify

clozapine: Clozaril

olanzapine: Zyprexa

quetiapine: Seroquel

risperidone: Risperdal

ziprasidone: Geodon

Atypical antipsychotic drugs are new agents that are designed to treat schizophrenia.

Pharmacokinetics

Atypical antipsychotics are absorbed after oral administration. Atypical antipsychotics are metabolized by the liver and eliminated in the urine, with a small portion eliminated in feces.

Pharmacodynamics

Atypical antipsychotics typically block the dopamine receptors (but not as effectively as the typical antipsychotics) in addition to blocking serotonin receptor activity. These combined actions account for the effectiveness of atypical antipsychotics against the positive and negative symptoms of schizophrenia with minimal side effects.

Pharmacotherapeutics

Atypical antipsychotics are indicated for schizophrenic patients whose conditions are unresponsive to typical antipsychotics. Because of the decreased instance of extrapyramidal effects with atypical antipsychotics, they are becoming widely prescribed.

MASSAGE IMPLICATIONS AND ASSESSMENT

Atypical antipsychotics are given orally. Therefore, massage has no effect on the rate of absorption. The same concerns exist with these drugs as with the typical antipsychotics. A physician release must be obtained for massage.

Side Effects

The side effects of atypical antipsychotics are the same as for typical antipsychotics. These side effects occur because of the effects of the drugs on dopamine and the nerve/muscle reactions. They are not as frequent or as severe as the side effects seen with typical antipsychotics, however. If present, they are approached by the massage therapist as discussed above with the typical antipsychotics. Any change or increase in symptoms must be reported to the physician immediately and massage withheld (see Sidebar: *Adverse Reactions to Atypical Antipsychotics*).

> **Adverse Reactions to Atypical Antipsychotics**
>
> - Agranulocytosis (an abnormal decrease in white blood cells)
> - Seizures
> - Extrapyramidal effects

Quick Quiz

1. A new client calls you and states that he is taking Haldol and Ativan for schizophrenia and anxiety. He has been hospitalized for psychotic episodes in the past but has been stable for the past 2 years. What should you do?

2. A 75-year-old woman comes to you for relaxation massage. She tells you she is taking Dalmane every night for sleep. You find that she falls asleep quickly on the table and is hard to rouse after the massage. She experiences dizziness upon rising. What should you do?

Endocrine Drugs

13

Drugs and the Endocrine System

The endocrine system consists of glands, which are specialized cell clusters, and hormones, the chemical transmitters secreted by the glands in response to stimulation. Together with the central nervous system, the endocrine system regulates and integrates the body's metabolic activities and maintains homeostasis (the body's internal equilibrium). The drug classes that treat endocrine system disorders include natural hormones and their synthetic analogs, hormonelike substances, and drugs that stimulate or suppress hormone secretion.

Antidiabetic Drugs and Glucagon

Insulin (a pancreatic hormone) and oral antidiabetic drugs are classified as hypoglycemic drugs because they lower blood glucose levels. Glucagon, another pancreatic hormone, is classified as a hyperglycemic drug because it raises blood glucose levels. Insulin is a hormone required for blood glucose (blood sugar) to enter the cells of the body and be used as fuel for energy.

Diabetes mellitus, or simply diabetes, is a chronic disease of insulin deficiency or resistance. It is characterized by disturbances in carbohydrate, protein, and fat metabolism. This leads to elevated levels of blood sugar (glucose) in the body. The disease comes in two primary forms: type 1, referred to as insulin-dependent diabetes mellitus, and type 2, referred to as non–insulin-dependent diabetes mellitus.

Insulin

Common Drug Names

combination insulins: Actraphane HM, Humulin 50/50, Humulin 70/30, Novolin 70/30

crystalline zinc insulin: Actrapid HM, Humulin R, Iletin, Novolin R, Velosulin

insulin analog: Humalog

insulin glargine: Lantus

insulin zinc suspension: Humulin L, Lente Iletin, Lente Insulin, Monotard HM, Novolin L

insulin zinc suspension extended: Humulin U, Ultralente Insulin, Ultratard HM

isophane insulin suspension (neutral protamine Hagedorn insulin [NPH]): Humulin N, Hypurin, Insulatard, Isophane, Novolin N, NPH Insulin, NPH Iletin, Protaphane HM

Patients with type 1 diabetes require an external source of insulin to control blood glucose levels. Insulin also may be given to patients with type 2 diabetes. Type 2 diabetics still produce some insulin and may require only diet changes and/or drugs (oral antidiabetic drugs) that stimulate insulin production and reduce insulin resistance in the cells.

Pharmacokinetics (how drugs circulate)

Insulin is not effective when taken orally because the gastrointestinal (GI) tract breaks down the protein molecule before it reaches the bloodstream. All insulins, however, may be given by subcutaneous injection. Absorption of subcutaneous insulin varies according to the injection site, the blood supply, and the degree of tissue hypertrophy at the injection site.

New techniques for the administration of insulin are being developed. Some diabetics are already using an infusion pump that contains their insulin and dispenses it in very small amounts throughout the day through a subcutaneous needle. After insertion, this needle can remain in tissue for up to 72 hours. Recent research has focused on a nasal spray form of insulin. Although not yet in use, study results are promising. Bronchial inhalation of insulin is also being studied.

After absorption into the bloodstream, insulin is distributed throughout the body. Insulin-responsive tissues are located in the liver, fatty tissue, and muscle. Insulin is metabolized primarily in the liver and, to a lesser extent, in the kidneys and muscle. It is excreted in the feces and urine.

Pharmacodynamics (how drugs act)

Insulin is an anabolic (or tissue building) hormone that promotes storing glucose as glycogen in the liver; increasing protein and fat synthesis; slowing the breakdown of glycogen, protein, and fat; and balancing fluids and electrolytes. Although it has no antidiuretic effect, insulin can correct the polyuria (excessive urination) and polydipsia (excessive thirst) associated with hyperglycemia by decreasing the blood glucose level. Insulin also facilitates the movement of potassium from the extracellular fluid into the cell (Fig. 13-1).

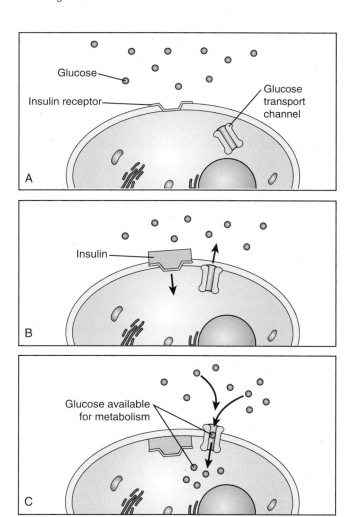

Figure 13-1. Insulin Aids Glucose Uptake. This illustration shows how insulin allows a cell to use glucose for energy. (**A**) Glucose cannot enter the cell without the aid of insulin. (**B**) Normally produced by the beta cells of the pancreas, insulin binds to the receptors on the surface of the target cell. Insulin and its receptor first move to the inside of the cell, which activates glucose transporter channels to move to the surface of the cell. (**C**) These channels allow glucose to enter the cell. The cell can then use the glucose for metabolism.

Pharmacotherapeutics (how drugs are used)

Insulin is indicated for type 1 diabetes, type 2 diabetes when other methods of controlling blood glucose levels have failed or are contraindicated, type 2 diabetes when blood glucose levels are elevated during periods of emotional or physical stress (such as infection and surgery), and type 2 diabetes when oral antidiabetic drugs are contraindicated because of pregnancy or hypersensitivity.

Insulin is also used to treat two complications of diabetes: diabetic ketoacidosis (more common with type 1 diabetes) and hyperosmolar hyperglycemic nonketotic syndrome (which is more common with type 2 diabetes). These are both the results of extremely high blood sugar levels or changes in the acidity of the blood. Both can lead to coma and death if not treated. Insulin is also used to treat severe hyperkalemia (elevated serum potassium levels) in patients without diabetes. Potassium moves with glucose from the bloodstream into the cell, lowering serum potassium levels.

MASSAGE IMPLICATIONS AND ASSESSMENT

Insulin has many far-reaching effects on the body. It is important to understand the disease, the drugs, the variety of peak times of action, and what all this information means for the massage therapist. Clients may take insulin injections anywhere from once to several times a day. They may have several types of insulin to take either together or at different times of the day. The insulin may have varying absorption and peak actions times. A good health history and complete drug screen are essential. All insulin is given by injection, most by the subcutaneous route. The local area of injection is a contraindicated site for massage for several hours up to 1 day after injection depending on the type of insulin used (Table 13-1).

Insulin acts directly in the bloodstream and cells of the body to allow breakdown and usage of glucose. Massage can act like exercise and use up the available glucose and insulin faster, leading to an insulin reaction or hypoglycemic episode. Several factors play into this, including how long since the client's last meal, how frequently the client has had problems with this at other times, how the client is feeling that day, how rapid or stimulating is the massage, and even the client's emotions. Whereas the action of insulin itself does not affect the application of massage, the lack of the body's ability to adapt to changing needs for glucose does. To prevent any reactions, some common sense precautions are followed. Although the client should not eat a large meal immediately before the massage, it is a good idea that he or she eats a meal within 2 to 3 hours or have a good snack no more than 1 hour before the massage. The therapist should always obtain both family and physician emergency numbers for the client. If the client carries glucose

Table 13-1   Onset, Peak, and Duration Times for Insulin Types

Type of insulin	Onset	Peak	Duration	Comment
Rapid (no designation)	0–15 minutes	30–90 minutes	Less than 5 hours	Used mostly in emergencies
Short-acting (Regular or R)	30–45 minutes	2–4 hours	5–7 hours	Often used with blood glucose readings
Intermediate-acting (Lente, L, or N)	1–4 hours	6–14 hours	18–24 hours	Most often part of regular dosages
Long-acting (Ultralente or U)	4–6 hours	18–26 hours	Approximately 30 hours	May require only once daily use

Clients may know the onset and peak action times of their insulin. If not, look it up in a drug book, *Physician's Desk Reference*, or call a pharmacist. These times will help determine how long you must avoid massaging the area of injection.

(sugar) tablets, the therapist should know where they are and be able to get to them quickly, or the therapist should keep some form of sugar in the office. Such forms include orange juice, regular soda, or regular (not diet) hard candies from which the sugar will be absorbed rapidly into the client's system in case of hypoglycemia. Although the symptoms of high blood sugar and low blood sugar are incredibly similar (see side effects below), it is more common for the diabetic client to have a low blood sugar incident. In either case, if giving the client sugar does not work to ease the symptoms quickly and/or the client becomes confused or lethargic, the therapist must call 911 immediately. There is nothing else for the therapist to do, and the quicker paramedics arrive the better.

Diabetes has many complications (such as neuropathies) that require alterations in how massage is given. This is for a pathophysiology book to describe. If the client with diabetes does not yet have any of the complications, massage can help to prevent some of them, reduce stress, and support the immune system. Massage is a very good health maintenance tool for the diabetic. All types of massage can be used with just a little common sense. However, physician approval must be obtained and open communications maintained regarding any changes in medication or condition.

Side Effects

The main side effects of insulin are those associated with insulin reaction or hypoglycemic reactions. They include dizziness, lethargy, confusion, blurred vision, slurred speech, weakness, fainting, shakiness, clammy cold skin, or increased sweating. If these occur, massage is stopped and the client given some form of easily absorbed sugar immediately. The therapist and the client can decide if they feel well enough to continue the massage if the symptoms improve. The client should get a more substantial snack as soon as possible after the incident. Therefore, if the incident occurred early in the massage or if the symptoms do not go away completely, it is better to stop and reschedule the massage.

Insulin injection sites may show bruising on occasion; light work over these areas is appropriate. Long-term diabetics sometimes have a hardening of the fascial tissue at injection sites used frequently. Vibration and friction strokes can help break this up.

The scope of practice of a massage therapist does not include using a blood glucose monitor to check blood sugar levels (even if client carries one) or injecting insulin. If the client cannot perform these activities, is confused, or is not responding to oral sugar, the therapist must call for help immediately (see Sidebar: *Adverse Reactions to Insulin*).

Adverse Reactions to Insulin

Side Effects

- Hypoglycemia
- Bruising at injection sites
- Hardening of skin at injection sites

Adverse Reactions

- Insulin shock
- Somogyi effect (hypoglycemia followed by rebound hyperglycemia)
- Hypersensitivity reactions
- Lipodystrophy (disturbance in fat deposition)
- Insulin resistance

Oral Antidiabetic Drugs

Common Drug Names

acarbose: Precose

acetohexamide: Dimelor, Dymilo

chlorpropamide: Diabinese, Apo-Chlorpropamide, Novo-Propamide *glimepiride:* Amaryl

glipizide: Glucotrol, Minidiab

glyburide: DiaBeta, Micronase, Euglucon, Apo-Glyburide, Gen-Glybe, Novo-Glyburide, Glynase

metformin: Glucophage

miglitol: Glyset

nateglinide: Starlix

pioglitazone: Actos

repaglinide: Prandin

rosiglitazone: Avandia

tolazamide: Tolinase

tolbutamide: Orinase, Mobenol, Apo-Tolbutamide, Novo-Butamide

Many oral antidiabetic drugs are approved for use in the United States. Types of oral antidiabetic drugs available include the following: (1) first-generation sulfonylureas, which include acetohexamide, chlorpropamide, tolazamide, and tolbutamide; (2) second-generation sulfonylureas, which include glipizide and glyburide; (3) nonsulfonylureas, thiazolidinedione antidiabetic drugs, pioglitazone and rosiglitazone; (4) a biguanide drug, metformin; (5) an alpha-glucosidase inhibitor, acarbose; (6) meglitinides; and (7) nateglinides.

Pharmacokinetics

Oral antidiabetic drugs are absorbed well from the GI tract and are distributed via the bloodstream throughout the body. Oral antidiabetic drugs are metabolized primarily in the liver and are excreted mostly in the urine, with some excreted in the bile. Glyburide is excreted equally in the urine and feces; rosiglitazone is largely excreted in both.

Pharmacodynamics

It is believed that oral antidiabetic drugs produce actions both within and outside the pancreas (extrapancreatic) to regulate blood glucose. Oral antidiabetic drugs probably stimulate pancreatic beta cells to release insulin in a patient with a minimally functioning pancreas. Oral antidiabetic drugs provide several extrapancreatic actions to decrease and control blood glucose. They can work in the liver and decrease glucose production (gluconeogenesis) there. Also, by increasing the number of insulin receptors in the peripheral tissues, they provide more opportunities for the cells to bind sufficiently with insulin, increasing movement of glucose into the cells for burning as fuel.

Other oral antidiabetic agents produce specific actions. Pioglitazone and rosiglitazone improve insulin sensitivity. Metformin decreases liver production of glucose and intestinal absorption of glucose and improves insulin sensitivity in the cells. Acarbose inhibits enzymes, delaying glucose absorption in the GI tract.

Pharmacotherapeutics

Oral antidiabetic drugs are indicated for patients with type 2 diabetes if diet and exercise cannot control blood glucose levels. These drugs are not effective in type 1 diabetes because the pancreatic beta cells are not functioning at a minimal level.

Combination oral antidiabetic drug and insulin therapy may be indicated for some patients whose disease does not respond to either drug alone.

MASSAGE IMPLICATIONS AND ASSESSMENT

Oral antidiabetic drugs act in the pancreas, liver, and insulin receptor sites. They do not affect how the body receives and reacts to massage. It is important to note that individuals diagnosed with type 2 diabetes often have other medical problems as well. It is prudent to have a physician's release to perform massage on any client taking these drugs.

Side Effects

Oral antidiabetic drugs do not have the high risk of hypoglycemic reactions or hyperglycemic reactions associated with insulin. However, the side effect of hypoglycemia is still a factor that may occur in some clients taking these medications. The same planning of the massage around a snack or meal takes place and the symptoms relieved with sugar pills, candy, or orange juice if they occur. Be aware if the client has any of the long-term complications of diabetes, such as neuropathy, that would contraindicate deep tissue work. Other adverse reactions must be reported to the client's physician (see Sidebar: *Adverse Reactions to Oral Antidiabetics*).

> ### Adverse Reactions to Oral Antidiabetics
>
> **Side Effects**
> - Hypoglycemia
> - Flushing
> - Gas
> - Heartburn
> - Diarrhea
> - Nausea/vomiting
> - Metallic taste in the mouth
> - Headache
> - Fatigue
> - Photosensitivity
>
> **Adverse Effects**
> - Gallbladder dysfunction
> - Rash
> - Megablastic anemia
> - Blood abnormalities

Glucagon

Common Drug Names

glucagon: GlucaGen

Glucagon, a hyperglycemic drug that raises blood glucose levels, is a hormone normally produced by the alpha cells of the islets of Langerhans in the pancreas (Fig. 13-2).

Pharmacokinetics

Glucagon is absorbed rapidly after subcutaneous, intramuscular, or intravenous injection. Glucagon is distributed throughout the body, although its effect occurs primarily in the liver. Glucagon is degraded extensively by the liver, kidneys, and blood. It is removed from the body by the liver and the kidneys.

Pharmacodynamics

Glucagon regulates the rate of glucose production through glycogenolysis (the conversion of glycogen back into glucose by the liver), gluconeogenesis (the formation of glucose from free fatty acids and proteins), and lipolysis (the release of fatty acids from adipose tissue for conversion to glucose).

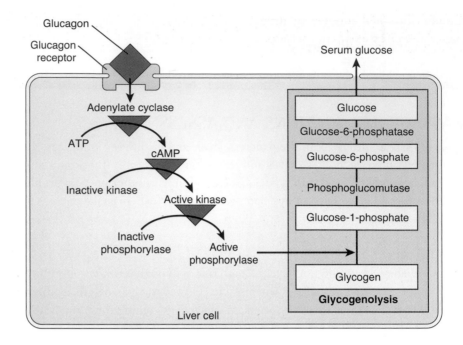

Figure 13-2. Glucagon Raises Glucose Levels. When adequate stores of glycogen are present, glucagon can raise glucose levels in patients with severe hypoglycemia. The process is as follows. (1) Initially, glucagon stimulates the formation of adenylate cyclase in the liver cell. (2) Adenylate cyclase then converts adenosine triphosphate (ATP) to cyclic adenosine monophosphate (cAMP). (3) This product initiates a series of reactions that result in an active phosphorylated glucose molecule. (4) In this phosphorylated form, the large glucose molecule cannot pass through the cell membrane. (5) Through glycogenolysis (the breakdown of glycogen, the stored form of glucose), the liver removes the phosphate group and allows the glucose to enter the bloodstream, raising blood glucose levels for short-term energy needs.

Pharmacotherapeutics

Glucagon is used for emergency treatment of severe hypoglycemia (low blood sugar). It is also used during radiologic examination of the GI tract to reduce GI motility.

Adverse Reactions to Glucagon

- Nausea
- Vomiting
- Hypersensitivity reactions

MASSAGE IMPLICATIONS AND ASSESSMENT

Glucagon is given parenterally in emergency situations and in certain medical tests. It is not appropriate to give massage at these times.

Side Effects

The main side effects of glucagon are nausea and vomiting (see Sidebar: *Adverse Reactions to Glucagon*).

Thyroid and Antithyroid Drugs

Thyroid and antithyroid drugs function to correct thyroid hormone deficiency (hypothyroidism) and thyroid hormone excess (hyperthyroidism).

Thyroid Drugs

Common Drug Names

desiccated thyroid extract: Armour Thyroid, Nature-Throid, Thyroid USP, Westhroid

levothyroxine sodium: Eltroxin, Levo-T, Levothroid, Levoxyl, Novothyrox, Synthroid, t_4, thyroxine, Unithroid,

liothyronine sodium: Cytomel, t_3, thyronine, Triostat

liotrix: t_3/t_4, Thyrolar

Thyroid drugs are natural or synthetic hormones. Natural thyroid drugs are made from animal thyroid and include thyroid USP (desiccated) and thyroglobulin. Synthetic thyroid drugs include levothyroxine sodium, liothyronine sodium, and liotrix.

Pharmacokinetics

Thyroid hormones are absorbed variably from the GI tract and are distributed in the blood. Thyroid drugs are metabolized primarily in the liver and are excreted unchanged in the feces.

Pharmacodynamics

The principal pharmacologic effect is an increased metabolic rate in body tissues. Thyroid hormones affect protein and carbohydrate metabolism and stimulate protein synthesis. They promote gluconeogenesis (the formation of glucose from free fatty acids and proteins) and increase the use of glycogen stores. Thyroid hormones also increase heart rate and cardiac output (the amount of blood pumped by the heart each minute). Finally, they may increase blood flow to the kidneys and increase urine output.

Pharmacotherapeutics

Thyroid drugs act as replacement or substitute hormones to treat the many forms of hypothyroidism, to prevent (with antithyroid drugs) goiter formation (an enlarged thyroid gland) and hypothyroidism, to differentiate between primary and secondary hypothyroidism during diagnostic testing, and to treat thyroid cancer

Levothyroxine is the drug of choice for thyroid hormone replacement and thyroid-stimulating hormone suppression therapy.

MASSAGE IMPLICATIONS AND ASSESSMENT

Thyroid drugs are given orally, so there are no implications with regard to absorption. They act on the tissues of the body in the same way as our own thyroid hormone does. All the actions of thyroid hormone are not fully understood. A client who has been taking thyroid drugs for a while and whose condition is well regulated may receive massage without any concerns. However, a client who is just starting drug therapy or has symptoms of thyroid disease is approached cautiously. Applications of massage may need to be altered depending on the symptoms of the disease more than the drug. A physician's input is appropriate in these cases.

Side Effects

The main side effects that are of concern to the massage therapist are nervousness and insomnia. Slow, rhythmic effleurage, rocking, and other strokes that are systemically reflexive are most helpful if these problems occur. Other adverse reactions must be reported to the physician and if severe, massage should be withheld (see Sidebar: *Adverse Reactions to Thyroid Drugs*).

Antithyroid Drugs

Common Drug Names

methimazole: Tapazole
propylthiouracil: Propyl-Thyracil
radioactive iodine: Iodotope, sodium iodide

A number of drugs act as antithyroid drugs or thyroid antagonists. Used for patients with hyperthyroidism (thyrotoxicosis), these drugs include thionamides (which include propylthiouracil and methimazole) and iodides (which include stable iodine and radioactive iodine).

Pharmacokinetics

Thionamides and iodides are absorbed through the GI tract, concentrated in the thyroid, and excreted in the urine.

Pharmacodynamics

Drugs used to treat hyperthyroidism work in different ways. Thionamides block thyroid hormone synthesis. Stable iodine inhibits hormone synthesis and release of thyroid hormone. Radioactive iodine reduces hormone secretion by destroying thyroid tissue.

Pharmacotherapeutics

Antithyroid drugs commonly are used to treat hyperthyroidism, especially in the form of Graves' disease (hyperthyroidism caused by autoimmunity). Graves' disease accounts for 85% of all cases.

To treat hyperthyroidism, the thyroid gland may be removed by surgery or destroyed by radiation. Before surgery, stable iodine is used to prepare the gland for surgical removal by firming it and decreasing its vascularity. Stable iodine is also used after radioactive iodine therapy to control symptoms of hyperthyroidism while the radiation takes effect.

Propylthiouracil, which lowers hormone levels faster than methimazole, is usually used for rapid improvement of severe hyperthyroidism. Propylthiouracil is preferred over methimazole in pregnant women because its rapid action reduces transfer across the placenta. Because methimazole blocks thyroid hormone formation for a longer time, it is better suited for administration once per day to patients with mild to moderate hyperthyroidism. Therapy may continue for 12 to 24 months before remission occurs.

MASSAGE IMPLICATIONS AND ASSESSMENT

Absorption rates of these oral drugs are not affected by massage. The drugs act by inhibiting thyroid hormone synthesis and/or by destroying thyroid tissue that creates the hormone. Although the drugs do not affect the action of the massage strokes, the disease itself may require alterations in the applications of massage. A physician must be consulted, especially in cases in which the client's condition is not regulated and the thyroid hormone production is unstable. Radioactive iodine requires special precautions. The amount of time that anyone is in close contact with the client (such as during massage) must be limited. Pregnant or nursing mothers should have no close contact at all with the client for 1 to 6 days. The physician can educate the therapist in the necessary precautions.

Side Effects

There are few side effects to these drugs that are of concern to the massage therapist, other than those associated with radioactive treatments. Adverse reactions can be severe and must be reported to the physician. Massage should be withheld (see Sidebar: *Adverse Reactions to Antithyroid Drugs*).

Adverse Reactions to Antithyroid Drugs

Side Effects
- Headache
- Drowsiness
- Vertigo
- Diarrhea
- Nausea/vomiting
- Cold intolerance
- Arthralgia
- Myalgia
- Enlarged lymph nodes
- Metallic taste in the mouth
- Burning in the mouth
- Salivary gland enlargement

Adverse Effects
- Hematologic disturbances
- Depression
- Hepatotoxicity
- Acute hypersensitivity reactions

Pituitary Drugs

Pituitary drugs are natural or synthetic hormones that mimic the hormones produced by the pituitary gland. Pituitary drugs consist of two groups. The anterior pituitary drugs are used diagnostically or therapeutically to control the function of other endocrine glands, such as the thyroid gland, adrenals, ovaries, and testes. Posterior pituitary drugs are used to regulate fluid volume and stimulate smooth muscle contraction in selected clinical situations.

Anterior Pituitary Drugs

Common Drug Names: Adrenocorticotropics

corticotropin: ACTH, Acthar

corticotropin repository: ACTH Gel, Acthar Gel

corticotropin zinc hydroxide

cosyntropin: Cortrosyn

Common Drug Names: Growth Hormone

somatrem: Protropin

Common Drug Names: Gonadotropics

chorionic gonadotropin: CG, Chorex, HCG, Novarel, Pregnyl, Profasi,

menotropin, Humegon, Pergonal

Common Drug Names: Thyrotropics

thyroid stimulating hormone: TSH

thyrotropin: Thyrogen, Thytropar

Pharmacokinetics

Anterior pituitary drugs are not given orally because they are destroyed in the GI tract. Some of these hormones can be administered topically, but most require injection. Usually, natural hormones are absorbed, distributed, and metabolized rapidly. Anterior pituitary hormone drugs are metabolized at the receptor site and in the liver and kidneys. The hormones are excreted primarily in the urine.

Pharmacodynamics

Anterior pituitary drugs exert a profound effect on the body's growth and development. The hypothalamus controls secretions of the pituitary gland. In turn, the pituitary gland secretes hormones that regulate secretions or functions of other glands.

The concentration of hormones in the blood helps determine hormone production rate. Increased pituitary hormone levels inhibit other organ hormone production. Decreased levels of pituitary hormones raise other organ production and secretion.

Pharmacotherapeutics

The clinical indications for anterior pituitary hormone drugs are diagnostic and therapeutic. Corticotropin and cosyntropin are used diagnostically to differentiate between primary and secondary failure of the adrenal cortex. Corticotropin is also used to treat adrenal insufficiency. Somatrem is used to treat pituitary dwarfism (growth hormone deficiency), chronic renal disease, and acquired immune deficiency syndrome (AIDS) wasting.

MASSAGE IMPLICATIONS AND ASSESSMENT

Because these drugs are most often given by injection (or topically), the site of administration is locally contraindicated for massage. The onset and peak action times for the drug in question determine how long massage is avoided in the area. The action of these drugs is that of replacing something that the body should be, but is not, making on its own. The drugs themselves will not interfere with the application of massage. However, because the disorders that require these treatments can be serious and complicated, a physician release must be obtained and the therapist must make sure he or she understands fully the effect the disease has on the body.

Side Effects

Side effects of these drugs that are of concern to the massage therapist occur with long-term use of corticotropins. Cushing's syndrome can develop as a result of the long-term use of corticotropins. The implications for massage in these cases are the same as for the long-term use of corticosteroids. See Chapter 11 for a complete discussion of corticosteroids (see Sidebar: *Adverse Reactions to Anterior Pituitary Drugs*).

Posterior Pituitary Drugs

Common Drug Names

antidiuretic hormone: ADH

desmopressin acetate: DDAVP, Octostim, Stimate

lypressin

oxytocin: oxytocin citrate, PIT, Pitocin, Syntocinon

vasopressin: Pitressin, Pressyn

Posterior pituitary hormones are synthesized in the hypothalamus and stored in the posterior pituitary, which in turn secretes the hormones into the blood. These drugs include all forms of antidiuretic hormone (ADH) (such as desmopressin acetate, lypressin, and vasopressin) and the oxytocic drugs oxytocin and oxytocin citrate.

Pharmacokinetics

Because enzymes in the GI tract can destroy all protein hormones, these drugs cannot be given orally. Posterior pituitary drugs may be given by injection or intranasal spray.

Like other natural hormones, oxytocic drugs usually are absorbed, distributed, and metabolized rapidly. Parenterally administered oxytocin is absorbed rapidly. However, absorption is erratic when it is administered intranasally.

Pharmacodynamics

Posterior pituitary hormones affect smooth muscle contraction in the uterus, bladder, and GI tract; fluid balance through kidney reabsorption of water; and blood pressure through stimulation of the arterial wall muscles. ADH increases reabsorption of water by the kidney. High dosages of ADH stimulate contraction of blood vessels, increasing the blood pressure. Desmopressin reduces increased urination and promotes clotting. In pregnant women, oxytocin may stimulate uterine contractions. It also can stimulate lactation (milk production by the breast) through its effect on mammary glands of the breasts.

Pharmacotherapeutics

ADH is prescribed for hormone replacement therapy in patients with neurogenic diabetes insipidus (an excessive loss of urine caused by a brain lesion or injury that interferes with ADH synthesis or release). However, it does not effectively treat nephrogenic diabetes insipidus (caused by renal tubular resistance to ADH).

Desmopressin and lypressin are the drugs of choice for chronic ADH deficiency and are administered intranasally. These drugs are particularly useful for patients allergic to a vasopressin of animal origin.

Short-term ADH treatment is indicated for patients with transient diabetes insipidus after head injury or surgery; therapy may be lifelong for patients with idiopathic hormone deficiencies. Used for short-term therapy, vasopressin elevates blood pressure in patients with hypotension caused by lack of vascular tone. It also relieves postoperative gaseous distention.

Oxytocics are used to induce labor and complete incomplete abortions; treat preeclampsia, eclampsia, and premature rupture of membranes surrounding the fetus in the womb; control bleeding and uterine relaxation after delivery; hasten uterine shrinking after delivery; and stimulate lactation (milk production in the breasts).

Adverse Reactions to Posterior Pituitary Drugs

Hypersensitivity reactions are the most common adverse reactions to posterior pituitary drugs.

Natural ADH
Anaphylaxis may occur after injection. Natural ADH can also cause:
- Ringing in the ears
- Anxiety
- Hyponatremia (low serum sodium levels)
- Proteins in the urine
- Eclamptic attacks
- Pupil dilation
- Transient edema

Synthetic ADH
Adverse reactions to synthetic ADH are rare. Synthetic oxytocin can cause adverse reactions for pregnant women, including:
- Bleeding after delivery
- GI disturbances
- Sweating
- Headache
- Dizziness
- Ringing in the ears
- Severe water intoxication

MASSAGE IMPLICATIONS AND ASSESSMENT

Because these drugs are given by injection, the site of injection is a local contraindication for massage. Absorption via intranasal administration is not affected by massage. The drugs themselves will not affect how the body receives massage strokes. However, a full understanding of the disease process is essential and may require some alteration in massage application. Physician consent must be obtained.

In the case of oxytocics, the muscles affected are mainly the mammary glands, uterus, bladder, and GI tract. Depending on the situation and why the drug is used, massage may not be appropriate. For example, for preeclampsia and eclampsia, massage may be completely contraindicated. In the use of oxytocics for inducing labor, however, massage that helps the client relax may help with delivering the baby.

Side Effects

Dizziness, hypotension, and anxiety are the main side effects about which the massage therapist is concerned. Care must be taken when the client is changing position. Systemic reflex strokes that stimulate are used at the end of the session. Other adverse reactions must be reported to the physician and contraindicate massage until they are under control (see Sidebar: *Adverse Reactions to Posterior Pituitary Drugs*).

Estrogens

Estrogens mimic the physiologic effects of naturally occurring female sex hormones. Estrogens are used to correct estrogen-deficient states and, in oral contraceptives, prevent pregnancy.

Estrogen Types

Common Drug Names: Synthetic Estrogens

conjugated estrogens: CES, Premarin

diethylstilbestrol: DES, Honvol, Stilbestrol, Stilphostrol

esterified estrogens: Estratab, Menest, Neo-Estrone

estradiol cypionate: depGynogen Injection (discontinued in the U.S.), Depo-Estradiol, Dura-Estrin, E-Cypionate, Estro-Cyp (discontinued in the U.S.), Estrofem

estradiol valerate: Delestrogen, Dioval, Duragen, Estadol LA, Estra-L (discontinued in the U.S.), Femogex, Gynogen L.A. Injection (discontinued in the U.S.), Menaval

estrone: Ogen, Ortho-Est

ethinyl estradiol: Estinyl

Common Drug Names: Bioidentical Estrogens

estradiol: Climara, Estrace, Estraderm, Estring, Vivelle

estriol: Estriol

estrone, estradiol, and estriol: Tri-Est, Triestrogen

Estrogens that treat endocrine system disorders include:

- Bioidentical products: conjugated estrogenic substances, estriol, estradiol, and estrone (these are chemically identical to the hormones produced in a woman's body)

- Synthetic estrogens: chlorotrianisene, dienestrol, diethylstilbestrol, diethylstilbestrol diphosphate (created in laboratories and chemically slightly different from the body's hormones—they have estrogen-like effects on the body)

- Esterified estrogens: estradiol cypionate, estradiol valerate, ethinyl estradiol, and quinestrol. (also synthetic).

Special Note: The chemically altered synthetic hormones have been the most widely used. Because they are not produced by nature, they can be patented and therefore cost more. They have been promoted widely by pharmaceutical companies. The natural or bioidentical hormones, because they occur in nature, cannot be patented and are less expensive. Women's groups are just now beginning to inform women of the many choices available to them; physicians are slowly becoming educated about them as well.

Pharmacokinetics

Estrogens are absorbed well and distributed throughout the body. Metabolism occurs in the liver, and the metabolites are excreted primarily by the kidneys.

Pharmacodynamics

The exact mechanism of action of estrogen is not clearly understood, but it is believed to increase synthesis of deoxyribonucleic acid (DNA), ribonucleic acid (RNA), and protein in estrogen-responsive tissues in the female breast, urinary tract, and genital organs.

Pharmacotherapeutics

Estrogens are prescribed primarily for hormone replacement therapy in postmenopausal women to relieve symptoms caused by loss of ovarian function. They are less commonly prescribed for hormonal replacement therapy in women with primary ovarian failure or female hypogonadism (reduced hormonal secretion by the ovaries) and in patients who have undergone surgical removal of the ovaries. Estrogens are used palliatively to treat advanced, inoperable breast cancer in postmenopausal women and prostate cancer in men.

Special Note: The National Institutes of Health study released in 2002 caused great concern about the use of synthetic estrogens and progestin hormones because it showed increased heart disease, cancer, strokes, and blood clots with their use. Use has declined and further studies are needed concerning synthetic versus bioidentical/natural hormones and their benefits and long-term effects. The study only used Prempro, a combination synthetic estrogen and progesterone pill. Most physicians still prescribe hormones for women with problems during perimenopause and menopause, but recommend use for shorter periods (less than 4 years). Hormone therapy is still recommended for women at high risk for serious osteoporosis.

Adverse Reactions to Estrogens

Side Effects
- Bilateral, pounding headache
- Recurrent vaginal yeast infections
- Breast swelling and tenderness
- Nausea/vomiting
- Leg cramps
- Bloating
- Yellow-tinged skin

Adverse Reactions
- Hypertension
- Thromboembolism (blood vessel blockage caused by a blood clot)
- Thrombophlebitis (vein inflammation associated with clot formation)
- Depression
- Excessive vaginal bleeding

MASSAGE IMPLICATIONS AND ASSESSMENT

The drugs themselves do not have any effect on how the body responds to massage. Any area of recent topical application is avoided for 2 to 4 hours.

Side Effects

Whereas the side effects of estrogens can be many and varied, they do not affect the application of massage. Assessing the client's needs determines how to best give a massage. In most cases, massage that is relaxing and utilizes systemic reflex strokes helps to balance the client and ease any side effects. One side effect that is of concern is that of increased incidence of blood clots and phlebitis. Signs of this include redness, heat, swelling, and pain, most often in the legs. If there is any symptom that is questionable, massage is completely contraindicated until a physician can determine if a clot is present (see Sidebar: *Adverse Reactions to Estrogens*).

Progesterones

Common Drug Names: Synthetic Progestins

medroxyprogesterone acetate: Amen (discontinued in the U.S.), Provera

medroxyprogesterone with conjugated equine estrogens (Provera and Premarin): Prempro

norethindrone acetate: Aygestin

Common Drug Names: Bioidentical Progesterones

micronized progesterone: Prometrium

progesterone: Crinone, Gesterol, Progestasert

Progesterone drugs are used to mimic the action of the hormone progesterone. This hormone is responsible for building up the uterine lining to prepare for a fetus. It is also a uterine muscle relaxant. Progesterone maintains a pregnancy. A drop in the progesterone level leads to the menstrual period and the sloughing off of the uterine blood in menstruation. Its effects balance out those of estrogen in the body. It is used, along with estrogen, to treat menopausal symptoms in women who have an intact uterus (estrogen alone increases the risk of uterine cancer). It also may be given for premenstrual syndrome (PMS) and in combination with estrogen in birth control pills.

Special Note: Like estrogens, progesterone is available in synthetic chemically altered forms with progesterone-like effects and in the bioidentical forms that are chemically identical to the hormone created by the body. Plant-based progesterones like yam creams are available over the counter. They vary greatly in their content of actual progesterone and some have none whatsoever. There are 2% progesterone creams available, however, that contain standardized amounts of progesterone USP. Labels must be checked carefully.

Pharmacokinetics

Progesterone is well absorbed and excreted in urine.

Pharmacodynamics

The mechanism of progesterone is not well understood. It targets the reproductive organs and stimulates them. It may have many other effects throughout the body.

Pharmacotherapeutics

Progesterone is prescribed for hormone replacement therapy for control of symptoms in perimenopausal and menopausal women, for fertility problems, for moderate to severe PMS, for excessive uterine bleeding, for birth control, and for amenorrhea (absence of menstrual flow).

Adverse Reactions to Progesterone

Side Effects
- Headache
- Lethargy
- Depression
- Nausea and vomiting
- Breakthrough bleeding
- Breast tenderness
- Weight gain and bloating
- Lack of sexual desire
- Moodiness

Adverse Effects
- Hypertension
- Thrombophlebitis
- Embolism
- Jaundice
- Hyperglycemia

MASSAGE IMPLICATIONS AND ASSESSMENT

The hormone does not affect how the body reacts to massage strokes. No change is needed in the application of massage. Any area of topical application is avoided for 2 to 4 hours. If the drug is being used to treat fertility problems and/or to maintain a high-risk pregnancy, massage is completely contraindicated unless physician approval is obtained.

Side Effects

Side effects of concern to the massage therapist are mainly caused by the synthetic hormones. They include breast tenderness, bloating, and increased risk of blood clots. The first two only require gentle approaches in massage, and the use of effleurage may help decrease these effects. Any concern or symptoms of blood clots (redness, swelling, pain, heat in extremities) is a complete contraindication, and the physician is notified immediately (see Sidebar: *Adverse Reactions to Progesterone*).

Quick Quiz

1. You have a new client who is 22 years old and has type 1 diabetes. She has been diabetic since she was 14 years old and states that her diabetes is well controlled, that she has very few incidents of hypoglycemia or hyperglycemia, and that she takes Novolin 70/30 twice a day. What will this mean for your massage?

2. A 46-year-old man comes to you for massage. He states that he has diabetes insipidus and he takes desmopressin three times a day intranasally. What should you do?

Drugs for Fluid and Electrolyte Balance

14

Drugs and Homeostasis

Illness can easily disturb the homeostatic mechanisms that help maintain normal fluid and electrolyte balance. Occurrences such as loss of appetite, medication administration, vomiting, surgery, and diagnostic tests can also alter this delicate balance. Fortunately, numerous drugs can be used to correct these imbalances and help bring the body back toward homeostasis.

Electrolyte Replacement Drugs

An electrolyte is a compound or element that carries an electrical charge when dissolved in water. Electrolyte replacement drugs are mineral salts that increase depleted or deficient electrolyte levels, thereby helping to maintain homeostasis (the stability of body fluid composition and volume). They include potassium, the primary intracellular fluid (ICF) electrolyte; calcium, a major extracellular fluid (ECF) electrolyte; magnesium, an electrolyte essential for homeostasis found in ICF; and sodium, another electrolyte necessary for homeostasis found in ECF.

Potassium

Common Drug Names

potassium bicarbonate: K Care, K-Ide, Klor-Con, K-Lyte

potassium chloride: Cena-K, Kaochlor, Kaon-Cl, K-Dur, K-Lease (discontinued in the U.S.), K-Lor, Slow-K, Micro-K

potassium gluconate: Glu-K, Kaon, Kaylixir, K-G Elixir (discontinued in the U.S.),
  Potassium-Rougier

potassium phosphate: Neutra-Phos-K

Potassium is the major positively charged ion (cation) in intracellular fluid (fluid inside the cell). Because the body cannot store potassium, adequate amounts must be ingested daily. If this is not possible, potassium replacement can be accomplished orally or intravenously with potassium salts, such as potassium bicarbonate, potassium chloride, potassium gluconate, or potassium phosphate.

Pharmacokinetics (how drugs circulate)

Oral potassium is absorbed readily from the gastrointestinal (GI) tract. After absorption into the extracellular fluid (fluid outside and surrounding the cells), almost all the potassium passes into the ICF. Normal serum levels of potassium are maintained by the kidneys, which excrete most of the excessive potassium intake. The rest is excreted in feces and sweat.

Pharmacodynamics (how drugs act)

Potassium moves quickly into ICF to restore depleted potassium levels and reestablish balance. Potassium is necessary for proper functioning of all nerve and muscle cells and for nerve impulse transmission. It is also essential for tissue growth and repair as well as for maintenance of acid-base balance.

Pharmacotherapeutics (how drugs are used)

Potassium replacement therapy corrects hypokalemia, low levels of potassium in the blood. Hypokalemia is a common occurrence in conditions that increase potassium excretion or depletion, such as vomiting or diarrhea, excessive urination, some kidney diseases, cystic fibrosis, burns, excess of antidiuretic hormone (ADH) or therapy with a potassium-depleting diuretic, alkalosis, insufficient potassium intake from starvation, and administration of a glucocorticoid, intravenous amphotericin B, or intravenous solutions that contain insufficient potassium.

Potassium is also used to decrease the toxic effects of digoxin. Because potassium inhibits the excitability of the heart, low potassium levels enhance the action of digoxin, which may result in toxicity.

MASSAGE IMPLICATIONS AND ASSESSMENT

Massage does not affect the absorption of potassium. The action of potassium actually helps the body to react appropriately to massage. Low levels of potassium can interfere with the reflex signals of the nervous system and make massage less effective on muscles. No change in application of massage needs to be made because of this drug.

Side Effects

There are no side effects of concern to the massage therapist. If adverse reactions occur, massage is withheld and a physician is notified (see Sidebar: *Adverse Reactions to Potassium*).

Calcium

Common Drug Names

calcium carbonate: Apo-Cal, Calci-Chew, Calcite, Cal-Plus, Caltrate, Fem Cal, Florical, Os-Cal, Oystercal, Rolaids Calcium, Tums

calcium chloride: Calciject

calcium citrate: Citracal

calcium glubionate: Calcium-Sandoz, Neo-Calglucon

calcium gluconate: Calfort, Cal-G

calcium lactate: Calbon, Cal-Lac, Ridactate

Calcium is a major cation (a positively charged ion) in ECF. (An ion is an atom that has lost one or more of its electrons; in the fluid of the body these are called electrolytes and can carry electricity.) Almost all the calcium in the body (99%) is stored in bone, where it can be released into the blood if necessary. When dietary intake is not enough to meet metabolic needs, calcium stores in bone are reduced. Calcium stores are reduced in osteoporosis. Chronic insufficient calcium intake can result in excess release of the mineral into the blood, causing weakening of the bone. Calcium is replaced orally or intravenously with calcium salts such as calcium carbonate, calcium chloride, calcium citrate, calcium glubionate, calcium gluconate, or calcium lactate.

Pharmacokinetics

Oral calcium is absorbed readily from the small intestine. A pH (blood acidity level) of 5 to 7, parathyroid hormone, and vitamin D all aid calcium absorption. Absorption also depends on dietary factors. Calcium is distributed primarily in bone. Calcium salts are eliminated primarily in feces; the rest is excreted in urine.

Pharmacodynamics

Calcium moves quickly into ECF to restore calcium levels and reestablish balance. Calcium has several important roles in the body. Extracellular ionized calcium plays an essential role in normal nerve and muscle excitability. Calcium is integral to normal functioning of the heart, kidneys, and lungs, and it affects the blood clotting rate. Calcium is a factor in neurotransmitter and hormone activity, amino acid metabolism, vitamin B_{12} absorption, and gastrin (the hormone that stimulates the stomach to release acid for digestion) secretion. Calcium also plays a major role in normal bone and tooth formation.

Adverse Reactions to Potassium

Most adverse reactions to potassium are related to the method of administration.

- Oral potassium sometimes causes nausea, vomiting, abdominal pain, and diarrhea. Enteric-coated tablets may cause small bowel ulceration, stenosis, hemorrhage, and obstruction.

- Intravenous infusion of potassium preparations can cause pain at the injection site and phlebitis (vein inflammation). Given rapidly, intravenous administration may cause cardiac arrest. Infusion of potassium in patients with decreased urine production increases the risk of hyperkalemia.

Pharmacotherapeutics

Calcium is helpful in treating excess magnesium (a condition that can slow the heart, lower blood pressure, and even lead to cardiac arrest). It is also helpful in strengthening myocardial tissue after defibrillation (electric shock to restore normal heart rhythm) or a poor response to epinephrine during resuscitation. Pregnancy and breast-feeding increase calcium requirements, as do periods of bone growth during childhood and adolescence.

The major clinical indication for intravenous calcium is acute hypocalcemia (low serum calcium levels), in which a rapid increase in serum calcium levels is needed. Conditions that create this need are tetany, cardiac arrest, vitamin D deficiency, parathyroid surgery, and alkalosis. Intravenous calcium is also used to prevent a hypocalcemic reaction during exchange transfusions.

Oral calcium is commonly used to supplement a calcium-deficient diet and prevent osteoporosis. Chronic hypocalcemia caused by such conditions as chronic hypoparathyroidism (a deficiency of parathyroid hormones), osteomalacia (softening of bones), rickets, and vitamin D deficiency is also treated with oral calcium.

Adverse Reactions to Calcium

Calcium preparations may produce hypercalcemia (elevated serum calcium levels). Early signs include:

- Drowsiness
- Lethargy
- Muscle weakness
- Headache
- Constipation
- Metallic taste in the mouth

Electrocardiogram changes that occur with elevated serum calcium levels include a shortened QT interval and heart block. Severe hypercalcemia can cause cardiac arrhythmias, cardiac arrest, and eventually coma.

MASSAGE IMPLICATIONS AND ASSESSMENT

With this replacement drug, no problems exist with the application of massage strokes. As with potassium, calcium improves the nerve and muscle reactions to the systemic and local reflex massage strokes.

Side Effects

Rarely, calcium causes drowsiness. Care needs to be taken to stimulate the client at the end of the massage if this side effect occurs. Adverse reactions must be reported to the physician and if severe, massage should be withheld (see Sidebar: *Adverse Reactions to Calcium*).

Magnesium

Common Drug Names

magnesium chloride: Slow-Mag

magnesium citrate: Citro-Mag

magnesium gluconate: Magonate

magnesium oxide: Mag-Ox, Mag-Gel

magnesium sulfate: Epsom salts

Magnesium is the most abundant cation (positively charged electrolyte) in ICF after potassium. It is essential in transmitting nerve impulses to muscle and activating enzymes necessary for carbohydrate and protein metabolism. Magnesium stimulates parathyroid hormone secretion, thus regulating ICF calcium levels. Magnesium also aids in cell metabolism and the movement of sodium and potassium across cell membranes.

Magnesium stores are depleted by malabsorption, chronic diarrhea, prolonged treatment with diuretics, nasogastric suctioning, prolonged therapy with intravenous fluids not containing magnesium, hyperaldosteronism, hypoparathyroidism or hyperparathyroidism, and excessive release of adrenocortical hormones. Magnesium is typically replaced in the form of magnesium sulfate.

Pharmacokinetics

Magnesium sulfate is distributed widely throughout the body. Intravenous magnesium sulfate acts immediately; intramuscular magnesium sulfate acts within 30 minutes of administration. Magnesium sulfate is not metabolized and is excreted unchanged in the urine; some is excreted in breast milk.

Pharmacodynamics

Magnesium sulfate replenishes and prevents magnesium deficiencies. It also prevents or controls seizures by blocking neuromuscular transmission.

Pharmacotherapeutics

Magnesium sulfate is the drug of choice for replacement therapy in magnesium deficiency. It is also used to treat seizures, severe toxemia, and acute nephritis in children.

MASSAGE IMPLICATIONS AND ASSESSMENT

As with the other electrolytes, there are no changes needed in the application of massage with the use of magnesium. It too improves the response of the muscles to reflex massage strokes, both local and systemic.

Side Effects

There are no side effects of concern to the massage therapist regarding magnesium. Some side effects can occur, as can some adverse effects. Any adverse effects must be reported to a physician and massage withheld (see Sidebar: *Adverse Reactions to Magnesium*).

> **Adverse Reactions to Magnesium**
>
> Adverse reactions to magnesium sulfate, which can be life-threatening, include:
> - Hypotension
> - Circulatory collapse
> - Flushing
> - Depressed reflexes
> - Respiratory paralysis
> - Diarrhea

Sodium

Common Drug Names

sodium chloride: normal saline, salt

Sodium is the major cation (positively charged electrolyte) in ECF. Sodium performs many functions. It maintains the pressure and concentration of ECF, acid-base balance, and water balance. It contributes to nerve conduction and neuromuscular function. It plays a role in glandular secretion.

Sodium replacement is necessary in conditions that rapidly deplete it, such as excessive loss of GI fluids and excessive perspiration. Diuretics and tap water enemas can also deplete sodium, particularly when fluids are replaced by plain water. Sodium also can be lost in trauma or wound drainage, adrenal gland insufficiency, cirrhosis of the liver with ascites, syndrome of inappropriate ADH, and prolonged intravenous infusion of dextrose in water without other solutes. Sodium is typically replaced in the form of sodium chloride.

Pharmacokinetics

Oral and parenteral sodium chloride are quickly absorbed and distributed widely throughout the body. Sodium chloride is not significantly metabolized. It is eliminated primarily in urine but also in sweat, tears, and saliva.

Pharmacodynamics

Sodium chloride solution replaces deficiencies of the sodium and chloride ions in the blood plasma.

Pharmacotherapeutics

Sodium chloride is used for water and electrolyte replacement in patients with hyponatremia from electrolyte loss or severe sodium chloride depletion. Severe symptomatic sodium deficiency may be treated with intravenous infusion of a solution containing sodium chloride.

Adverse Reactions to Sodium

Adverse reactions to sodium include:
- Pulmonary edema (if given too rapidly or in excess)
- Hypernatremia
- Potassium loss

MASSAGE IMPLICATIONS AND ASSESSMENT

The use of the drug sodium does not affect the application of massage in any way. It enhances the reaction of nerves and muscles to the massage strokes.

Side Effects

There are no side effects of concern with sodium. Adverse reactions must be reported to the physician and massage withheld (see Sidebar: *Adverse Reactions to Sodium*).

Alkalinizing and Acidifying Drugs

Alkalinizing and acidifying drugs act to correct acid-base imbalances in the blood. These acid-base imbalances include metabolic acidosis, a decreased serum pH (level of acidity/alkalinity) caused by excess hydrogen ions in the ECF, which is treated with alkalinizing drugs, and metabolic alkalosis, an increased serum pH (level of acidity/alkalinity) caused by excess bicarbonate in the ECF, which is treated with acidifying drugs.

Alkalinizing and acidifying drugs have opposite effects. An alkalinizing drug will increase the pH of the blood (making it more alkaline). An acidifying drug will decrease the pH (making it more acidic). (The normal pH of blood is 7.4, which is slightly acidic. Below 7.4 means more acid and above 7.4 means less acid and more alkaline.)

Some of these drugs also alter urine pH, making them useful in treating some urinary tract infections and drug overdoses.

Alkalinizing Drugs

Common Drug Names

sodium bicarbonate: Citrocarbonate, Neut

sodium citrate: Polycitra

sodium lactate

These drugs are used to increase blood pH. Sodium bicarbonate is also used to increase urine pH.

Pharmacokinetics

All alkalinizing drugs are absorbed well when given orally. Sodium citrate and sodium lactate are metabolized to the active ingredient, bicarbonate. Sodium bicarbonate is not metabolized. Tromethamine undergoes little or no metabolism and is excreted unchanged in the urine.

Pharmacodynamics

Sodium bicarbonate separates in the blood to provide bicarbonate ions that are used in the blood buffer system to decrease the hydrogen ion concentration and raise blood pH (acid/alkaline levels). As the bicarbonate ions are excreted in the urine, urine pH rises. Sodium citrate and lactate, after conversion to bicarbonate, alkalinize the blood and urine in the same way.

Pharmacotherapeutics

Alkalinizing drugs are commonly used to treat metabolic acidosis. Other uses include raising the urine pH to help remove certain substances, such as phenobarbital, after an overdose. Sodium bicarbonate may be used as an antacid.

MASSAGE IMPLICATIONS AND ASSESSMENT

Alkalinizing drugs are used in a very serious condition of acidosis. Massage is not appropriate at this time or until the client is stabilized. If used as an antacid, it does not affect the reaction of the body to any massage strokes (see Sidebar: *Adverse Reactions to Alkalinizing Drugs*).

Adverse Reactions to Alkalinizing Drugs

Adverse reactions to alkalinizing drugs vary.

Sodium Bicarbonate
- Bicarbonate overdose
- Cerebral dysfunction, tissue hypoxia, and lactic acidosis (with rapid administration for diabetic ketoacidosis)
- Water retention and edema

Sodium Citrate
- Metabolic alkalosis, tetany, or aggravation of existing heart disease (with overdose)
- Laxative effect (with oral administration)

Sodium Lactate
- Metabolic alkalosis (with overdose)
- Extravasation
- Water retention or edema (in patients with kidney disease or heart failure)

Acidifying Drugs

Common Drug Names

ammonium chloride
ascorbic acid and ammonium chloride
hydrochloric acid

Ammonium chloride and hydrochloric acid are used to correct metabolic alkalosis. Ascorbic acid, along with ammonium chloride, is a urinary acidifier.

Pharmacokinetics

The action of most acidifying drugs is immediate. Orally administered ammonium chloride is absorbed completely in 3 to 6 hours. It is metabolized in the liver to form urea, which is excreted by the kidneys, and hydrochloric acid, the acidifying drug. After intravenous administration, hydrochloric acid is broken down into hydrogen and chloride ions. The hydrogen ions are used as the acidifying drug. Orally administered ascorbic acid usually is absorbed well, distributed widely in body tissues, and metabolized in the liver. It is excreted in the urine along with excess ascorbic acid, which is excreted unchanged.

Pharmacodynamics

Acidifying drugs have several actions. Ammonium chloride lowers the blood pH. Hydrochloric acid lowers blood pH directly by acidifying the blood with hydrogen ions. Ascorbic acid directly acidifies the urine, providing hydrogen ions and lowering urine pH.

Pharmacotherapeutics

A patient with metabolic alkalosis requires therapy with an acidifying drug that provides hydrogen ions; such a patient may need chloride ion therapy as well. Although the patient can receive both in a hydrochloric acid infusion, this infusion is difficult to prepare, and an overdose can produce severe adverse reactions. Most patients receive both types of ions in oral or parenteral doses of ammonium chloride, a safer drug that is easy to prepare.

Adverse Reactions to Acidifying Drugs

Adverse reactions to acidifying drugs are usually mild, such as GI distress. Overdose may lead to acidosis.

Ammonium Chloride
- Metabolic acidosis and loss of electrolytes, especially potassium (with large doses)
- Hydrochloric acid
- Metabolic acidosis (with an overdose)

Ascorbic Acid
- GI distress (with high doses)
- Hemolytic anemia (in a patient with glucose-6-phosphate dehydrogenase deficiency)

MASSAGE IMPLICATIONS AND ASSESSMENT

Acidifying drugs are used to treat alkalosis. This is a serious condition, and massage is contraindicated until the client's condition is stabilized. On occasion, hydrochloric acid may be used as a digestive aide. In these cases, the drug itself would not affect how the body reacts to massage strokes (see Sidebar: *Adverse Reactions to Acidifying Drugs*).

Quick Quiz

1. An elderly female client tells you she is taking Slow-K. She does not know why. She is also taking a diuretic for high blood pressure. Will this be a problem for massage?

2. A client tells you she is taking Os-Cal by doctor's order for her osteoporosis. Can you give her massage?

Cancer Drugs

15

Drugs and Cancer

In the 1940s, antineoplastic (chemotherapeutic) drugs were used to treat cancer when all other therapeutic measures failed. However, most antineoplastic drugs commonly had serious adverse effects. Today, many of these effects can be minimized so they are not as devastating to the patient. In fact, many childhood cancers are now considered curable because of the advent of chemotherapeutic drugs, many of which are now the drug of choice for different types of cancer. In addition, drugs such as interferons are being used to treat patients with cancer. The massage implications for clients taking these drugs are numerous, complex, and similar no matter which drugs are being taken. Massage implications are discussed in one section at the end of this chapter, after the various types of cancer drugs are examined in depth.

Alkylating Drugs

Alkylating drugs, given alone or with other drugs, act effectively against various malignant neoplasms. These drugs fall into one of six classes: nitrogen mustards, alkyl sulfonates, nitrosoureas, triazenes, ethyleneimine, and alkylating-like drugs.

All of these drugs produce their antineoplastic effects by deactivating deoxyribonucleic acid (DNA). They halt DNA's replication process.

Nitrogen Mus tards

Common Drug Names

chlorambucil: Leukeran

cyclophosphamide: Cytoxan, Neosar, Procytox

estramustine: Emcyt

ifosfamide: Ifex

mechlorethamine hydrochloride: Mustargen

melphalan: Alkeran

uracil mustard

Nitrogen mustards represent the largest group of alkylating drugs. Mechlorethamine hydrochloride was the first nitrogen mustard introduced and is still the most rapid-acting.

Pharmacokinetics (how drugs circulate)

The absorption and distribution of nitrogen mustards, as with most alkylating drugs, vary widely. Nitrogen mustards are metabolized in the liver and excreted by the kidneys. Mechlorethamine undergoes metabolism so rapidly that no active drug remains after a few minutes. Most nitrogen mustards possess longer half-lives than mechlorethamine.

Pharmacodynamics (how drugs act)

Nitrogen mustards form bonds with DNA molecules in a chemical reaction known as alkylation. Alkylated DNA cannot replicate properly, thereby resulting in cell death. Unfortunately, cells may develop resistance to the cytotoxic effects of nitrogen mustards (Fig. 15-1).

Pharmacotherapeutics (how drugs are used)

Because they produce leukopenia (reduced number of white blood cells [WBCs]), the nitrogen mustards are effective in treating cancers, such as Hodgkin's disease (cancer causing painless enlargement of the lymph nodes, spleen, and lymphoid tissues) and leukemia (cancer of the blood-forming tissues), that have an associated elevated WBC count.

Nitrogen mustards also are effective against malignant lymphoma (cancer of the lymphoid tissue), multiple myeloma (cancer of the marrow plasma cells), melanoma (malignancy that arises from melanocytes), and cancers of the breast, ovaries, uterus, lung, brain, testes, bladder, prostate, and stomach (see Sidebar: *Adverse Reactions to Nitrogen Mustards*).

Alkyl Sulfonate

Common Drug Names

busulfan: Busulfex, Myleran

The alkyl sulfonate busulfan is commonly used to treat chronic myelogenous leukemia and less commonly to treat polycythemia vera (increased red blood cell mass and increased number of WBCs and platelets) as well as other myeloproliferative (pertaining to the bone marrow) disorders.

Pharmacokinetics

Busulfan is absorbed rapidly and well from the gastrointestinal (GI) tract. Little is known about its distribution. Busulfan is metabolized extensively in the liver before urinary excretion. Its half-life is 2 to 3 hours.

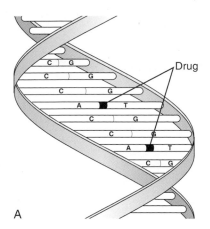

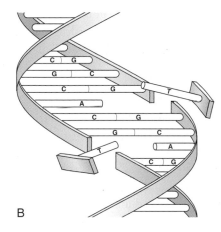

Figure 15-1 Mechanism of Action of Alkylating Drugs. Alkylating drugs attack deoxyribonucleic acid (DNA) in two ways. **(A)** Some drugs become inserted between two base pairs in the DNA chain, forming an irreversible bond between them. This is called bifunctional alkylation, which causes cytotoxic effects capable of destroying or poisoning cells. **(B)** Other drugs react with just one part of a pair, separating it from its partner and eventually causing it and its attached sugar to break away from the DNA molecule. This is called monofunctional alkylation, which eventually causes permanent cell damage.

Pharmacodynamics

As an alkyl sulfonate, busulfan forms bonds with the DNA molecules in a process called alkylation. This prevents cell replication and causes cell death.

Pharmacotherapeutics

Busulfan primarily affects granulocytes (a type of WBC) and, to a lesser degree, platelets. Because of its action on granulocytes, it is the drug of choice for treating chronic myelogenous leukemia. Busulfan is also effective in treating polycythemia vera (excessive amounts of red blood cells). However, other drugs are usually used to treat polycythemia vera because busulfan can cause severe myelosuppression (halting of bone marrow function) (see Sidebar: *Adverse Reactions to Busulfan*).

> ### *Adverse Reactions to Busulfan*
>
> The major adverse reaction to busulfan is bone marrow suppression, producing severe leukopenia, anemia, and thrombocytopenia (reduced white blood cells, red blood cells, and platelets, respectively), which is usually dose-related and reversible.

Nitrosoureas

Common Drug Names

carmustine: BiCNU, Gliadel

lomustine: CCNU, CeeNU

streptozocin: Zanosar

Nitrosoureas are alkylating agents that work by halting cancer cell reproduction.

Pharmacokinetics

The drug carmustine is poorly absorbed when used topically. After oral administration, lomustine is absorbed adequately, although incompletely. Streptozocin, which is administered intravenously, does not undergo absorption.

Nitrosoureas are lipophilic (attracted to fat), distributing to fatty tissues and cerebrospinal fluid (CSF). They are metabolized extensively before urine excretion.

Pharmacodynamics

During a process called bifunctional alkylation, nitrosoureas interfere with amino acids, purines, and DNA needed for cancer cells to divide, thus halting their reproduction.

Pharmacotherapeutics

The nitrosoureas are highly lipid (fat) soluble, which allows them or their metabolites to cross the blood–brain barrier easily. Because of this ability, nitrosoureas are used to treat brain tumors and meningeal leukemias (cancer of the meninges, which are the coverings of the brain and spinal cord) (see Sidebar: *Adverse Reactions to Nitrosoureas*).

Triazenes

Common Drug Names

dacarbazine: DIC, DTIC, DTIC-Dome

The triazene dacarbazine functions as an alkylating drug after it has been activated by the liver.

Pharmacokinetics

After intravenous injection, dacarbazine is distributed throughout the body and metabolized in the liver. Within 6 hours, 30% to 46% of a dose is excreted by the kidneys. In patients with kidney or liver dysfunction, the drug's half-life may increase to 7 hours.

Pharmacodynamics

Dacarbazine first must be metabolized in the liver to become an alkylating drug. It seems to inhibit ribonucleic acid (RNA) and protein synthesis, thus stopping cell replication.

Pharmacotherapeutics

Dacarbazine is used primarily to treat patients with malignant melanoma but also is used with other drugs to treat patients with Hodgkin's disease (see Sidebar: *Adverse Reactions to Triazenes*).

Ethyleneimine

Common Drug Names

thiotepa: TESPA, Thioplex, TSPA

Thiotepa, an ethyleneimine derivative, is a multifunctional alkylating drug.

Pharmacokinetics

After intravenous administration, thiotepa is 100% bioavailable. Significant systemic absorption may occur when thiotepa is administered into pleural (around the lungs) or peritoneal (abdominal) spaces or is instilled into the bladder.

Thiotepa crosses the blood–brain barrier and is metabolized extensively in the liver. Thiotepa and its metabolites are excreted in the urine.

Pharmacodynamics

Thiotepa exerts its cytotoxic activity by interfering with cell replication. Ultimately, it disrupts nucleic acid function and causes cell death.

Pharmacotherapeutics

Thiotepa is used to treat bladder cancer. This alkylating drug is also prescribed for palliative (symptom relief) treatment of lymphomas and ovarian or breast carcinomas.

The Food and Drug Administration (FDA) has approved thiotepa for the treatment of intracavitary effusions (accumulation of fluid in a body cavity). It may also prove useful in the treatment of lung cancer (see Sidebar: *Adverse Reactions to Ethyleneimine*).

Alkylating-Like Drugs

Common Drug Names

carboplatin: CBDCA, Paraplatin, Paraplatin-AQ
cisplatin: CDDP, Platinol, Platinol-AQ

Carboplatin and cisplatin are heavy metal complexes that contain platinum. Because their action resembles that of alkylating drugs, these drugs are also referred to as alkylating-like drugs.

Pharmacokinetics

The distribution and metabolism of carboplatin are not defined clearly. After intravenous administration, carboplatin is eliminated primarily by the kidneys. The elimination of

---

Adverse Reactions to Triazenes

Dacarbazine may cause some adverse reactions, including:

- Leukopenia
- Thrombocytopenia
- Nausea and vomiting (which begin within 1 to 3 hours after administration in most patients and may last up to 12 hours)
- Phototoxicity
- Flulike syndrome
- Hair loss

Adverse Reactions to Ethyleneimine

The major adverse reactions to thiotepa are blood-related and include:

- Leukopenia
- Anemia
- Thrombocytopenia
- Pancytopenia (deficiency of all cellular elements of the blood), which may be fatal

Other adverse reactions include:

- Nausea and vomiting (commonly)
- Stomatitis and ulceration of the intestinal mucosa (especially at bone marrow transplant doses)
- Hives, rash, and pruritus (occasionally)

carboplatin is biphasic. It has an initial half-life of 1 to 2 hours and a terminal half-life of 2.5 to 6 hours.

When administered intrapleurally (into the pleural space around the lung) or intraperitoneally (into the peritoneum), cisplatin may exhibit significant systemic absorption. Highly protein-bound, cisplatin reaches high concentrations in the kidneys, liver, intestines, and testes but has poor central nervous system (CNS) penetration. The drug undergoes some liver metabolism, followed by excretion through the kidney. Platinum is detectable in tissue for at least 4 months after administration.

Pharmacodynamics

Like alkylating drugs, carboplatin and cisplatin inhibit DNA synthesis and cell replication.

Pharmacotherapeutics

These alkylating-like drugs are used in the treatment of several cancers. Carboplatin is used primarily to treat ovarian and lung cancer. Cisplatin is prescribed to treat bladder and metastatic ovarian cancer. Cisplatin is also the drug of choice for metastatic testicular cancers and may also be used to treat head, neck, and lung cancer (see Sidebar: *Adverse Reactions to Alkylating-Like Drugs*).

Antimetabolite Drugs

Because antimetabolite drugs structurally resemble natural metabolites (products of metabolism—the physical and chemical changes that take place within the body), they can become involved in processes associated with the natural metabolites, that is, the synthesis of nucleic acids and proteins. Antimetabolites differ sufficiently from the natural metabolites in how they interfere with this synthesis. The antimetabolites affect cells that actively synthesize DNA. Normal cells that are reproducing actively as well as the cancer cells are affected by the antimetabolites.

These drugs are subclassified according to the metabolite affected and include folic acid analogs, pyrimidine analogs, and purine analogs.

Folic Acid Analogs

Common Drug Names

methotrexate: MTX, methotrexate LPF, Rheumatrex

Although researchers have developed many folic acid analogs, the early compound methotrexate remains the most commonly used.

Pharmacokinetics

Methotrexate is absorbed well and distributed throughout the body. At usual dosages, it does not enter the CNS readily. Although methotrexate is metabolized partially, it is excreted primarily unchanged in the urine. Methotrexate has a terminal half-life that is 3 to 10 hours for a low dose and 8 to 15 hours for a high dose.

Adverse Reactions to Alkylating-Like Drugs

Carboplatin and cisplatin produce many of the same adverse reactions as the alkylating drugs.

- Carboplatin can produce bone marrow suppression
- Kidney toxicity may occur with cisplatin, usually after multiple courses of therapy; carboplatin is less toxic to the kidneys
- Neurotoxicity can occur with long-term cisplatin therapy but is less common with carboplatin
- Tinnitus (ringing in the ears) and hearing loss, which is often permanent, may occur with cisplatin and much less commonly with carboplatin
- Cisplatin also produces significant nausea and vomiting

Pharmacodynamics

Methotrexate reversibly inhibits the action of the enzyme dihydrofolate reductase, thereby blocking normal biochemical reactions and inhibiting DNA and RNA synthesis. The result is cell death.

Pharmacotherapeutics

Methotrexate is especially useful in treating acute lymphoblastic leukemia (abnormal growth of lymphocyte precursors, the lymphoblasts) in children, choriocarcinoma (cancer that develops from the chorionic portions of the products of conception), osteogenic sarcoma (bone cancer), malignant lymphomas (cancer of the lymph nodes), and carcinomas of the head, neck, bladder, testis, and breast. This drug is also prescribed in low doses to treat severe psoriasis and rheumatoid arthritis that resist conventional therapy (see Sidebar: *Adverse Reactions to Folic Acid Analogs*).

Pyrimidine Analogs

Common Drug Names

cytarabine: DepoCyt

floxuridine: FUDR

fluorouracil: Adrucil, Carac, Efudex, 5-FU, Fluoroplex

gemcitabine: Gemzar

Pyrimidine analogs are a diverse group of drugs that inhibit production of pyrimidine nucleotides necessary for DNA synthesis.

Pharmacokinetics

Because pyrimidine analogs are absorbed poorly when they are given orally, they are usually administered by other routes. With the exception of cytarabine, pyrimidine analogs are distributed well throughout the body, including CSF. They are metabolized extensively in the liver and are excreted in the urine.

Pharmacodynamics

Pyrimidine analogs kill cancer cells by interfering with DNA synthesis (see Box 15–1).

Pharmacotherapeutics

Pyrimidine analogs may be used to treat many tumors. However, they are primarily indicated in the treatment of acute leukemias, GI tract adenocarcinomas (malignant epithelial cell tumors of the glands and organs), carcinomas

---

Adverse Reactions to Folic Acid Analogs

Adverse reactions to methotrexate include:

- Bone marrow suppression
- Stomatitis
- Pulmonary toxicity, exhibited as pneumonitis or pulmonary fibrosis
- Skin reactions, such as photosensitivity and hair loss

With high doses, kidney toxicity can also occur with methotrexate use. During high-dose therapy, leucovorin (folinic acid) may be used to minimize adverse reactions.

Adverse reactions to intrathecal administration (through the spinal cord into the subarachnoid space) of methotrexate may include seizures, paralysis, and death. Other less severe adverse reactions may also occur, such as headaches, fever, neck stiffness, confusion, and irritability.

Box 15-1

Mechanism of Action of Pyrimidine

To understand how pyrimidine analogs work, it helps to consider the basic structure of deoxyribonucleic acid (DNA).

Climbing the Ladder to Understanding

DNA resembles a ladder that has been twisted. The rungs of the ladder consist of pairs of nitrogenous bases: adenine always pairs with thymine, and guanine always pairs with cytosine. Cytosine and thymine are pyrimidines; adenine and guanine are purines.

One Part Sugar . . .

The basic unit of DNA is the nucleotide. A nucleotide is the building block of nucleic acids. It consists of a sugar, a nitrogen-containing base, and a phosphate group. It is on these components that pyrimidine analogs do their work.

In the Guise of a Nucleotide

After pyrimidine analogs are converted into nucleotides, they are incorporated into DNA, where they may inhibit DNA and ribonucleic acid synthesis as well as other metabolic reactions necessary for proper cell growth.

of the breast and ovaries, and malignant lymphomas (see Sidebar: *Adverse Reactions to Pyrimidine Analogs*).

Adverse Reactions to Pyrimidine Analogs

Like most antineoplastic drugs, pyrimidine analogs can cause:

- Fatigue and lack of energy
- Inflammation of the mouth, esophagus, and throat, leading to painful ulcerations and tissue sloughing
- Bone marrow suppression
- Nausea and anorexia

Diarrhea may occur with fluorouracil administration. Hair loss commonly occurs with fluorouracil.

Purine Analogs

Common Drug Names

cladribine: 2-CdA, Leustatin

fludarabine phosphate: Fludara

mercaptopurine: 6-MP, Purinethol

thioguanine: Lanvis, 6-TG, TG

Purine analogs are incorporated into DNA and RNA, interfering with nucleic acid synthesis and cell replication.

Pharmacokinetics

The pharmacokinetics of purine analogs are not defined clearly. They are largely metabolized in the liver and excreted in the urine.

Pharmacodynamics

Like the other antimetabolites, fludarabine, mercaptopurine, and thioguanine first must be converted to a nucleotide level to be active. The resulting nucleotides are then incorporated into DNA, where they may inhibit DNA and RNA synthesis as well as other metabolic reactions necessary for proper cell growth.

Pharmacotherapeutics

Purine analogs are used to treat acute and chronic leukemias and may be useful in the treatment of lymphomas (see Sidebar: *Adverse Reactions to Purine Analogs*).

Adverse Reactions to Purine Analogs

Purine analogs can produce:

- Bone marrow suppression
- Nausea and vomiting
- Anorexia
- Mild diarrhea
- Stomatitis
- Rise in uric acid levels (a result of the breakdown of purine)

Fludarabine, when used at high doses, may cause severe neurologic effects including blindness, coma, and death.

Antibiotic Antineoplastic Drugs

Common Drug Names

bleomycin: Blenoxane, BLM

dactinomycin: Actinomycin D, Cosmegen

daunorubicin: Cerubidine, daunomycin, Daunorubicin, DNR, rubidomycin

doxorubicin hydrochloride: ADR, Adriamycin, Caelyx, Doxil, Doxorubicin, Rubex

idarubicin hydrochloride: 4dmdr, Idamycin (discontinued in the U.S.)

mitomycin: MTC, Mutamycin

mitoxantrone hydrochloride: DHAD, Novantrone

pentostatin: DCF, Nipent

plicamycin: Mithracin, mithramycin

Antibiotic antineoplastic drugs are antimicrobial products that produce tumoricidal (tumor-destroying) effects by binding with DNA. These drugs inhibit the cellular processes of normal and malignant cells.

Pharmacokinetics

Because antibiotic antineoplastic drugs are usually administered intravenously, absorption is immediate. Some of the drugs are also administered directly into the body cavity being treated. Bleomycin, doxorubicin, and mitomycin are sometimes given as topical bladder instillations in which significant systemic absorption does not occur. When bleomycin is injected into the pleural space for malignant effusions, up to one-half of the dose is absorbed. Distribution of antibiotic antineoplastic drugs throughout the body varies, as do their metabolism and elimination.

Pharmacodynamics

With the exception of mitomycin and pentostatin, antibiotic antineoplastic drugs insert themselves between adjacent base pairs of a DNA molecule, physically separating them. The overall effect is cell death.

Although the exact mechanism of pentostatin's antitumor effect is unknown, it inhibits the enzyme adenosine deaminase, blocking DNA synthesis and inhibiting RNA synthesis. Mitomycin produces single-strand breakage of DNA. It also cross-links DNA, leading to cell death.

Pharmacotherapeutics

Antibiotic antineoplastic drugs act against many cancers, including Hodgkin's disease and malignant lymphomas; testicular carcinoma; squamous cell carcinoma of the head, neck, and cervix; Wilms' tumor (a malignant neoplasm of the kidney, occurring in young children); osteogenic sarcoma (bone cancer) and rhabdomyosarcoma (malignant neoplasm composed of striated muscle cells); Ewing's sarcoma (a malignant tumor that originates in bone marrow, typically in long bones or the pelvis) and other soft tissue sarcomas; breast, ovarian, bladder, and bronchogenic carcinomas; melanoma; carcinomas of the GI tract; and choriocarcinoma (a rare cancer at the site of fetal implantation). These drugs are also effective against acute leukemias and hypercalcemia (see Sidebar: *Adverse Reactions to Antibiotic Antineoplastic Drugs*).

Adverse Reactions to Antibiotic Antineoplastic Drugs

- The primary adverse reaction to these drugs is bone marrow suppression
- Irreversible cardiomyopathy and acute electrocardiogram changes can also occur as well as nausea and vomiting
- An antihistamine and antipyretic should be given before bleomycin to prevent fever and chills; anaphylactic reactions can occur in patients receiving bleomycin for lymphoma, so test doses should be given first
- Plicamycin may produce hypotension and kidney toxicity as well as bleeding, such as nose bleed, blood during vomiting or coughing, bruising, and prolonged clotting and bleeding times
- Doxorubicin may color urine red; mitoxantrone may color it blue-green

---

Hormonal Antineoplastic Drugs

Hormonal antineoplastic drugs are prescribed to alter the growth of malignant neoplasms or to manage and treat their physiologic effects. Hormonal therapies are effective against hormone-dependent tumors, such as cancers of the prostate, breast, and uterus. Lymphomas and leukemias are usually treated with therapies that include corticosteroids because of their potential for affecting lymphocytes.

Antiestrogens

Common Drug Names

anastrozole: Arimidex

exemestane: Aromasin

letrozole: Femara

tamoxifen citrate: Apo-Tamox, Gen-Tamoxifen, Nolvadex, Tamofen, tamoxifen

The antiestrogen tamoxifen citrate has been the drug of choice for advanced breast cancer involving estrogen receptor–positive tumors in postmenopausal women and is still used extensively. Tamoxifen citrate is also used as an adjunct treatment for breast cancer and to reduce its incidence in woman at high risk. Newer drugs recently approved are now being used for these purposes.

Pharmacokinetics

After oral administration, antiestrogens are absorbed well and undergo extensive metabolism in the liver before being excreted in the feces.

Pharmacodynamics

Estrogen receptors, found in the cancer cells of half of premenopausal and three-fourths of postmenopausal women with breast cancer, respond to estrogen to induce tumor growth. The antiestrogen tamoxifen binds to the estrogen receptors and inhibits estrogen-mediated tumor growth. The newer drugs, letrozole, anastrozole, and exemestane are aromatase inhibitors. They stop conversion of androgens (masculine hormones that are the precursors to estrogen) to estrogen and decrease estrogen levels in the body by 85% to 95%. This stops the estrogen stimulation that increases tumor growth.

Pharmacotherapeutics

The antiestrogens are used in the palliative treatment of metastatic breast cancer that is estrogen receptor–positive. Tamoxifen is also used as an adjunct to surgery in postmenopausal women with axillary lymph nodes that contain cancer cells and estrogen receptor–positive tumors (see Sidebar: *Adverse Reactions to Antiestrogens*).

Adverse Reactions to Antiestrogens

Tamoxifen is a relatively nontoxic drug. The most common adverse reactions include:

- Hot flashes
- Nausea
- Diarrhea
- Fluid retention
- Vomiting

Leukopenia or thrombocytopenia (reduced white blood cell and platelets, respectively) may also occur.

In patients with bone metastasis, hypercalcemia (elevated serum calcium levels) may occur as well.

Androgens

Common Drug Names

fluoxymesterone: Halotestin

testolactone: Teslac

testosterone: Andronaq, Histerone, Testamone, Testaqua, Testoject

testosterone cypionate: Andronate, Cypionate, depAndro Injection (discontinued in the U.S.), Depotest Injection (discontinued in the U.S.), Depo-Testosterone, Duratest, T-Cypionate, Testred, Virilon

testosterone enanthate: Andro-LA, Andropository (discontinued in the U.S.), Andryl, Delatest, Delatestryl, Durathate, Everone

The therapeutically useful androgens are synthetic derivatives of naturally occurring testosterone.

Pharmacokinetics

The pharmacokinetic properties of therapeutic androgens resemble those of naturally occurring testosterone. Oral androgens, fluoxymesterone and testolactone, are absorbed well. The parenteral ones, testosterone enanthate and testosterone propionate, are designed specifically for slow absorption.

Androgens are distributed well throughout the body, metabolized extensively in the liver, and excreted in the urine. The duration of the parenteral forms is longer because the oil suspension is absorbed slowly. Parenteral androgens are administered one to three times per week.

Pharmacodynamics

Androgens may inhibit estrogen synthesis or competitively bind at estrogen receptors. These actions prevent estrogen from affecting estrogen-sensitive tumors.

Pharmacotherapeutics

Androgens are indicated for the palliative treatment of advanced breast cancer, particularly in postmenopausal women with bone metastasis (see Sidebar: *Adverse Reactions to Androgens*).

Antiandrogens

Common Drug Names

bicalutamide: Casodex

flutamide: Apo-Flutamide, Euflex, Eulexin, Novo-Flutamide

nilutamide: Nilandron

Antiandrogens are used as an adjunct therapy with gonadotropin-releasing hormone analogs (GRHAs) (see below) in treating advanced prostate cancer.

Pharmacokinetics

After oral administration, antiandrogens are absorbed rapidly and completely. Antiandrogens are metabolized rapidly and extensively and excreted primarily in the urine.

Pharmacodynamics

Flutamide, nilutamide, and bicalutamide exert their antiandrogenic action by inhibiting androgen uptake or preventing androgen binding in cell nuclei in target tissues, decreasing the stimulating effect of androgens on tumor growth.

Pharmacotherapeutics

Antiandrogens are used with a GRHA, such as leuprolide, to treat metastatic prostate cancer. Concomitant administration of antiandrogens and a GRHA may help prevent

---

Adverse Reactions to Androgens

Nausea and vomiting are the most common adverse reactions to androgens. Fluid retention caused by sodium retention may also occur.

Women taking androgens may develop:

- Acne
- Clitoral hypertrophy
- Deeper voice
- Increased facial and body hair
- Increased sexual desire
- Menstrual irregularity

Males taking androgens may experience the following effects as a result of conversion of steroids to female sex hormone metabolites:

- Gynecomastia
- Prostatic hypertrophy
- Testicular atrophy

Children taking androgens may develop:

- Premature epiphyseal closure
- Secondary sex characteristic developments (especially in boys)

the disease flare that occurs when the GRHA is used alone (see Sidebar: *Adverse Reactions to Antiandrogens*).

Progestins

Common Drug Names

hydroxyprogesterone caproate: Hylutin, Prodox

medroxyprogesterone acetate: Alti-MPA, Depo-Provera, Gen-Medroxy, Novo-Medrone, Provera

megestrol acetate: Apo-Megestrol, Megace (discontinued in the U.S.), Nu-Megestrol

Progestins are hormones used to treat various forms of cancer.

Pharmacokinetics

When taken orally, megestrol acetate is absorbed well. After intramuscular injection in an aqueous or oil suspension, hydroxyprogesterone caproate and medroxyprogesterone are absorbed slowly from their deposit sites. These drugs are distributed well throughout the body and may be stored in fatty tissue. Progestins are metabolized in the liver and excreted as metabolites in the urine.

Pharmacodynamics

The mechanism of action of progestins in treating tumors is not completely understood. Researchers believe the drugs bind to a specific receptor to act on hormonally sensitive cells.

Because progestins do not exhibit a cytotoxic activity (destroying or poisoning cells), they are considered cytostatic (they keep the cells from multiplying).

Pharmacotherapeutics

Progestins are used for the palliative treatment of advanced uterine, breast, and renal cancers. Of these drugs, megestrol is used most often (see Sidebar: *Adverse Reactions to Progestins*).

Gonadotropin-Releasing Hormone Analogs

Common Drug Names

goserelin acetate: Zoladex

leuprolide acetate: Eligard, Lupron, Lupron Depot, Viadur

triptorelin: Trelstar

GRHAs are used for treatment of advanced prostate cancer.

Pharmacokinetics

Goserelin is absorbed slowly for the first 8 days of therapy and rapidly and continuously thereafter. After subcutaneous injection, leuprolide and triptorelin are absorbed well. These drugs have unclear distribution, metabolism, and excretion.

Pharmacodynamics

GRHAs act on the male's pituitary gland to increase luteinizing hormone (LH) secretion, which stimulates testosterone production. The peak testosterone level is reached approximately 72 hours after daily administration. With long-term administration, however,

---

Adverse Reactions to Antiandrogens

When an antiandrogen is used with a gonadotropin-releasing hormone analog, the most common adverse reactions are:

- Hot flashes
- Decreased sexual desire
- Impotence
- Diarrhea
- Nausea
- Vomiting
- Breast enlargement

Adverse Reactions to Progestins

Mild fluid retention is probably the most common reaction to progestins. Other reactions include:

- Thromboemboli
- Breakthrough bleeding, spotting, and changes in menstrual flow
- Breast tenderness
- Liver function abnormalities

Patients who are hypersensitive to the oil carrier used for injection (usually sesame or castor oil) may have a local or systemic hypersensitivity reaction.

they inhibit LH release from the pituitary and subsequently inhibit testicular release of testosterone. Because prostate tumor cells are stimulated by testosterone, the reduced testosterone level inhibits tumor growth.

Pharmacotherapeutics

Goserelin and leuprolide are used for the palliative treatment of metastatic prostate cancer. The drugs lower the testosterone level without the adverse psychological effects of castration or the adverse cardiovascular effects of diethylstilbestrol (see Sidebar: *Adverse Reactions to Gonadotropin-Releasing Hormone Analogs*).

Natural Antineoplastic Drugs

A subclass of antineoplastic drugs known as natural products includes vinca alkaloids and podophyllotoxins.

Vinca Alkaloids

Common Drug Names

vinblastine: VLB, Velban

vincristine: Oncovin, VCR, Vincasar

vinorelbine: Navelbine

Vinca alkaloids are nitrogenous bases derived from the periwinkle plant.

Pharmacokinetics

After intravenous administration, the vinca alkaloids are distributed well throughout the body. Vinca alkaloids undergo moderate liver metabolism before being eliminated through different phases, primarily in the feces with a small percentage eliminated in the urine.

Pharmacodynamics

Vinca alkaloids may disrupt normal function, and cells cannot complete mitosis (cell division). Cell division is arrested, causing cell death.

Pharmacotherapeutics

Vinca alkaloids are used in several therapeutic situations. Vinblastine is used to treat metastatic testicular carcinoma, lymphomas, Kaposi's sarcoma (a cancer of the blood vessels which is the most common acquired immunodeficiency syndrome [AIDS]-related cancer), neuroblastoma (a highly malignant tumor originating in the sympathetic nervous system), breast carcinoma, and choriocarcinoma.

Vincristine is used in combination therapy to treat Hodgkin's disease, malignant lymphoma (lymph node cancer), Wilms' tumor (a type of kidney cancer), rhabdomyosarcoma (cancer of skeletal muscle), and acute lymphocytic leukemia.

Adverse Reactions to Gonadotropin-Releasing Hormone Analogs

Hot flashes, impotence, and decreased sexual desire are commonly reported reactions to goserelin and leuprolide, two gonadotropin-releasing hormone analogs. Other adverse effects include:

- Peripheral edema
- Nausea and vomiting
- Constipation
- Anorexia

Disease symptoms and pain may worsen or flare during the first 2 weeks of goserelin or leuprolide therapy. The flare can be fatal in patients with bony vertebral metastasis.

Vinorelbine is used to treat non–small-cell lung cancer. It may also be used in the treatment of metastatic breast carcinoma, cisplatin-resistant ovarian carcinoma, and Hodgkin's disease (see Sidebar: *Adverse Reactions to Vinca Alkaloids*).

Podophyllotoxins

Common Drug Names

etoposide: EPEG, Etopophos, Toposar, VePesid, VP-16
teniposide: EPT, VM-26, Vumon

Podophyllotoxins are semisynthetic glycosides. Teniposide has demonstrated some activity in treating Hodgkin's disease, lymphomas, and brain tumors.

Pharmacokinetics

When taken orally, podophyllotoxins are only moderately absorbed. Although the drugs are distributed widely throughout the body, they achieve poor CSF levels. Podophyllotoxins undergo liver metabolism and are excreted primarily in the urine.

Pharmacodynamics

Although their mechanisms of action are not completely understood, podophyllotoxins produce several biochemical changes in tumor cells that block replication and cause cell death.

Pharmacotherapeutics

Etoposide is used to treat testicular cancer and small-cell lung cancer. It may also be used to treat various lymphomas and leukemias, although these indications have not yet been approved by the FDA. Teniposide is used to treat acute lymphoblastic leukemia (see Sidebar: *Adverse Reactions to Podophyllotoxins*).

Unclassifiable Antineoplastic Drugs

Many other antineoplastic drugs cannot be included in existing classifications. These drugs include asparaginase, procarbazine, hydroxyurea, interferon, aldesleukin, altretamine, paclitaxel, and docetaxel.

Asparaginases

Common Drug Names

asparaginase: colaspase, Elspar, Kidrolase
pegaspargase: Oncaspar, PEG-L-asparaginase

Asparaginases are cell cycle–specific and act during the G_1 phase.

Adverse Reactions to Vinca Alkaloids

- Nausea, vomiting, constipation, and stomatitis (mouth inflammation) may occur in patients taking vinca alkaloids
- Vinblastine and vinorelbine toxicities occur primarily as bone marrow suppression
- Neuromuscular abnormalities frequently occur with vincristine and vinorelbine and occasionally with vinblastine therapy
- Vinblastine may produce tumor pain described as an intense stinging or burning in the tumor bed, with an abrupt onset 1 to 3 minutes after drug administration; the pain usually lasts 20 minutes to 3 hours
- Reversible alopecia occurs in up to half of patients receiving vinca alkaloids; it is more likely to occur with vincristine than with vinblastine

Adverse Reactions to Podophyllotoxins

The majority of patients receiving podophyllotoxins experience hair loss. Other adverse reactions include:
- Nausea and vomiting
- Anorexia
- Stomatitis
- Bone marrow suppression, causing leukopenia and, less commonly, thrombocytopenia
- Acute hypotension (if a podophyllotoxin is infused too rapidly intravenously)

Pharmacokinetics

Asparaginase is administered parenterally. After administration, asparaginase remains inside the blood vessels, with minimal distribution elsewhere. The metabolism of asparaginase is unknown; only trace amounts appear in urine.

Pharmacodynamics

Asparaginase and pegaspargase capitalize on the biochemical differences between normal cells and tumor cells. Most normal cells can synthesize asparagine, but some tumor cells depend on other sources of asparagine for survival. Asparaginase and pegaspargase help to degrade asparagine to aspartic acid and ammonia. Deprived of their supply of asparagine, the tumor cells die.

Pharmacotherapeutics

Asparaginase is used primarily to induce remission in patients with acute lymphocytic leukemia. Pegaspargase is used to treat acute lymphocytic leukemia in patients who are allergic to the native form of asparaginase (see Sidebar: *Adverse Reactions to Asparaginase Drugs*).

Procarbazine

Common Drug Names

procarbazine: Matulane, MIH, Natulan

Procarbazine hydrochloride is used to treat Hodgkin's disease as well as primary and metastatic brain tumors.

Pharmacokinetics

After oral administration, procarbazine is absorbed well. It readily crosses the blood–brain barrier and is well distributed into the CSF. Procarbazine is metabolized rapidly in the liver. It is excreted in urine, primarily as metabolites. Respiratory excretion of the drug occurs as methane and carbon dioxide gas.

Pharmacodynamics

An inert drug, procarbazine must be activated metabolically in the liver before it can produce various cell changes. It can cause chromosomal damage, suppress mitosis (cell division and replication), and inhibit DNA, RNA, and protein synthesis. Cancer cells can develop resistance to procarbazine quickly.

Pharmacotherapeutics

Used with other antineoplastic drugs, procarbazine is most effective in the MOPP regimen for Hodgkin's disease. The MOPP regimen consists of *m*echlorethamine, *O*ncovin (vincristine), *p*rocarbazine, and *p*rednisone.

Procarbazine is used to treat primary and metastatic brain tumors. The drug may also be useful against small-cell lung cancer, malignant lymphoma, myeloma, melanoma, and CNS tumors (see Sidebar: *Adverse Reactions to Procarbazine*).

Adverse Reactions to Asparaginase Drugs

- Many patients receiving asparaginase and pegaspargase develop nausea and vomiting; fever, headache, abdominal pain, and liver toxicity may also occur
- Asparaginase and pegaspargase can cause anaphylaxis, which is more likely to occur with intermittent intravenous dosing than with daily intravenous dosing or intramuscular injections; the risk of a reaction rises with each successive treatment
- Hypersensitivity reactions may also occur

Adverse Reactions to Procarbazine

- Late-onset bone marrow suppression is the most common dose-limiting toxicity associated with procarbazine; interstitial pneumonitis (lung inflammation) and pulmonary fibrosis (scarring) may also occur
- Initial procarbazine therapy may induce a flulike syndrome, including fever, chills, sweating, lethargy, and muscle pain
- GI reactions include nausea, vomiting, stomatitis, and diarrhea

Hydroxyurea

Common Drug Names

hydroxyurea: Droxia, Hydrea, Mylocel

Hydroxyurea is used most commonly for patients with chronic myelogenous leukemia. Hydroxyurea is also used for solid tumors as well as head and neck cancer.

Pharmacokinetics

Hydroxyurea is absorbed readily and distributed well into the CSF after oral administration. It reaches a peak serum level 2 hours after administration. Approximately half of a dose is metabolized by the liver to carbon dioxide, which is excreted by the lungs, or to urea, which is excreted by the kidneys. The remaining half is excreted unchanged in the urine.

Pharmacodynamics

Hydroxyurea exerts its effect by inhibiting the enzyme ribonucleotide reductase, which is necessary for DNA synthesis. Hydroxyurea kills cells and holds cells where they are most susceptible to irradiation.

Pharmacotherapeutics

Hydroxyurea is used to treat selected myeloproliferative (bone marrow cancers) disorders. It may produce temporary remissions in some patients with metastatic malignant melanomas as well. Hydroxyurea also is used in combination therapy with radiation to treat carcinomas of the head, neck, and lung (see Sidebar: *Adverse Reactions to Hydroxyurea*).

Adverse Reactions to Hydroxyurea

Treatment with hydroxyurea leads to few adverse reactions. Those that do occur include:

- Bone marrow suppression
- Drowsiness
- Headache
- Nausea and vomiting
- Anorexia
- Elevated uric acid levels, which require some patients to take allopurinol to prevent kidney damage

Interferons

Common Drug Names

interferon alfa-2a: IFLrA, rIFNA, Roferon-A,
interferon alfa-2b: INF-alpha 2, Intron
interferon alfa-2b and ribavirin: Rebetron
interferon alfa-n3: Alferon
interferon beta-1a: Avonex, Rebif
interferon beta-1b: Betaseron
interferon gamma-1b: Actimmune

A family of naturally occurring glycoproteins, interferons are so named because of their ability to interfere with viral replication.

Pharmacokinetics

After intramuscular or subcutaneous administration, interferons are usually absorbed well. Information about their distribution is unavailable. Interferons are filtered by the kidneys, where they are broken down.

Pharmacodynamics

Although their exact mechanism of action is unknown, interferons appear to bind to specific membrane receptors on the cell surface. When bound, they initiate a sequence of intracellular events that includes the induction of certain enzymes. This process may account for the ability of interferons to inhibit viral replication, suppress cell proliferation, enhance macrophage activity (engulfing and destroying microorganisms and other debris), and increase cytotoxicity of lymphocytes making them better able to destroy target cells.

Pharmacotherapeutics

Interferons have shown their most promising activity in treating blood malignancies, especially hairy cell leukemia. Their approved indications currently include hairy cell leukemia and AIDS-related Kaposi's sarcoma. Interferons also demonstrate some activity against chronic myelogenous leukemia, malignant lymphoma, multiple myeloma, melanoma, and renal cell carcinoma (see Sidebar: *Adverse Reactions to Interferons*).

Aldesleukin

Common Drug Names

aldesleukin: interleukin-2, Proleukin

Aldesleukin is a human recombinant interleukin-2 derivative (made from human DNA) that is used to treat metastatic renal cell carcinoma.

Pharmacokinetics

After intravenous administration of aldesleukin, about 30% is absorbed into the plasma and about 70% is absorbed rapidly by the liver, kidneys, and lungs. The drug is excreted primarily by the kidneys.

Pharmacodynamics

The exact antitumor mechanism of action of aldesleukin is unknown. The drug may stimulate an immunologic reaction against the tumor.

Pharmacotherapeutics

Aldesleukin is used to treat metastatic renal cell carcinoma. It may also be used in the treatment of Kaposi's sarcoma and metastatic melanoma (see Sidebar: *Adverse Reactions to Aldesleukin*).

Altretamine

Common Drug Names

altretamine: Hexalen

Altretamine is a synthetic cytotoxic antineoplastic drug that is used as palliative treatment for patients with ovarian cancer.

Adverse Reactions to Interferons

- Blood toxicity occurs in up to half of patients taking interferons and may produce leukopenia, neutropenia, thrombocytopenia, and anemia
- Adverse gastrointestinal reactions include anorexia, nausea, and diarrhea
- The most common adverse reaction to interferons is a flulike syndrome that may produce fever, fatigue, muscle pain, headache, chills, and joint pain
- Coughing, difficulty breathing, hypotension, edema, chest pain, and heart failure have also been associated with interferon therapy

Adverse Reactions to Aldesleukin

During clinical trials, adverse reactions to aldesleukin developed in more than 15% of patients. These include:
- Pulmonary congestion and difficulty breathing
- Anemia, thrombocytopenia, and leukopenia
- Elevated bilirubin, transaminase, and alkaline phosphate levels
- Hypomagnesemia and acidosis
- Reduced or absent urinary output
- Elevated serum creatinine levels
- Stomatitis
- Nausea and vomiting

Pharmacokinetics

Altretamine is absorbed well after oral administration. It is metabolized extensively in the liver and excreted by the liver and kidneys.

Pharmacodynamics

The exact mechanism of action of altretamine is unknown.

Pharmacotherapeutics

Altretamine is used as palliative treatment of persistent or recurring ovarian cancer (see Sidebar: *Adverse Reactions to Altretamine*).

Taxines

Common Drug Names

docetaxel: Taxotere

paclitaxel: Onxol, Taxol

Taxine antineoplastics are used to treat metastatic ovarian and breast carcinoma after chemotherapy has failed.

Pharmacokinetics

Paclitaxel is metabolized primarily in the liver with a small amount excreted unchanged in the urine. Docetaxel is excreted primarily through feces.

Pharmacodynamics

Paclitaxel and docetaxel exert their chemotherapeutic effect by disrupting the microtubule network in the cell that is essential for mitosis (cell division and replication) and other vital cellular functions.

Pharmacotherapeutics

Paclitaxel is used when first-line or subsequent chemotherapy has failed in treating metastatic ovarian carcinoma as well as metastatic breast cancer. The taxines may also be used for the treatment of head and neck cancer, prostate cancer, and non–small-cell lung cancer (see Sidebar: *Adverse Reactions to Taxines*).

New and Experimental Antineoplastic Drugs

There is a continuous flow of new and more cancer-cell specific drugs that are being introduced for use with cancer patients.

Common Drug Names

docetaxel: Taxotere

gefitinib: Iressa

imatinib: Gleevec

infliximab: monoclonal antibodies, Remicade

oxaliplatin: Eloxatin

rituximab: anti-CD20 monoclonal antibodies, C2B8 monoclonal antibody, Pan-B antibodies, Rituxan

The drugs infliximab and rituximab are being used for B-cell and non-Hodgkin's lymphomas. The drug imatinib is used to treat chronic myeloid leukemia. Oxaliplatin is used for colorectal cancer, and gefitinib treats non–small-cell lung cancer. In many cancers that have not responded to other therapies, docetaxel is considered a last chance treatment.

MASSAGE IMPLICATIONS AND ASSESSMENT FOR CLIENTS RECEIVING CHEMOTHERAPY AND CANCER TREATMENTS

The implications for the massage therapist in providing massage to a client receiving cancer treatments are many and complex. After all, the chemotherapy drugs are truly poisons, toxic to cells, both cancerous and otherwise. Many research studies have been done and are being done to determine the effect of massage on the chemotherapy and cancer client. The results have mostly shown that massage can increase the effectiveness and decrease the side effects of chemotherapy. However, the jury is still out and there are still those with concerns about massage spreading cancer through blood and lymph and moving the toxins through the body. Everyone—the therapist, the client, and the physician—need to feel comfortable going ahead with massage during chemotherapy.

The complexity of drug regimens for cancer patients requires a close working relationship with the physician. The interactions of the drugs, how quickly they are excreted from the body, how they are excreted from the body, how often they are being given, what other drugs are being used to prevent side effects, and the client's on-going changes in condition all need to be discussed with the physician. Each client will be affected differently.

Any surgical sites are contraindicated for massage until full healing of the incision has been achieved. If the client is receiving radiation treatments, the site of radiation is completely contraindicated for massage, and no oils or lotions are to be put on or near the site. This could increase the burn effect of the radiation. If the client has had radioactive treatments or implants, the massage therapist needs to know the radiation protocol. Is there a time limit to how close you can be to the patient before being affected by the radioactive implants? The action of these drugs is to kill cells. This affects the whole body, not just the cancer sites. The more invasive types of massage, such as deep tissue and even strong myofascial work, are contraindicated.

Massage that helps relax and bring the client into balance is the best focus. The systemic reflex strokes that increase endorphins and enkephalins and balance neuroendocrine secretions include rocking, shaking, gentle friction at the muscle-tendon junctures, and effleurage. If the client is receiving chemotherapy frequently, effleurage may need to be limited so as not to move the toxins through the blood system any faster than the body can handle. The physician can tell you how long it takes for the chemicals to be excreted from the body. Massage is usually best given before chemotherapy treatment, although this may vary from client to client. Areas of tension may be worked with local mechanical strokes such as pétrissage. Energy therapies are also very beneficial.

Side Effects

The side effects and adverse effects of chemotherapy and radiation are numerous. Often, a variety of drugs is given in conjunction with the chemotherapy to prevent or lessen these effects. All are of concern to the massage therapist. Fatigue is a frequent effect and may require that sessions be short. Dizziness, low blood pressure, and weakness can occur and require the massage practitioner to take precautions when turning and getting a client off the table. Hair loss is frequent. Scalp massage should only be done gently and if the client and practitioner are not upset by the hair that can come out while doing this work. Peripheral neuropathies may make it even more important to modify depth and pressure applied. In those who have decreased WBC counts and/or red blood cell counts, extra care needs to be taken to prevent exposure to infection. It may not be appropriate for the client to come out to the office, and extra care in handwashing is needed. Massage can be an important adjunct in the client's treatment, but it must be approached with care and with knowledge.

Quick Quiz

The reader is referred to case studies 1 and 2 in Appendix A.

Herbs, Supplements, and Alternative Medicine

16

This text is primarily written to provide concise information about pharmaceuticals used in traditional Western medicine. However, no book on pharmacology is complete without at least some mention and explanation of the alternative treatments that are so popular and available today. Although it is not possible to do an in-depth study in one chapter, the most common alternatives and herbals are discussed.

It is important to remember that the definition of a drug is any substance that will change the chemical processes of the body. All these alternatives fit that description and should therefore be taken with care. All these supplements that are sold over the counter in health food stores, drug stores, and grocery stores are not regulated by the Food and Drug Administration (FDA), as are Western pharmaceuticals. They do not have to undergo any of the rigorous testing and research or even have standardized and consistent amounts of the active components of the item being sold. They all fall under the Dietary Supplement Health Education Act. This requires that no medical claims be made, that they state clearly that the FDA has not evaluated the effects of the supplements, and that appropriate warnings be placed on the labels.

The definition of a dietary supplement according to this law is, "a product (other than tobacco) intended to supplement the diet or that bears or contains one or more of the following ingredients: a vitamin, a mineral, an herb or other botanical, an amino acid, a dietary supplement for use by man to supplement diet by increasing the total dietary intake, a concentrate, metabolic, constituent, extract, or combination of any of the former ingredients." This is a very broad definition, and just about everything outside of FDA pharmaceuticals falls in this category. Some herbals and alternatives have undergone extensive research, and others have undergone practically none. There is a great deal of controversy over this lack of regulation. Many of the herbals especially have serious interactions with other drugs, both prescription and over the counter. They can have side effects, and self-treatment can prevent the customer from seeking medical help for a serious condition. Whether further regulation of these items occurs is yet to be seen. All drugs in whatever form need to be respected and taken carefully.

There is also a long history of the use of many of these herbal and other supplements. There are very reputable companies manufacturing and selling them who do standardize their products for consistency, and many people have been aided in improving their health and wellness by the use of these products (see Sidebar: *Information Sources for Herbals and Supplements*).

The common alternatives to Western pharmaceuticals in favor today discussed in this chapter are homeopathy, flower essence therapy, vitamin supplements, and herbals. (Ayurveda, Chinese Medicine, and naturopathy also use alternatives to Western pharmaceuticals but are complex systems beyond the scope of this chapter.)

Homeopathy

Common Homeopathic Remedies

arsenicum albums: hives with chills, for frequent awakenings in the night

apis mellifica: fever, sore throat, hives, inflammation

arnica montana: sore muscles

calms forte: anxiety, insomnia

cantharis: sunburn, burns

chamomilla: toothache

colulus indicus: motion sickness

engystol-N: antiviral

hypericum: toothache

magphos: bruxism, temporomandibular joint dysfunction

nux vomica: morning sickness, early morning awakenings

oscillocoxum: influenza

phosphorus: diarrhea

pulsatilla: morning sickness

rhus toxicodendum: heel pain, plantar fascitis, hives, shingles

sepia: nausea and vomiting

staphisagria: urinary tract infection

urtica urens: stinging, burning hives, or rash

veratrum: diarrhea

These are just a few; there are hundreds of homeopathics remedies.

Western medicine is based for the most part on allopathic principles. The substances given to patients are used to suppress the symptoms the patient is experiencing. This requires fairly strong doses of the prescribed medication, often with side effects. Homeopathy is based on the homeopathic principle that "like heals like." Homeopathic medicines are extremely diluted amounts of natural substances from plant, animal, and mineral sources. Homeopathic physicians believe symptoms are the result of the body's own healing efforts. These symptoms need to be supported and strengthened, not suppressed. The body's own healing ability will then be able to overcome the illness.

The homeopathic medicine given to the patient is a dilute amount of a substance that will actually cause the same symptoms the patient is experiencing if given to a healthy individual. For example, arnica montana is a homeopathic medicine. When given to a healthy individual with no symptoms, it causes bruising and sore, achy muscles. When taken in diluted form by a patient who has fallen and is bruised and sore, the symptoms are quickly relieved.

The dilution of the plant, animal, or mineral substance is made with milk sugar or alcohol at either 1:100 (C) or 1:10 (D or X) strengths. That means one part medicine substance to either 99 or 9 parts of the diluting solution. This is then dried and the dilution repeated over and over again until the substance can barely be detected. A label will state "30C," for example, which means that the substance is diluted 1:100 parts 30 times.

Homeopathic physicians are rigorously trained in taking a complete, holistic history of all symptoms and circumstances to choose the correct remedy. They should always be consulted for serious or complex illnesses or issues. However, many homeopathic remedies are readily available and safe for use by consumers without consultation with a homeopathic physician.

Pharmacokinetics, Pharmacodynamics, and Pharmacotherapeutics

Most homeopathic medicines are in the form of tablets taken by mouth or dissolved under the tongue. They can, however, be given as liquids, sprays, ointments, suppositories, or even injections. The action of most homeopathic remedies is unknown. Homeopaths believe they strengthen the body's own healing abilities. Some believe that there is an energetic component, that the substance changes the vibration of the body at a cellular level. Homeopathic medicines can be used for acute and chronic illnesses, mental and emotional problems, infections, and day-to-day transient health issues like insomnia and sore muscles. These medicines are considered extremely safe and non-toxic because they are so dilute.

MASSAGE IMPLICATIONS AND ASSESSMENT

No cautions or contraindications for massage exist for homeopathic medicines. They may actually be complemented by massage because both enhance the body's own healing properties and balance. It would be important, however, for the massage therapist to encourage any client with a serious, complex illness to consult a homeopathic physician rather than self-medicate.

Side Effects

In general, there are no side effects noted from taking homeopathic remedies.

Flower Essence Therapy

Common Flower Essence Remedies

agrimony: worry

aloe vera: "burned out" feeling

angelica: spiritual crises

arnica: trauma

chamomile: lack of emotional control, oversensitive

dandelion: muscle tension from stress

rescue remedy: emergencies, calm anxiety

walnut: transition times in life

There are many remedies; these are just a few of those that are commonly used.

This therapy form brings highly refined qualities from flowering plants that act on both the physical and psychological aspects of the client. Although similar to homeopathy, flower essence therapy uses only fresh flowering plants harvested at precise moments of flowering. A unique solar extraction method is used to preserve the "essence" or energy of the plants in creating the solutions for these remedies.

Pharmacokinetics, Pharmacodynamics, and Pharmacotherapeutics

Flower essences are taken orally or topically and are in liquid form. As with homeopathy, they are small amounts of dilute substances, in this case from flowers. They can be taken singly or in combination for synergistic effects.

The flower essence remedies seem to act as catalysts. They are not used for suppression of symptoms; however, on an energetic level, they seem to open consciousness to new thoughts, ideas, and expression. They touch on the emotional aspects that practitioners believe underlie all illness and symptomology. As the emotional and psychological aspects of the illness are brought to the consciousness, the body can then act to heal itself on all levels, both physical and emotional.

Flower essences are used for everything from learning disorders, family issues, allergies, stress, and grief to acute illnesses and chronic disorders. As with homeopathy, practitioners are trained in thorough, holistic assessment of all symptoms and issues to choose the appropriate remedies. Flower essence remedies are readily available in health food stores for self-medication by consumers.

MASSAGE IMPLICATIONS AND ASSESSMENT

Flower essences are very dilute and gentle. There are no cautions or contraindications for massage therapy for clients using these remedies. Because massage brings clients into balance and supports healing, it can work with these remedies for the benefit of the client.

Side Effects
There are little to no side effects from the use of flower essence remedies. On occasion, an increased emotional sensitivity may be noted. Clients may safely use these remedies themselves. If the issue or illness is serious or complex, the massage therapist should encourage the client to consult a trained flower essence therapist.

Vitamin Supplements

Common Vitamin Supplements: Fat-Soluble Vitamins

vitamin A

vitamin D

vitamin E

vitamin K

Common Vitamin Supplements: Water-Soluble Vitamins

all B-complex vitamins

vitamin C

Vitamins are essential to the healthy functioning of the human body. They are found in nature and are ingested in food. They are precursors or components of all the vital chemicals that allow our bodies to function. They can also act as or be part of enzymes, which are catalysts for proper chemical reactions in the body.

The recommended daily allowance (RDA) for vitamins created years ago is based on the amounts of the vitamin needed to *prevent* deficiency diseases. Many believe that optimal health requires much larger amounts of these vitamins than proposed by the RDA. There is no clear consensus about just what levels are needed for optimum health.

Some vitamins are water-soluble; that is, they must be taken into the body regularly because they cannot be stored. The body uses what it needs and then excretes the rest, most often in the urine. These vitamins are vitamin C and all the B vitamins. Vitamins A, D, E, and K are all fat-soluble. They can be stored in the body for longer periods in the fatty tissue and the liver. Fat-soluble vitamins can have toxic effects if taken in very high dosages over long periods because of the body's ability to store them in the tissues.

Pharmacokinetics, Pharmacodynamics, and Pharmacotherapeutics

Vitamins are mostly absorbed through the gastrointestinal (GI) tract. Some are synthesized by the body, such as vitamin K. Vitamin D is synthesized by the body from the action of ultraviolet light from the sun on the skin. Vitamins are metabolized by the liver and most are excreted through the urine and feces. Vitamins are used therapeutically to treat nutritional deficiencies and widely used to supplement diets for health and wellness.

Vitamin A

Vitamin A is a fat-soluble vitamin important for eye, skin, and GI health. It is needed for tissue regeneration and protein metabolism. It is also an antioxidant with cancer-fighting properties and immune system support. Large amounts in a pregnant woman (more than 25,000 IU) may cause fetal abnormalities.

B-Complex Vitamins

B vitamins are water-soluble; they must be taken in very regularly in the diet. They act as a team for nerve health. They are precursors for neurotransmitters and enzymes and can themselves act as coenzymes in cellular energy production. They are important in eye, skin, hair, liver, muscle, and blood health. The B vitamins are as follows:

- B_1: thiamine
- B_2: riboflavin
- B_3: niacin
- B_5: pantothenic Acid
- B_6: pyridoxine
- B_{12}: cyanocobalamin
- biotin
- choline
- folic acid
- inositol

Vitamin C

Vitamin C is a water-soluble vitamin. It is essential for tissue growth and repair, adrenal function, and blood clotting. It also is an antioxidant with immune-enhancing and cancer-fighting properties. Large amounts may cause false-positive readings in occult blood tests of the feces.

Vitamin D

Vitamin D is a fat-soluble vitamin essential for calcium and phosphorus metabolism for bone and teeth maintenance as well as growth. It can be obtained through food but must be activated by the liver. The body can create it from the sun's ultraviolet light on the skin surface in its active form.

Vitamin E

Another fat-soluble vitamin, Vitamin E is a strong antioxidant and immune supporter. It is essential for cardiovascular health and blood clotting.

Vitamin K

Vitamin K is a fat-soluble vitamin that is essential in blood clotting, bone formation, and the ability of the body to store and use glucose. Large doses can be toxic to the fetus in a pregnant woman, especially in the last trimester.

MASSAGE IMPLICATIONS AND ASSESSMENT

There are no cautions or contraindications for massage in clients who are taking vitamin supplements.

Side Effects

Side effects from vitamin therapies are rare. Increased bruising may occur with large doses of vitamins E, C, or K and must be reported to the client's physician and massage withheld. The B vitamin niacin and large doses of vitamin K may cause flushing but massage may still be given.

Herbal Supplements

Common Herbal Medicines

aloe: skin irritation and wound healing

black cohosh: menopausal symptoms, fluid retention

capsicum or capsaicin: muscle pain and arthritis

cascara sagrada: constipation

chamomile: sedative, stomach problems, headache, cramps

chaste tree: PMS, heavy menstrual bleeding

cranberry extract: urinary tract infections

dandelion: liver cleanse, kidney function, diuretic

dong quai: PMS, menopausal symptoms

echinacea: immune support

eucalyptus: nasal congestion

evening primrose oil: PMS, fibrocystic breast disease, skin disorders, perimenopausal symptoms, dry skin, hair loss in women, general anti-inflammatory

garlic: asthma, antibacterial, to lower cholesterol

ginger: digestion aide

ginkgo: circulation, diuretic, memory and brain function

ginseng: increased memory, increased stamina and energy

green tea: energy, anticancer, vascular health, and for atherosclerosis

kava kava: anxiety, insomnia, muscle spasms

lavender: insomnia, headache, muscle spasm, anxiety, and cramps

licorice: stomach disorders

pau d'arco: antibacterial, allergies, immune support, headache, sore throat, or as a general tonic *peppermint:* digestion

saw palmetto: prostate health, benign prostatic hypertrophy

senna: constipation

St. John's wort: depression, insomnia

stinging nettles: allergies, skin problems

tea tree: acne, fungal infections and antibacterial

valerian: insomnia, anxiety, tension, muscle spasms, cramps

Potentially Dangerous Herbal Medicines

- Bloodroot: an expectorant and purgative; can cause death from excessive vomiting
- Chan su: a topical aphrodisiac also known as stone, love stone, and rockhard; can cause death if taken internally
- Chaparral tea: used for pain relief; can cause liver failure
- Coltsfoot: for respiratory problems; can cause liver failure
- Comfrey: for wound healing and gastric ulcers; can cause liver failure
- Jin bu huan: sedative; can cause addiction and hepatitis
- Kombucha tea: a general cure-all; can cause acidosis and death
- Lobelia: for respiratory problems; can cause respiratory paralysis and death
- Ma huang (also known as ephedra): for weight loss; can cause psychotic behavior, seizures, irregular heartbeats, heart attack, stroke, and death
- Pennyroyal: to induce menstruation and to treat flu; can cause liver or kidney failure
- Sassafras: a diuretic; can cause liver damage and miscarriage
- Yohimbe bark: an aphrodisiac; can cause psychotic behavior

Herbs have been used medicinally for thousands of years. The use of herbs formed the basis of today's Western pharmaceuticals. True traditional herbal medicine uses the whole plant. Often, these herbs are gathered at specific times of the day or night in keeping with certain phases of the moon or sun. These traditions, handed down for centuries, were thought to be superstitions or "magical" principles in modern times. However, recent research has shown some real scientific reasoning for these precise harvesting times. Alkaloid activity in plants fluctuates with changes in the moon cycle and/or over 24-hour periods. Thus, picking a plant at a certain time, when an activity is at its highest, helps ensure the potency of the properties that the herbalist wishes to use. Herbal medicine is allopathic in principle, just like Western pharmaceuticals. They seek to suppress symptoms.

Pharmacokinetics, Pharmacodynamics, and Pharmacotherapeutics

Many herbs that were used for centuries have been studied and researched thoroughly. For example, foxglove was used for cardiac conditions. It is now the source of the cardiac prescriptions based on digitalis (more often than not it is now synthesized in the laboratory rather than gathered from the plant). Others have had some research performed on how they work and whether they work for the traditional uses. Many herbals have not been studied. There is no proof of their efficacy other than centuries of anecdotal stories.

Herbs may be taken as tablets, capsules, ointments, tinctures, or teas. They can be used in compresses or in baths and even as inhalants. Herbs are generally thought to be safe for use by the general consumer and are widely used to self-medicate. However, these are drugs in the true sense of the word and have side effects. They can be dangerous when used improperly or mixed with other pharmaceuticals. Care must be taken to follow directions closely, inform health care providers of all medicines being taken, and report all adverse effects. Any serious or complex problem should be addressed by a qualified herbalist (see Sidebar: *Potentially Dangerous Herbal Medicines*).

Herbs are used for just about any type of physical ailment or symptom as well as for mental and emotional disorders. Herbals have become the most popular form of alternative and complimentary medicine used today. Billions of dollars are spent yearly on their purchase.

MASSAGE IMPLICATIONS AND ASSESSMENT

Massage implications vary with the type of herb, the reason it is being used, and the actions of the herbs. In general, there are no cautions or contraindications for massage with a client taking herbal medicines. Use of reference books that show the use and actions of the various herbs may be helpful in deciding if there are any effects on the application of massage. In many cases, the action of the herb will not be known.

Side Effects

Each herb has its own side effects. The massage therapist should report any unusual effects to a physician, and reference books will help to show if any special care should be taken when giving massage. Any client using multiple herbs or with serious or complex problems should be referred to an herbal practitioner.

- Chamomile: used mostly for relaxation and stomach problems; can increase the effects of anticoagulant drugs and lead to bleeding
- Kava kava: used for relaxation and anxiety; can lead to liver toxicity and addiction
- Pau d'arco: used for immune system support; can interact with anticoagulants and lead to bleeding

These and other herbs can be safe to use but may have serious effects if used in inappropriate ways or at too high a dosage. Always check with your pharmacist for drug interactions.

Non-Herbal Alternative Supplements

Common Non-Herbal Remedies

acidophilus: diarrhea, (especially with antibiotic use) yeast infections

bee pollen: allergies, asthma, energy, circulation

chondroitin: arthritis, joint pain

coenzyme Q: heart health

glucosamine: arthritis, cartilage damage

melatonin: insomnia, jet lag

Non-herbal supplements are animal and plant items taken for specific health benefits that are not traditional plant-based herbal remedies. They are used for a variety of illnesses.

MASSAGE IMPLICATIONS AND ASSESSMENT

There are no implications for massage with these supplements. No cautions or contraindications are known for clients taking these supplements. They are generally thought to be safe.

Side Effects

Very few side effects are known. If any unusual effects are noted, the physician must be alerted and massage withheld.

Quick *Quiz*

1. Your 64-year-old client is taking Coumadin for atrial fibrillation. When she comes in for her massage, she tells you that she has started taking ginkgo for her memory and vitamin E for her heart. You note that she has numerous bruises and that she cannot remember how she got them. What do you do?

Case Studies

Case Study 1

Your client has stage III non-Hodgkin's lymphoma. He is receiving Cytoxan, vincristine, prednisone, and Rituxan every 3 weeks. Cytoxan is an alkylating drug with a half-life of 4 to 6.5 hours. Vincristine is a vinca alkaloid that has a half-life initially of 4 minutes, then of 2.5 hours, and then of 8.5 hours. Prednisone is a corticosteroid that your client takes for 5 days after each chemotherapy treatment. It has a half-life of 18 to 36 hours. The Rituxan is monoclonal antibodies whose half-life is unknown. Clearly, a physician's input and permission to perform massage are required. The first two drugs act by destroying the fast-growing cancer cells; the Rituxan is antibodies that are very specific for destroying lymph tissue, especially cancerous, fast-growing tissue. The prednisone is an adrenal hormone used to decrease inflammation. All these drugs are excreted in urine and feces.

Massage the week of the chemotherapy should be done before the chemotherapy is given. The next massage should be given 8 days after the chemotherapy session. That will give time for the drugs to exit the body. No deep tissue can be done because side effects of the drugs include altered sensation. The goal is for relaxation, stress reduction, and pain relief. The best strokes to use are the systemic reflex strokes of rocking, gentle friction at the tendons, and mechanical local strokes such as pétrissage. Effleurage should be limited, especially the first week after the chemotherapy, because vincristine and Rituxan may still be in the body and you do not want to push the toxins through the system. For areas of tightness and tension, myofascial work or the local reflex stroke of vibration can be done. Be aware that side effects of fatigue, dizziness, and hypotension could be problems, and assist the client on and off the table. Energy therapies, such as Reiki, healing touch, and some craniosacral, could also be used.

Case Study 2

Your client has breast cancer. She has had a left modified radical mastectomy and is going through chemotherapy. She receives mitoxantrone, 5-FU, and leucovorin calcium every 3 weeks. The chemotherapy agent mitoxantrone is an antineoplastic antibiotic excreted through the urine with a half-life of 5.8 days. 5-FU is an antimetabolite that stops cancer cell replication. It is metabolized into carbon dioxide, which is excreted through the lungs, and its half-life is unknown. Leucovorin calcium is a folic acid derivative that also affects life and replication of cancer cells. It is excreted in urine and has a half-life of 6.2 hours.

The surgical site should not be massaged until completely healed and the physician has given permission. Massage also requires physician approval for the duration of chemotherapy treatment as well. No effleurage should be done for 2 weeks following the chemotherapy treatment due to the long half-life of the drugs. In the third week, some effleurage may be done if massage is given prior to the next scheduled chemotherapy treatment. There is no limitation to any of the other types of massage strokes. Effleurage is limited because it moves fluids throughout the body and could overtax the liver and kidneys as they deal with moving the chemotherapy agents out of the client's system. Deep tissue should not be used on the side of the mastectomy. Strokes on that side should always go distal to proximal. If there is any significant lymphedema, someone trained in manual lymph drainage should work on that arm and shoulder. Myofascial work will help with tight areas and scar tissue. Side effects of the drugs include fatigue, hair loss, nausea, dizziness, and hypotension. If necessary, sessions should be kept short. Avoid turning the client over more than absolutely necessary (client will not be able to lie on the stomach for a while) and take safety precautions when getting the client on and off the table.

Case Study 3

Your client is a hospice patient (receiving only comfort measures and having 6 months or less to live). She has pancreatic and liver cancer with metastasis to the brain. She is taking Reglan, Dilantin, Phenobarbital, and Valium. She is experiencing some nausea and fatigue and has both jaundice (yellow color of the eyes and skin) and ascites (fluid build up in the abdominal cavity). The Reglan increases gastrointestinal motility, working directly on the gastric muscles. The other drugs are all central nervous system depressants with a variety of possible actions on the brain. The client denies any pain. Side effects of the drugs include sleepiness, dizziness, and hypotension.

The goal of the session is for comfort and increased feeling of well-being. Because of the client's condition, short sessions of 15 to 20 minutes only should be used. Deep strokes should not be used. No rocking or shaking should be used because they may increase nausea. The client should not try to lie on the stomach and may not be able to lie on either side because of ascites. Use systemic reflex strokes, such as friction to muscle/tendon junctions, to increase endorphins; a good site for this would be the hands and feet. Otherwise, use mechanical strokes—gentle pétrissage and light effleurage. Very light effleurage over the abdomen may bring some comfort.

Energy therapy may also be used. As the client's condition deteriorates, sessions may need to be decreased to 5 minutes or even discontinued. Energy work may be used up to the time of death, again in short sessions.

Case Study 4

Your client is a man in his 70s. He has arthritis of the spine, coronary artery disease, high blood pressure, and high cholesterol. He is taking Prevacid for gastric reflux, Norvasc and metoprolol for his cardiac condition, and Feldene for arthritis pain. The client is looking for relief from muscular tension and pain in the neck and low back.

Prevacid works at the gastric cells to decrease acid production. Norvasc is a drug that inhibits calcium transport in the cardiac and smooth muscle cells. This dilates arteries and reduces demand on the heart muscle. Side effects are dizziness, flushing, fatigue, and sleepiness. The beta-blocker metoprolol blocks the stimulation of the sympathetic nervous system. This decreases heart rate, contraction, and oxygen need of the heart and lowers blood pressure. Side effects are dizziness, hypotension, and fatigue. Feldene is a nonsteroidal anti-inflammatory drug that probably acts by decreasing prostaglandin production. This, in turn, decreases pain and inflammation. Side effects are dizziness, peripheral edema, and drowsiness.

Because of the beta-blocker, this client will be less easy to stimulate and go into relaxation states quickly. The side effects of several of the drugs will increase this effect. Because pain control and muscle relaxation are the goals, systemic reflex strokes that will increase endorphins, yet not be too relaxing, are best. This includes friction and slightly more rapid effleurage than usual. For the muscles, mechanical strokes such as pétrissage will work best. If muscles are very tight, myofascial work can be done. Deep tissue should not be used or only used with extreme caution both because of the arthritis (especially on the back) and the reduction in pain sensation from the Feldene. With multiple drugs and a cardiac condition, physician approval for massage must be obtained.

Case Study 5

Your client is a 40-year-old woman who has an anxiety disorder, depression, gastroesophageal reflux disease, and hypothyroidism. She works full-time and has two teenage children. She is coming for massage to help control stress in her life. She takes Paxil, trazodone, Aciphex, and Synthroid. Paxil is a selective serotonin reuptake inhibitor. It acts to increase serotonin (a neurotransmitter) levels in the brain. This seems to help with the symptoms of depression and anxiety. Side effects include hypotension, tremor, and paresthesia. The action of trazodone is unknown, but it is also believed to increase the levels of serotonin in the brain and relieve depression. Its side effects are sleepiness, dizziness, hypotension, and increased sweating. Aciphex affects the gastric cells and decreases the production of acid in the stomach. There are little or no side effects. Synthroid is a replacement drug. It provides the body with thyroid hormone, which is a naturally occurring hormone in the body, and stimulates metabolism on a cellular level. When dosages are well regulated, little or no side effects occur.

None of these drugs affect the action of massage strokes on the body. Care should be taken if the client is sleepy or dizzy; side effects and stimulation at the end of the massage can help prevent this.

Because the goal is stress reduction, systemic reflex strokes should predominate the massage. These are effleurage, friction, rocking, and tapotement. These will entrain the client into parasympathetic nervous system relaxation and increase endorphins (the "feel good" hormone).

Medication Assessment Form for Massage Therapy

Medication Assessment Form for Massage Therapy

Client Name:_____ Date:_____

Name of Drug:_____

Action of Drug in the Body:_____

_____

Side Effects of Drug:_____

_____

Does drug raise any red flags or require MD approval for massage therapy?

____ no   ____ yes:

            ____ Massage contraindicated

            ____ MD approval received: Date:_____

               Physician Name:_____

Are any massage stroke actions affected by the drug actions?

____ no   ____ yes:

            ____ Massage strokes or types of massage contraindicated

                  _____

            ____ Types of massage strokes affected

            ____ Local Mechanical: ____ increased effects ____ decreased effects

            ____ Local Reflex: ____ increased effects ____ decreased effects

            ____ Systemic Reflex: ____ increased effects ____ decreased effects

            ____ Systemic Mechanical: ____ increased effects ____ decreased effects

Goal of sessions: _____

Client experiencing any side effects?

____ no   ____ yes:_____

_____

Best strokes to use for this client: _____

_____

Strokes to reduce side effects:_____

Summary of massage protocol: _____

_____

_____

_____

Massage Strokes Action Summary

Local Mechanical: Effleurage, Pétrissage, Friction, Myofascial, Swedish (mechanically brings blood and lymph to the local area, softens tissue and increases cellular exchange of wastes and nutrients in the area being worked)

Local Reflex: Touch/Compression, Vibration/Shaking, Friction, Stretching/Traction, Deep Tissue, Sports, Thai Massage (uses neurological feedback from the muscle/tendons being massaged to change or adjust the tonus—amount of contraction/relaxation of muscle fibers—of the muscles being worked)

Systemic Reflex: Effleurage, Rocking, Friction, Tapotement, Swedish, Sports Massage (stimulates chemical/hormonal changes in the whole of the body mediated through the central nervous system neurotransmitters and hormones that affect relaxation and stimulation)

Systemic Mechanical: Effleurage, Tapotement (mechanically affects a whole body system; effleurage increases blood flow and blood pressure and heart rate in the cardiovascular system; tapotement increases general stimulation of the nervous system)

Answers to Quick Quizzes

Chapter 1

1. You look up her insulin and discover that the absorption of this insulin occurs by the drug crystallizing in the tissue and being slowly absorbed over 10 to 24 hours with no clear onset or peak of action. Massage of the area will affect the rate of absorption and is therefore locally contraindicated in the left thigh. The time element would be 24 hours, because the absorption could take up to 24 hours. Also, the special element of the crystallization of the insulin in the tissue at the site of injection is a further contraindication to massage in that area. No massage should be done at the site of injection for this client. Ask her to be sure and use another site for injection for her next massage so that the left thigh could be massaged at her next session; then avoid the area of that injection (e.g., the right thigh) for that session.

2. Apply the deductive process to this client. (1) The goal is relaxation. (2) Massage strokes used could be effleurage (for both mechanical and reflexive effects), pétrissage (for mechanical and somatic reflex effects), and rocking (for reflexive effects) with some friction and deep compression (for somatic and systemic reflex effects) on areas of tightness and constriction. (3) Massage would not affect the rate of absorption of any of the medications, and no immediate "red flags" regarding safety are apparent. (4) Synthroid is a replacement drug and acts on the rate of metabolism. None of the side effects or the actions of the drug increase or decrease the desired massage effect or interfere with the effects of the massage strokes. (5) Birth control pills are hormones that suppress ovulation. This action does not affect nor is affected by massage. Side effects that could be of concern are increased blood clotting and increased blood pressure. If the client has not had any of these side effects, then massage effects of relaxation will not be increased or decreased. If these side effects have been present, discussion with the client's physician is required. (6) Multivitamins are replacement nutrients and do not affect the massage goal or application. Generally, proceeding with the massage as planned is indicated.

Chapter 2

1. A. Pharmacokinetics discusses the movement of drugs through the body and involves absorption, distribution, metabolism, and excretion.

2. C. Maintenance therapy seeks to maintain a certain level of health in patients who have chronic conditions.

3. C. Pharmacodynamics studies the mechanisms of action of drugs and seeks to understand how drugs work in the body.

Chapter 3

1. First consider the action of the drug, a cholinergic. It mimics the parasympathetic nervous system. However, because this drug is given in eye drop form, systemic absorption is limited, as are the side effects. This means that no change will be needed in the type of strokes or type of massage you will give.

2. Aricept is an anticholinesterase drug that stimulates the parasympathetic activity. The client may be drowsier or more easily relaxed during the massage. Also, side effects of concern are orthostatic hypotension and muscle cramps. Using direct mechanical and somatic reflex strokes (such as compression and friction) will work to ease muscle tightness, but systemic reflex strokes (such as rocking and slow effleurage) may cause a drop in blood pressure. Using more rapid effleurage throughout the massage and tapotement at the end will help the client to feel relaxed but not too sedated. Stay with the client until he or she is seated on the edge of the table and assure that he or she is not dizzy from the position change.

3. Transderm Scōp is a cholinergic blocker; it stops the action of the parasympathetic nervous system by blocking acetylcholine at specific muscarinic sites. They have mixed and paradoxical effects. In this case, the target organ is the gastrointestinal tract. Decreasing parasympathetic action slows the motility and decreases the secretions of the stomach and intestines. Massage strokes over the gastrointestinal tract are contraindicated—you do not want to stimulate it mechanically! The systemic effects of these drugs are harder to classify. Ask the client about any side effects. Most people find a depressant effect on the central nervous system and sedation to be a problem. More stimulating strokes would then be indicated. Others may feel restless and nervous; in such cases, more relaxing strokes could be used. In all cases, check for safety when getting the client off the table.

4. Primatene Mist is an epinephrine inhalant used to dilate the bronchioles to stop an acute asthma attack. Because the route is inhalation, only small amounts are absorbed systemically. The drug stimulates the sympathetic nervous system (fight or flight). Massage does not affect the absorption of the drug or its action. Ask the client about any side effects. Most common ones are some nervousness, restlessness, and increased heart rate. If she is experiencing any of these, start massage with rocking and rhythmic effleurage to get the systemic reflex relation response going. Avoid any strokes (such as tapotement, deep tissue, or prolonged friction) that would stimulate too much and exacerbate the symptoms.

5. Lopressor is a beta-blocker. It stops the actions of the sympathetic nervous system. Its action is selective to the heart in this case and will work to decrease blood pressure. Because massage also can decrease blood pressure, caution needs to be used. Utilize a little more rapid effleurage stroke and tapotement at the end of a session. Systemic actions and side effects of the drug may increase sedation and relaxation. This can be handled as above. Safety at the end of the session when the client is changing position to sit up is important.

Chapter 4

1. Because of the age and instability of this patient, no massage should be done before receiving more information and approval from the physician. Any stimulation of the nervous system, such as that which occurs at the beginning of any massage, may set off a seizure. Although relaxation massage—using gentle effleurage and pétrissage as well as rocking to entrain the nervous system—may be useful, physician consent must be received.

2. Because Depakene works by slowing the transmission of nerve impulses in the motor cortex, the use of strokes that work with the local and systemic reflexes may be slower or less effective in some patients. A patient who has been taking medication for a long time, however, is less likely to have this problem. For relaxation, reflex systemic strokes may be used. For the knots in her shoulders, the use of myofascial techniques may be more effective. Deep tissue should be used with caution until her ability to give feedback is determined.

3. Drowsiness is one of the common side effects as well as constipation. Effleurage of the abdomen may help, and tapotement at the end of the session may be indicated as well.

Chapter 5

1. For the goal of decreased pain and increased range of motion, the systemic and somatic reflex strokes would work well. Systemic reflex strokes to increase endorphins could be effleurage and friction at the attachment sites of the muscles. Somatic reflex strokes could be compression, stretching, and deep tissue to the gluteated neck and shoulder muscles. The action of the drug is to decrease the synthesis of prostaglandins, thus decreasing the pain sensation and inflammation. This will not affect the systemic or somatic reflex action of the chosen strokes of effleurage, friction, and stretching. However, decreased pain sensation makes deep work a contraindication. Compression could still be used but with caution as to depth. Deep tissue should be replaced by another type of stroke that will loosen gluteated tissue without a great deal of depth needed. The local effects of pétrissage and the myofascial stretch techniques are the better choice for this session.

2. The goal of this session is specific muscle group relaxation. Normally, the planned strokes would be effleurage and pétrissage to warm up the sites locally and mechanically, and deep tissue compression at the muscle bellies and attachment sites to bring in the somatic reflex arcs. Tylenol #3 is a combination pain relief product made up of acetaminophen and codeine. Acetaminophen acts to decrease pain perception by unknown mechanisms, whereas codeine blocks the peripheral opiate receptors to decrease sensation transmission including pain. Deep tissue is not a good choice here because pain and sensation are diminished. Depth needs to be approached with caution. Also, somatic reflex arcs may be slower and these strokes less effective. Choosing other strokes that focus locally on the muscles and tissue in question is more appropriate. Effleurage and pétrissage to locally and mechanically warm and bring blood to the areas, then lighter myofascial work to soften tissues and bring healing fluids to the area are good substitutions. Some deep tissue might be done after the above are used to increase the effects of the massage, but always with caution concerning depth. Side effects of this drug include drowsiness,

dizziness, and low blood pressure. Counter these effects by gentle but rapid effleurage strokes for systemic stimulation at the end of the session.

Chapter 6

1. Being flushed and red-faced is a common side effect of Isordil because of its vasodilating effects. If the client is not experiencing any other side effects (such as dizziness or low blood pressure), you can proceed with massage and suggest that she speak with her physician about the side effects she is experiencing. Avoid effleurage strokes that may increase vasodilation mechanically.

2. The combination of two drugs that have side effects of hypotension and the blocking of the sympathetic nervous system have increased the effects of the massage relaxation. You could have done slightly more rapid work, mostly with pétrissage, and used tapotement at the end of the session to prevent the effect. Have the client lay on her side if possible, or elevate the legs. Do some rapid friction strokes to the feet and hands and offer some juice if available. Let the client lie on her side for a while, then assist her to a sitting position. Have her sit with legs dangling for a while until the feelings of dizziness and nausea pass. Then assist her in getting off the table.

Chapter 7

1. The presence of a blood clot is a contraindication for massage. Even if the client says that the clot has dissolved, no massage should be given and the physician should be contacted. Only the physician can indicate when it is safe to give massage again, and this may not be for several months (up to 10) after the diagnosis. If you are not certain the physician understands the implications for massage, always use caution and when in doubt, do not massage.

2. The massage should be postponed until you can speak with the physician and determine if the client's condition is stable. If it is, deep tissue would be used only with caution and circulatory massage limited.

Chapter 8

1. Because Primatene is a topical decongestant, there will be minimal systemic effects from this sympathetic system agonist drug. However, both guaifenesin and codeine have sedation and drowsiness as side effects and therefore have implications for your massage. Increased stimulation at the end of the session is needed so the client does not continue to feel sedated and fatigued after the session.

2. Both of the inhalers being used are sympathetic system agonists. Inhalation usually means that there is mostly local action and not as much systemic absorption or effects. However, because your client is taking these inhalers regularly (ask how often she needs to use the acute asthma attack inhaler Combivent), she may be absorbing the drugs systemically and may have some sympathetic stimulation. Try using rocking to start the relaxation process for this client, or use slow effleurage throughout the session.

Chapter 9

1. Lactulose is a hyperosmolar laxative that pulls fluid into the intestines to allow easy evacuation of stool. It takes anywhere from 24 to 48 hours for onset of action. Therefore, you can proceed with the massage as planned and may additionally give gentle abdominal massage in the direction of the intestinal path to aid in the efficacy of the drug.

2. Lomotil is an opioid-related antidiarrheal with strong effects on the smooth muscle of the bowel. The presence of pain and constipation are red flags for possible bowel obstruction, and you should instruct the client to call his physician immediately. No massage can be done until serious adverse reactions have been ruled out.

Chapter 10

1. Because the client is having little or no symptoms and the drug does not affect application of massage strokes, you can proceed with the massage as usual. Encourage the client to drink extra fluids after the massage.

2. A client with active TB must get clearance from a physician before starting massage. There is no risk of disease spread after approximately 10 to 14 days of treatment, and the drugs do not affect the massage stroke response. If the physician agrees, proceed with the massage, focusing on systemic reflex strokes that can help support the immune system. If the client has side effects of peripheral neuropathy, do not use deep tissue massage.

3. You may give the client massage but completely avoid the affected areas. Be sure to change sheets and wash hands thoroughly after the massage.

Chapter 11

1. Your client is still having some symptoms of the allergic reaction. Rubbing the area may increase blood flow to the area and exacerbate her symptoms again. You should not do massage until all symptoms have abated. You could offer her energy therapies or use rocking and shaking techniques to relax her. Scalp, face, hand, and foot massage may also be an option if these areas were not affected.

2. This client should not receive a massage until you have obtained a release from the physician.

Chapter 12

1. Your client has a controlled psychotic disorder. You should get the client's permission to speak with his physician and get a release before doing any massage. Discuss any symptoms that should be reported to the physician. Be aware that both drugs will increase the relaxation effects of the massage, so stimulate the client at the end of the massage. Also, Haldol can slow local reflex strokes, so use mechanical strokes and stimulating systemic reflex strokes.

2. The client is experiencing long-term effects of the drug that increase the relaxant effects of the massage. Try to schedule your massage later in the day and use more

stimulating systemic reflex strokes throughout the massage. Stay with the client when she sits up after the massage until you are both certain that she is steady.

Chapter 13

1. All clients with diabetes must have a release from their physician for massage. For this client, there are no contraindications to any kind of massage. After receiving physician approval, be sure the client has had a snack within 1 hour before the massage and avoid massaging the site of the last injection of insulin. Keep a source of sugar on hand just in case the client has a hypoglycemic reaction.

2. You must obtain a physician release for massage and talk with the physician about any cautions and complications regarding the disease. After doing so for this client, massage may be given without any need to change it related to the drug. Be aware that the client may need to go to the bathroom more frequently; limit effleurage that moves fluid through the body to avoid this if possible. Do not have anything that could stimulate the need to go to the bathroom, such as a water fountain, in the area. Ask if the client has a "water prescription" because sometimes such patients have a specific amount of water they must drink. If such a prescription exists, inform the client that he or she must adhere to it.

Chapter 14

1. She is taking Slow-K as a replacement because potassium can be depleted by the use of diuretics. In this case, if her blood pressure is stable (you may need to contact her physician to be sure), there is no reason you could not give massage. There is no effect on the massage strokes caused by the medication.

2. Although the calcium itself will not require that you do anything to change your massage, the osteoporosis might. Contact the physician and find out if the disease is mild, moderate, or severe and change your massage accordingly. Moderate to severe osteoporosis is a contraindication for deep tissue, and pressure (especially on the ribs and back) should be very light.

Chapter 16

1. You know that Coumadin is an anticoagulant used to prevent blood clotting. When you look up vitamin E, you see it also has functions related to blood clotting and is a fat-soluble vitamin that can be stored in the body. You also see that ginkgo can interact with anticoagulants and *increase* their action in the body. You should not do massage. Instruct your client to call her physician and tell him or her about the supplements and the bruising. The client may be at risk for bleeding and need her medication adjusted.

Antitussive: a drug used to suppress a cough.

Aphrodisiac: drug or food that is said to stimulate sexual desire and/or increase arousal.

Aplastic anemia: deficiency in red blood cell production because of bone marrow disorders.

Apnea: periods when a patient stops breathing.

Arrhythmias: any abnormality in the rate or rhythm of the heart.

Asthma: a disease caused by increased sensitivity of the trachea and bronchia of the lungs, leading to bronchospasm and constriction of the airways and increased inflammation.

Ataxia: defect in muscle coordination that manifests when voluntary muscular movements are attempted.

Atherosclerosis: buildup of plaque and fatty deposits in blood vessels.

Athetosis: a condition of slow, irregular twisting movements occurring in the extremities.

Atria: the two upper chambers of the heart. When they contract, they push blood into the ventricles or lower chambers of the heart.

Atrioventricular node: area of the heart that controls electrical impulses across the atria and ventricles of the heart and regulates heart rate and rhythm.

Atrophy: a wasting or abnormal decrease in size of an organ or tissue.

Attention deficit disorder: persistent pattern of inability to maintain focus or attention, often with hyperactivity.

Atypical depression: depression manifesting in symptoms that are not usually seen in this disorder and/or that will not respond to the usual antidepressant drugs.

Atypical psychosis: psychosis not showing the usual symptoms and not responding to the usual antipsychotic drugs.

Autism: developmental disorder in which connection to and communication with the outside world are altered, causing isolation and problems with daily functioning.

Autoimmune: caused by one's own immune system.

Autonomic nervous system: part of the nervous system that controls involuntary bodily functions.

A-V node: see atrioventricular node.

Benign prostatic hypertrophy: abnormal but noncancerous enlargement of the male prostate gland.

Beta receptors: one type of receptor of the sympathetic nervous system.

Biliary colic: pain caused by stones in the bile duct.

Bipolar disorder: mental disorder that manifests two sets of emotional symptoms (i.e., mania and depression) in a cyclic manner.

Blood urea nitrogen: blood test that measures kidney function.

Bone marrow: soft substance found in the cavity of many of the bones of the body that produces many other cells needed by the body, such as red blood cells.

BPH: see Benign prostatic hypertrophy.

Bradycardia: a slower than normal heart rate.

Brief reactive psychosis: psychosis caused by severe physical or mental trauma or ingestion of drugs or alcohol; is usually temporary.

Bronchitis: inflammation of the mucous membranes of the bronchus of the lungs.

Bronchospasm: spasm and constriction of the bronchus and bronchioles of the lungs, which causes difficulty breathing.

Buffalo hump: excess fat deposits in the shoulders and upper back.

Buffered: having a substance added to a medication that maintains acid/base balance, thus preventing increased acidity and stomach upset.

BUN: see Blood urea nitrogen.

Cachexia: extreme emaciated condition; very poorly nourished.

Carcinoma: cancer of epithelial tissues.

Catalyst: substance that speeds the rate of chemical reaction while not itself being changed.

Catecholamine: biologically active amines (norepinephrine and epinephrine) that regulate many aspects of metabolism and affect the cardiac and nervous systems. Catecholamines stimulate the sympathetic nervous system effects in the body.

Cation: positively charged ion.

Caution: any symptom or circumstance indicating the need for care in applying an otherwise advisable treatment.

Cellular metabolism: the physical and chemical changes taking place within a cell.

Cerebral hemorrhage: bleeding in the brain.

Cerebral palsy: a motor function disorder caused by damage to the brain.

Cerebrovascular accident: see Stroke.

Cholinergic: liberating acetylcholine, or a drug that produces the same effects as acetylcholine.

Cholinergic agonist: drug that mimics the effects of acetylcholine and the parasympathetic nervous system.

Cholinergic blockers: drugs that block the effects of the parasympathetic nervous system, especially the action of acetylcholine.

Cholinesterase: an enzyme that breaks down the neurotransmitter acetylcholine in the nerve synapse and thus stops or limits parasympathetic nervous system stimulation.

Chorea: involuntary muscular twitching or movements of the limbs and face.

Choriocarcinoma: cancer of the tissues of conception such as placental or fetal cells left in the uterus.

Chronic bronchitis: inflammation of the mucosal lining of the bronchus and bronchioles of the lungs that persists despite treatment.

Chronotropic: affecting heart rate.

Clitoral hypertrophy: abnormal enlargement of the clitoris.

Clitoris: small erectile body found in the female labia that responds to sexual stimuli.

CMV: see Cytomegalovirus.

Complimentary medicine: use of non-Western medicine in conjunction with Western medicine to enhance the effects of both.

Congestive heart failure: condition in which the heart muscle is so weakened it cannot effectively circulate blood in the body.

Connective tissue: tissue that supports and connects other tissues and parts of the body.

Contraindication: any symptom or circumstance indicating the inappropriateness of an otherwise advisable treatment.

Coronary arteries: series of arteries that bring oxygen-rich blood to the heart muscle.

Coryza: profuse discharge from the nose.

Cushing's disease: condition of abnormally high secretion of glucocorticoids, such as cortisol, from the adrenal glands.

Cushingoid symptoms: symptoms of Cushing's disease or syndrome.

CVA: see Stroke.

Cyanosis: blue color to the skin usually caused by decreased oxygen.

Cytomegalovirus: a herpes-like virus causing no or mild flu-like symptoms in healthy individuals; however, the virus may be deadly in immunocompromised patients. It is also a cause of severe birth defects in the fetus of a mother infected with the virus at the time of pregnancy.

Cytotoxic: deadly to a cell.

Deductive reasoning: the process of reasoning from the general to the particular.

Defibrillation: use of an external electrical shock to the heart muscle to stop fibrillation and return the heart rate and rhythm to normal.

Delirium: extreme confusion usually with agitation

Delusion: false belief not in keeping with reality or caused by any external input.

Dementia: a broad term that refers to cognitive deficits, including memory impairment.

Demineralization: the loss of minerals such as calcium and phosphorus from a bone, weakening the bone.

Deoxyribonucleic acid: complex structure arranged in two twisted chains found in the nucleus of a cell that carries the entire genetic code of the organism or cell.

Dependence: see Drug dependence.

Desiccated: dried.

Diaphoresis: increased sweating.

Dilution: process of weakening a substance, usually with water or alcohol.

Diplopia: double vision; seeing double.

Diuresis: increased urine output.

Diverticulitis: condition in which diverticuli—sacs or pouches along the colon wall—become inflamed and/or infected.

Diverticulosis: condition in which small sacs or pouches form along the colon.

DNA: see Deoxyribonucleic acid

Dopaminergic: drug that mimics the effects of the neurotransmitter dopamine in the sympathetic nervous system.

Dromotropic: affecting the speed of electrical conduction in the heart.

Drug dependence: a psychologic craving for a drug with or without actual physiologic dependency.

Duration: amount of time a drug will continue to have its effects in the body.

Dysarthria: difficulty in or inability to speak related to problems with muscle control of the tongue and/or face.

Dyskinesia: defect in the ability to perform voluntary muscle movements.

Dyspepsia: burning in the stomach, or indigestion.

Dysphagia: difficulty in swallowing.

Dyspnea: difficulty breathing.

Dystonia: prolonged muscle contractions that cause rhythmic jerking movements that are not under voluntary control.

Eclamptic: condition of or related to pregnancy-induced hypertension causing seizures and coma if not treated.

Ectopic: outside the normal area or rhythm.

Edema: local or generalized condition in which the tissues contain an excessive amount of fluid.

Electrolyte: a substance that in fluid can conduct electricity; an ionized (positively or negatively charged) salt in the blood, tissue fluids, and cells of the body.

Emaciated: the state of being extremely thin because of a lack of nourishment or disease process.

Emphysema: chronic pulmonary disease marked by an abnormal increase in size and loss of elasticity in the alveoli and/or destruction of the alveoli.

Encephalopathy: inflammation of the brain and ensuing scar tissue formation.

Endocrine substance: an internal secretion from a gland directly into the blood stream; also called a hormone.

Endometriosis: the presence of cells of the endometrium outside the uterus; these cells still respond to hormonal changes and can cause severe pain and bleeding.

Endometrium: the mucous membrane of the uterus that cyclically builds up with blood in preparation for possible pregnancy.

Endorphins: a polypeptide produced in the brain that acts to reduce pain perception at the opiate receptors in the body; it also gives a feeling of euphoria.

Enkephalin: a pentapeptide produced in the brain that reduces pain perception at the opiate receptors in the body; it can also give a feeling of euphoria.

Enteral: route by which drugs enter the body through the gastrointestinal system.

Entrained: to alter the biologic rhythms to a different cycle.

Epinephrine: a hormone secreted by the adrenal glands in response to sympathetic nervous system stimulation.

EPS: see Extrapyramidal symptoms.

Erythema: reddening of the skin.

Erythropoietin: a substance produced by the kidneys that stimulates the production of red blood cells in the bone marrow.

Essence: the spirit or principle of a thing; that which makes it what it is.

Euphoria: state of extreme elation often with decreased inhibitions and poor decision-making abilities.

Extracellular fluid: fluid that bathes the outside of the cells in the tissues of the body.

Extrapyramidal symptoms: uncontrolled movements of the head, neck, arms, and legs, often because of drug side effects.

Extravasation: escape of fluids into surrounding tissue. Can occur when intravenous needles or catheters become dislodged or blocked.

Extremities: legs and arms, hands and feet.

Fasciculations: involuntary contraction of muscle fibers that do not cause movement of a joint often visible under the skin.

Fascitis: inflammation of fascial tissue.

Fecal impaction: condition in which feces are hard and dry and wedged in the rectum. Most often requires manual removal.

Ferritin: an iron-phosphorus protein complex formed in the intestinal mucosa and a means of storing iron until it is needed.

Fibrillation: extremely rapid and incomplete contractions of the atria or ventricles of the heart that are ineffective in pumping blood.

Flatulence: condition of having and expelling excess gas from the gastrointestinal tract.

GABA: see Gamma-aminobutyric acid.

Gamma-aminobutyric acid: a neurotransmitter in the central nervous system that inhibits certain amino acids and decreases neuron activity.

Gastroesophageal reflux disease: disorder in which the stomach contents flow backward into the esophagus, causing heartburn and other symptoms.

GERD: see Gastroesophageal reflux disease

Glaucoma: a group of eye diseases characterized by increased intraocular (inside the eye) pressure, resulting in atrophy of the optic nerve that can lead to blindness.

Globulin: a type of simple protein insoluble in water but soluble in solutions of salts of strong acids.

Glossitis: inflammation of the tongue

Glycogen: form of sugar when stored in liver cells.

Gonadotropin-releasing hormone: hormone released by the hypothalamus to stimulate the pituitary gland to release its hormones regulating some sexual characteristics and cycles.

Ground substance: the matrix or intercellular substance in which the cells of an organ or tissue are imbedded.

Gynecomastia: abnormal enlargement of the breasts.

H. pylori: see *Helicobacter pylori.*

Half-life: time it takes for half of a drug dose to be eliminated from the body.

Hay fever: hypersensitivity or allergic reaction in which the mucous membranes of the nose and upper air passages become inflamed and produce watery discharge from the nose, eyes, and sinuses.

HDL: see High-density lipoproteins.

Helicobacter pylori: bacteria that causes some stomach ulcers.

Helper T-cells: immune system cells that help to "turn on" or stimulate other immune cells to action in the body.

Hemolytic anemia: anemia caused by the destruction of red blood cells in the body.

Hemosiderin: iron-containing pigment derived from hemoglobin from the disintegration of red blood cells. It is where iron is stored in the body until it is needed to make new red blood cells.

Hepatitis: inflammation of the liver.

Herb: plant with soft stem and little or no wood that produces seeds and then dies at the end of one season.

Herbal: made from an herb.

Hernia: protrusion or bulging out of an organ or part of an organ through the wall of the cavity that usually holds it in.

Herpes zoster: acute viral infection affecting the peripheral nerves and causing pain and fluid-filled skin esions.

High-density lipoproteins: lipoproteins that contain more protein than fat and are "better" for decreasing plaque formation in blood vessels and cardiovascular disease.

Histamine: substance found in the body that causes flushing and swelling of tissues especially in response to trauma/injury or allergens.

Hodgkin's disease: a specific type of cancer of the lymphatic system.

Homeopathy: school of medicine based on the theory that drugs that cause certain symptoms will actually cure those symptoms when given in extremely diluted form. "Like heals like."

Homeostasis: state of dynamic equilibrium in the internal environment of the body; ability of the body to react appropriately to changing internal and external conditions.

Hypercholesterolemia: condition of extremely high levels of cholesterol and lipids in the blood.

Hyperkalemia: excessive levels of potassium in the blood.

Hypernatremia: excessive levels of sodium in the blood.

Hypertrophic cardiomyopathy: a disease of the heart muscle characterized by enlargement of the heart and decreased effectiveness of the heart; often leads to congestive heart failure.

Hyperventilation: abnormally rapid breathing.

Hypnosis: a subconscious condition.

Hypnotic: pertaining to sleep.

Hypochondriasis: mental condition marked by excessive concern over one's health often with a false belief that one is suffering from one or more diseases.

Hypoglycemia: low blood sugar.

Hypokalemia: low potassium levels in the blood.

Hyponatremia: too low levels of sodium in the blood.

Hypotension: low blood pressure, often causing dizziness, weakness, and fainting.

Hypothalamus: portion of the brain that secretes hormones and has regulatory functions over the pituitary, body temperature, and sympathetic and parasympathetic nervous system balance.

Hypotonia: abnormal decrease in the tone of muscles.

Hypoxia: condition in which insufficient oxygen is reaching the cells of the body.

Iatrogenic effects: adverse reaction to drug that mimics a disease or pathological disorder.

IM: see Intramuscular.

Immunocompromised: patient who is known to have a poorly functioning immune system and is unable to fight infections.

Immunosuppressants: drugs used to decrease the activity of the immune system.

Impotence: the inability to achieve and maintain erection of the penis.

Impulse control disorder: mental disorder in which the patient has little or no rational control over the emotions and acts on them without thought to the consequences.

Incontinence: inability to control bowel and/or bladder, leading to accidents in urination and defecation.

Increased intracranial pressure: condition in which fluid or tumor growth in the head causes increased pressure on the brain.

Inhalation: route by which drugs enter the body by being taken into the lungs by breathing them in.

Inotropic: affecting the strength of contraction of the heart muscle.

Insomnia: inability to sleep

Insulin reaction: sudden drop in blood sugar level related to taking too much insulin by injection or not eating after taking an insulin injection.

Intracellular fluid: fluid that is inside the cell and contained by the cell membrane.

Intramuscular: injection of drug into the muscles tissue for systemic absorption directly into the bloodstream.

Intravenous: injection of a drug directly into a vein and therefore directly into the bloodstream.

Intrinsic factor: substance secreted by the gastric cells of the stomach; essential for the absorption of vitamin B_{12}.

Ion: an atom or group of atoms that has lost or gained one or more electrons and therefore is charged and can conduct an electrical impulse.

IV: see Intravenous.

Joint receptors: receptors in the joint that are sensitive to increased pressure and use a feedback loop in the nervous system to increase relaxation of the muscles.

Kaposi's sarcoma: cancer of the blood vessels. Often the tumors are seen as purple lesions on the skin and mucous membranes.

Ketoacidosis: acidosis caused by increased ketones in the blood that may occur in diabetics when the body cannot burn blood sugar; may cause coma and death.

LDL: see Low-density lipoproteins.

Lennox-Gastaut syndrome: see Seizure, atypical absence.

Leukemia: a group of cancers of the blood-forming cells in the bone marrow.

Leukopenia: abnormally low number of white blood cells.

Limbic system: a group of brain structures that interpret emotional significance of sensory input and regulate endocrine and autonomic nervous system responses.

Lipoproteins: proteins combined with fat circulating in the blood.

Low-density lipoproteins: lipoproteins with more fat than protein that are the "bad" form of cholesterol; increase plaque formation in the blood vessels and increase the risk of cardiovascular disease.

Lupus erythematosus: an autoimmune disease that affects multiple body systems. It causes inflammation and often affects the joints, kidneys, heart, lung, and skin.

Lymphomas: cancer of the lymph nodes and lymph tissue.

Macrocytic: cell size that is larger than normal.

Malignant hyperthermia: a rare but potentially fatal complication of anesthesia characterized by skeletal muscle rigidity and high fever.

Malignant melanoma: cancer of the melanocytes (pigment-containing cells); usually starts in the skin and spreads rapidly throughout the body.

Manic: mood state characterized by excessive energy, poor impulse control, psychosis, agitation, frenzied movement, and decreased sleep.

Mast cells: large tissue cells containing enzymes present around blood vessels and in the skin and bone marrow. Mast cells can produce histamine.

Melanoma: see Malignant melanoma.

Metabolism: the sum of all physical and chemical changes taking place within an organism.

Metabolites: the products of chemical and physiologic activity in the cells of the body.

Metastatic cancer: cancer that has spread from its original site and started growing at other sites in the body.

Microcytic: cell size that is smaller than normal.

Mineral: an inorganic compound, not of animal or plant origin.

Mitral stenosis: a narrowing of the mitral valve in the heart.

Moon face: excess fat deposits in the face and jaw.

Multiple sclerosis: a disease in which progressive demyelination or destruction of the sheath that protects the nerve cells causes multiple neurologic dysfunction.

Muscle spindles: a specialized sensory fiber within a muscle that is sensitive to tension and changes in the length of the muscle. When stimulated they cause the muscle to contract strongly and then relax.

Myasthenia gravis: an autoimmune disease marked by skeletal muscle fatigability caused by the destruction of acetylcholine receptors at the nerve–muscle junction.

Myeloproliferative disorders: disorders of the bone marrow and its products.

Necrosis: death of tissue and cells.

Neuroleptic malignant syndrome: possible side effect of antipsychotic drugs marked by muscle rigidity, paralysis, coma, high blood pressure, high fever, and respiratory distress.

Neurotransmitter: substance that is released when the axon terminal of a presynaptic neuron is excited. The substance then travels across the synapse to act on the target cell to either inhibit or excite it.

Neutropenia: abnormally low numbers of neutrophils (a type of white blood cell) in the blood.

Neutrophils: a type of white blood cell responsible for much of the body's protection against infection.

Noncatecholamines: synthetic substances that stimulate the sympathetic nervous system effects.

Nonsteroidal anti-inflammatory drugs: group of drugs that inhibit prostaglandin production; used to decrease inflammation, pain, and fever.

Norepinephrine: a hormone secreted by the adrenal glands that is similar to epinephrine, or a neurotransmitter released by the sympathetic nervous system to produce its effects.

Normocytic: cell size that is normal.

NSAIDs: see Nonsteroidal anti-inflammatory drugs.

Nystagmus: constant, involuntary, cyclical movement of the eyeball.

Occult blood test: laboratory test to detect blood that is not visible to the eye, usually in feces.

Onset: amount of time it takes for a drug to start having its effects in the body.

Opiate receptor: a specific site on a cell surface that interacts with narcotic drugs and hormones to mediate the perception of pain.

Orthostatic hypotension: sudden drops in blood pressure caused by a change in body position, such as going from lying down to standing.

Osteomalacia: disease in which the bones become increasingly soft, causing increased flexibility, brittleness, and deformities.

OTC: see Over the counter.

Over the counter: medication/drugs sold without a physician prescription required.

Palliative: treatment with the goal of alleviating symptoms, not curing, stopping, or controlling a disease process.

Palpitations: an abnormally rapid, throbbing, or fluttering of the heart perceptible to the patient.

Panic disorder: anxiety disorder with sudden intense attacks of irrational fear.

Paradoxical: not the usual or expected response.

Paralytic ileus: paralysis of the intestines with distention of the abdomen and blockage of the movement of feces through the system.

Parasympathetic nervous system: a division of the autonomic nervous system that brings about a relaxing state in the body for rest and repair, digestion, and other restorative actions.

Parenteral: route by which drugs enter the body directly into the bloodstream.

Parkinson's disease: a disease in which a deficiency of the neurotransmitter dopamine in the basal ganglia of the brain causes movement disorders affecting muscle actions and coordination.

Paroxysmal atrial tachycardia: sudden, periodic attacks of increased rate of atrial contraction.

Paroxysmal supraventricular tachycardia: sudden, periodic attacks of rapid heart rate starting in the atria and moving into the ventricles of the heart.

Peak: amount of time it takes for a drug to have its strongest effects in the body.

Peptic ulcer: an ulcer in the mucosal lining of the lower esophagus or the stomach.

Perforation: an abnormal hole in any organ wall.

Pericardial effusion: abnormal amount of fluid in the lining around the heart; can cause serious heart problems.

Peripheral neuropathy: loss of or change in sensation in the extremities.

Peripheral resistance: pressure opposition to the flow of blood through the arteries and capillaries.

Peripheral vascular insufficiency: condition in which the peripheral blood flow is not sufficient to bring oxygen and nutrients to the cells or take waste and fluid away from the cells. Can lead to non-healing wounds and ulcers.

Peripheral vascular resistance: amount of resistance to the flow of blood through the arteries and capillaries. High peripheral vascular resistance requires the heart to work harder, use more oxygen, and increases blood pressure.

Peristalsis: the muscle movement of the gastrointestinal tract.

Pernicious anemia: type of anemia caused by the lack of intrinsic factor in the stomach.

Personality disorder: pathologic disturbance in cognitive, emotional, and interpersonal abilities.

Pharmacodynamics: the study of drugs and how they act on living organisms.

Pharmacokinetics: the study of the metabolism and action of drugs with particular emphasis on absorption, duration of action, distribution in the body, and method of excretion.

Pharmacology: the study of drugs and their origin, nature, properties, and effects on living organisms.

Pharmacotherapeutics: the study of the use of drugs in the treatment of disease.

Pheochromocytoma: tumor-secreting catecholamines that cause severe high blood pressure.

Phlebitis: inflammation of a vein without the presence of a blood clot.

Phobias: irrational fear of a specific object or activity.

Photophobia: fear of light or an unusual sensitivity to light.

Phototoxicity: condition in which exposure to light causes serious skin lesions, fever, and other symptoms.

Plantar fascitis: inflammation of fascial tissue of the heel and foot.

Pneumonia: the presence of excess fluid in the lungs; can be caused by many different factors including infection, irritation, and heart problems.

Polycythemia vera: a condition in which too many red blood cells are produced too rapidly by the bone marrow. This can lead to clotting and poor circulation.

Potency: relative amount of a drug required to produce a desired response.

Precursor: substance that precedes another substance or from which another substance is synthesized.

Premature epiphyseal closure: in children, the too early closure of the growth plates at the ends of the long bones of the body, resulting in stoppage of normal growth in height.

Premature ventricular contractions: contraction of the ventricles before the normal time because of abnormalities in the electrical conduction system of the heart.

Preterm labor: going into labor for childbirth before the full 9 months of pregnancy is completed.

Prinzmetal's angina: chest pain occurring during rest caused by spasms of the coronary arteries (arteries that serve the heart muscle itself).

Prostaglandin: any of a large number of substances produced by the body and having many different physiologic effects, including increased inflammation and increased sensitivity to pain.

Prostatic hypertrophy: see Benign prostatic hypertrophy.

Psychogenic disorders: illnesses of mental origin.

Psychotic disorders: any mental disorder in which there is a profound loss of contact with reality.

Purgative: an agent or drug that causes a bowel movement or emptying of the bowel.

Purkinje fibers: an intricate web of fibers that carry electrical impulses into the ventricles of the heart and regulate heart rate and rhythm.

PVCs: see Premature ventricular contractions.

Radioactive: substance that emits damaging rays or particles.

Raynaud's disease: an disorder characterized by intermittent abnormal constriction of the blood vessels of the extremities, probably caused by nervous system problems.

Receptor: a cell component that combines with a drug or with neurotransmitters and hormones to alter the function of that cell.

Reflex: an involuntary response to a stimulus that is specific, predictable, and takes place through the nervous system; may have local effects only or may have systemic effects on the whole body.

Reflex arcs: fast and predictable responses to change in the environment inside and outside the body (i.e., pulling hand away from extreme heat before you even realize you are being burned).

Replication: creating new, identical cells from a parent cell.

Respiratory syncytial virus: a virus that can cause severe illness and even respiratory failure in children.

Reticuloendothelial system: a part of the immune system that filters blood and body fluid and creates the phagocytic cells that destroy debris, pathogens, and foreign substances in the body.

Reye's syndrome: encephalopathy associated with use of aspirin in children with any kind of viral infection.

Rhabdomyosarcoma: cancer of muscle tissue.

Rheumatic fever: serious inflammatory and febrile (causing fever) disease that is a complication of Strep throat and can affect the heart and/or kidneys.

Rheumatoid arthritis: autoimmune disease causing inflammation of joints but that can also affect heart, lungs, kidneys, and other body systems.

Rhinitis: inflammation of the mucosal lining of the nose and sinuses.

Ribonucleic acid: a structure in cells that controls the protein synthesis of that cell and therefore cell reproduction.

Ribosomes: in a cell, the site of RNA attachment necessary for cell replication.

RNA: see Ribonucleic acid.

RSV: see Respiratory syncytial virus.

S-A node: see Sinoatrial node.

Sarcoma: cancers of connective tissue.

SC: see Subcutaneous.

Schizoaffective disorder: personality disorder in which the patient has an inability to feel and express appropriate emotions, often causing disconnection from others.

Schizophrenia: mental disorder with severe loss of contact with reality, hallucinations, and inability to function.

Seizure, absence: consciousness is lost for several seconds to several minutes without any change in muscle contraction. Also called petit mal.

Seizure, atonic: seizure that causes a brief loss of consciousness and a fall with no muscle contractions occurring.

Seizure, atypical absence: consciousness is lost for several seconds to several minutes without any change in muscle contraction and the patient also has other forms of seizures that occur frequently. Usually starts in childhood and does not respond well to antiseizure drugs. Also called Lennox-Gastaut syndrome.

Seizure, febrile: seizure caused by the presence of a very high body temperature.

Seizure, grand mal: see Seizure, tonic-clonic.

Seizure, myoclonic: sudden and brief seizure with contraction of a single muscle group or of the entire body.

Seizure, partial: seizure or uncontrolled electrical activity in the brain that only affects a portion of the body with or without loss of consciousness.

Seizure, petit mal: see Seizure, absence.

Seizure, tonic-clonic: uncontrolled electrical activity in the brain causing sudden onset of muscle contractions affecting the whole body with loss of consciousness. Also called grand mal.

Sensory: conveying impulses from the sense organs to the reflex or higher centers of the nervous system.

Shingles: see Herpes zoster.

Side effect: an action or effect of a drug other than that desired.

Sinoatrial node: area of the heart that controls electrical impulses across the atria of the heart and regulating heart rate and rhythm.

Sinusitis: inflammation in the mucosal lining of the sinuses.

Sjögren's syndrome: a chronic progressive autoimmune disorder characterized by dry eyes and mouth and salivary gland enlargement.

SLE: see Systemic lupus erythematosus.

Sloughing: process of dead tissue being separated from healthy tissue and cast off the body by the body's healing processes.

Somatic: pertaining to the structures of the body wall, such as skin, muscles, and tendons.

Spasticity: increased tone and contraction of muscles causing stiff and awkward movements.

Status epilepticus: a series of grand mal seizures during which the patient does not regain consciousness between the attacks; may be fatal if not treated immediately.

Stevens-Johnson syndrome: widespread and severe systemic lesions of the skin, eyes, mouth, and mucous membranes with fever.

Stomatitis: inflammation of the mouth.

Stroke: circulation problem in the brain that deprives the brain of oxygen and causes damage to brain tissue. Also called cerebrovascular accident or CVA.

Stupor: level of consciousness in which the patient cannot be fully aroused to consciousness. Usually responds to pain stimulus, vigorous movement.

Subcutaneous injection: injection of drug into the subcutaneous layer of the skin for systemic absorption directly into the bloodstream.

Suppressor T-cells: immune system cells that "turn off" or suppress the action of other immune cells.

Sympathetic nervous system: a division of the autonomic nervous system that stimulates the body generally to alertness and to cope with the activities and stress of daily life. It also initiates the fight or flight response to situations perceived as severely stressful or life-threatening.

Syndrome of inappropriate antidiuretic hormone: condition in which the pituitary gland secretes antidiuretic hormone in excess or when it is not needed, causing fluid retention and electrolyte imbalances.

Synthesis: the union of elements to form a compound; the process of building up or creating.

Synthetic analog: a substance that is chemically similar to another naturally occurring substance but that is created in a laboratory.

Systemic lupus erythematosus: a chronic autoimmune disease causing inflammation in multiple body systems.

Tachycardia: a heartbeat that is more rapid than normal.

Tardive dyskinesia: condition of slow, rhythmic, uncontrolled movements especially of the head, tongue, neck, and arms.

Tendon organ: also called Golgi tendon organ, it is a spindle-shaped structure at the junction of a muscle and a tendon. When stimulated by tension or stretch to the muscle or tendon, it inhibits muscle contraction and increases muscle relaxation through a feedback loop in the nervous system.

Thrombocytopenia: abnormally low numbers of platelets.

Thromboembolism: part of a blood clot moving through the circulatory system that broke off from a stationary blood clot elsewhere in the body.

Thrombophlebitis: inflammation of a vein caused by the presence of a stationary blood clot.

Tic douloureux: see Trigeminal neuralgia.

Tinnitus: ringing in the ears.

Topical: route by which drugs placed on the skin are only absorbed into the top layers of the skin and not into the entire body.

Tourette's syndrome: disorder characterized by involuntary movements, tics, and sounds.

Transdermal: route by which drugs enter the bloodstream by being absorbed into the fluid surrounding the cells of the skin.

Transferrin: a globulin in blood that binds and transports iron.

Trigeminal neuralgia: disorder characterized by excruciating pain along the trigeminal nerve serving the side of the face. Also called tic douloureux.

Triglycerides: combination of glycerol with fatty acids circulating in the blood.

Trimester: a 3-month period associated with stages of pregnancy.

Unipolar disorder: mental disorder that manifests only one set of emotional symptoms.

Urate: a salt of uric acid that is a waste product of protein metabolism (breakdown) in the body; in excess, urate can crystalize and cause inflammation, especially in the smaller joints.

Urine retention: inability to empty the bladder of urine.

Uterus: female reproductive organ for containing and nourishing the embryo, fetus, and infant from conception to birth.

Vagal nerve: the 10th cranial nerve that has both sensory and motor functions that affects the heart and lungs.

Vasomotor rhinitis: inflammation of the mucosal lining of the nose caused by the dilation of blood vessels in the area.

Ventricles: the two lower chambers of the heart. When they contract, they push blood out of the heart and into the body.

Vertigo: dizziness.

Vitamin: group of organic substances other than carbohydrates, proteins, and fats, essential for growth, development, and metabolism of the body.

Wasting: loss of strength or size, emaciated.

Wilms' tumor: type of cancer of the kidneys found in infants and children.

Withdrawal: symptoms that occur when stopping drugs or alcohol on which a person is physically or psychologically dependent.

INDEX

Pages numbers in *italics* denote figures; those followed by a t denote tables.

Drug Index